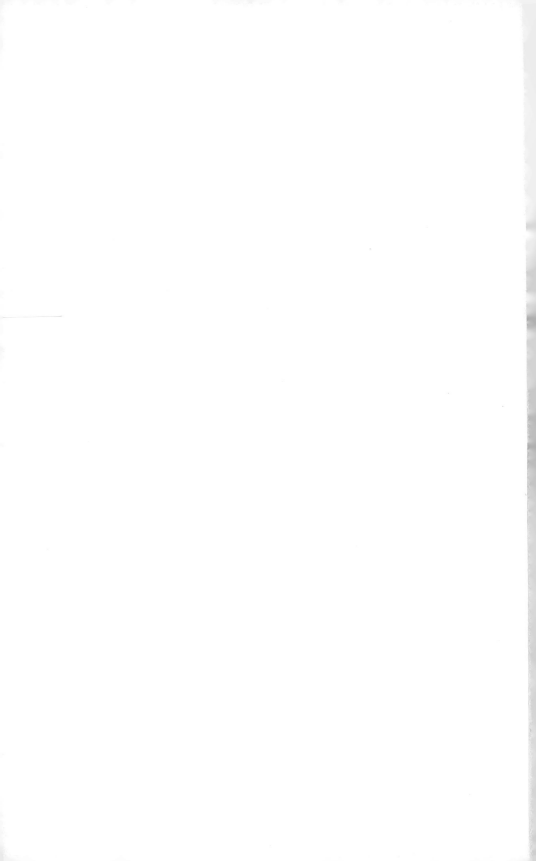

THE HEALTHCARE LABYRINTH

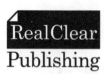

www.amplifypublishing.com

The Healthcare Labyrinth:
A Guide to Navigating Health Plans and Fixing American Health Insurance

For more information, please contact:
Amplify Publishing, an imprint of Mascot Books
620 Herndon Parkway, Suite 320
Herndon, VA 20170
info@amplifypublishing.com

Library of Congress Control Number: 2021906318

CPSIA Code: PBANG1221A

ISBN-13: 978-1-64543-993-6

Printed in the United States

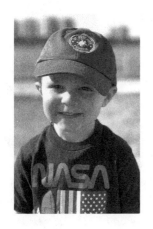

Dedicated to Owen Scott Ryan, my grandson, and all the children who deserve worry-free, affordable, and quality healthcare in their future.

THE

HEALTHCARE

LABYRINTH

A Guide to Navigating
Health Plans and Fixing
American Health Insurance

Marc S. Ryan

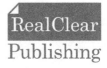
RealClear
Publishing

CONTENTS

PART ONE: Why This Book?

PART TWO: Fundamentals of U.S. Health Insurance

PART THREE: Where We Are Today

PART FOUR: The Future of U.S. Healthcare

Why This Book?

I n Part One, I tell you why I wrote this book as well as about my own transformation in terms of how I think about healthcare. Healthcare in America is a maze that few can comprehend. That means finding solutions is that much harder. I also tell you how the concept of social welfare policy and health coverage emerged and about the origins and growth of healthcare in America.

CHAPTER 1

My Journey through the Labyrinth

So, why did I write this book? It's simple: because the American health-care system is a complex maze—like Daedalus's labyrinth from Greek mythology. As economist Uwe Reinhart characterized healthcare in his book *Priced Out*, it is "almost beyond human comprehension."[1-1] It frustrates millions of Americans as they attempt to obtain quality healthcare coverage for themselves and their families. It, too, is one of the leading reasons for financial stress and bankruptcy. In fact, most of those who have to declare bankruptcy due to mammoth medical expenses actually have health coverage.[1-2]

With that in mind, I set out to break down how the health insurance system operates in America to demystify at least part of accessing healthcare and help Americans make more educated decisions.

I admit that this book will only educate at best. It won't stop most of the frustration or the financial stress. But I hope it does help Americans think differently and become wiser consumers. I, too, wanted to give hope by explaining that, despite the dysfunction we see today, we seem to be headed in a better direction—one that hopefully brings us to value-based care and a quality-focused system. That is if parties can set aside their political differences and forge responsible compromise. I offer thoughts on how we can reform the system by getting our arms around price/cost, promoting affordable universal access, as well as emphasizing wellness, prevention, and care management.

So why are we so dysfunctional? America's healthcare system is absolutely unique. It is the only predominantly employer-based healthcare system in the developed world. And as you will learn, relying on an employer-based system alone will not cover all Americans. To cover those that fall through the cracks, a patchwork system has been built over the years. This promotes inefficiency, waste, fraud, abuse, poor quality, lack of consistent coverage, and healthcare spending (as a percentage of gross domestic product or GDP) that is a huge outlier compared to other developed nations. Costs are so massive that if our healthcare system were its own country, it would rank fifth in the world—behind only the United States, China, Japan, and Germany. We also have not arrived at a consensus on offering affordable universal access to everyone. The United States is the only developed country in the world without it.

Over the years, we have put a series of dirty Band-Aids on our healthcare system. The problem is that the system is not just cut and bruised. We cannot treat our system as if there is just a small infection. In fact, the patient is hemorrhaging, and the system cannot survive as we know it.

Some say the solution must be a government-run, socialized system. Well, you will learn from this book that I don't view national socialized medicine as something that would represent quality in the United States. At the very least, it is not likely to meet Americans' expectations of instantaneous access to high-quality, technology-driven healthcare (if you can afford it).

There also is a single-payer approach. But based on the latest proposals out there, I think single-payer in the United States would likely be very inefficient and of poor quality. I am also a relative pragmatist when it comes to where we should go. I don't see us abandoning employer-sponsored healthcare any time soon.

Thus, at least for the foreseeable future, we will have more fragmentation than not. But I do think that ensuring affordable, universal access or coverage for all Americans is one of the solutions to begin to right the healthcare ship of state. With price reform and focus on care management, this would bring down overall expenditures and move the quality needle. Stressing affordable universal access is heresy in many political parts, but I don't mind pushing back on conventional wisdom—even in my own Republican Party.

On healthcare issues, I am clearly a moderate and a bit unconventional for my party. I drive a bit up the middle on healthcare issues largely because of my background, one that has seen my philosophy morph over time. While I am a fiscal conservative, I support federal subsidies for affordable universal access. I am also a supporter of expanded Medicaid and the Exchanges (at least until we have a better solution). I think my support for affordable universal access is based on sound policy and fiscal analysis—something often lacking from both parties on healthcare.

So, who am I? You probably want to know a bit about my mindset as we wind and wend our way through healthcare in these coming pages.

I was born in Albany, New York. My middle-class parents were both public employees, so we were blessed, as healthcare was never an issue. They made huge sacrifices for me to go to Georgetown University. I spent time in my college days in the then Soviet Union and Poland. I traveled extensively during that time throughout Eastern Europe. It remains a passion for me. While at Georgetown, I transitioned from my deep Democratic roots (my father was a leader in the relatively conservative Albany Democratic machine) to the Republican Party and worked on Ronald Reagan's re-election campaign in 1984.

Reagan inspired me for a number of reasons. He had an extraordinary ability to communicate. He had simple, yet inspired messages. He had the ability to move political mountains, such as tax reform. Perhaps most importantly, I studied his ability to compromise and get things done with his friend, House Speaker Tip O'Neill of Massachusetts. (He was from a Democratic machine background, too.) These men were so different, yet they made things work. Reagan's hidden-from-the-public-eye pragmatism was something I used later in life.

During my college years and after graduating from Georgetown, I got caught up in the conservative political movement. I became infatuated with William Buckley, who was L. Brent Bozell III's (my boss's) uncle. My political philosophy was a mix of hardcore conservative politics and Catholic conservative religious philosophy. I was a commentator/writer/editor on liberal media bias as well as executive director of a foundation centered on bringing down communism and the Iron Curtain. One of our proudest moments was crafting a bipartisan blueprint for free and fair elections in Nicaragua. I was also associated with a political action committee devoted to electing conservative candidates. I was actually in Vice President Dan Quayle's office the day the Iron Curtain fell in 1989, a remarkable memory for me.

After the Iron Curtain fell, I was looking for new opportunities. This led me to a position as an editorial writer, editor, and political columnist at the Waterbury *Republican-American*. At that time, I started graduate school for public administration.

My political columns on Connecticut politics led me to become the deputy communications director for Connecticut Governor John Rowland. Given my budding interest in public administration, I moved to the Connecticut Office of Policy and Management (the state budget and management agency), where I worked myself up through various policy and budget positions while attending graduate school. I landed the deputy secretary/deputy budget director spot in 1997 and the number one job in the agency in late 1998. I was just thirty-four years old.

My healthcare knowledge began to grow in 1997 when the then budget director told me that he was focusing on the general government side of things (his forte), and I would need to learn healthcare to oversee social services, Medicaid, mental health, foster care and child protection, developmental disabilities, and more. This led to a crash course on healthcare policy and budgeting, while learning the ins and outs of Medicaid, state waivers, and federal financing of numerous healthcare and social services programs.

While I was known as a fiscal conservative, I did begin to soften my relative animus toward government programs. I oversaw the creation of the Children's Health Insurance Program, supportive and affordable housing, alternatives to nursing home institutionalization, and new HIV and AIDS investments. Our transformation of long-term care in the state to focus on community supports for the poor and middle income won national plaudits and awards.

Despite challenges, being budget director remains the best job I've ever had. My years were not without political theatrics and controversies as we sometimes battled the Democrats who largely dominated the legislature. But as the governor's chief negotiator on most matters, I quickly learned that compromise is needed and is a benefit to overall public policy. We were able to work with the opposing party to balance our budgets, increase our bond rating, weather various fiscal storms, and preserve and enhance the state's social safety net and other programs. It was a model that worked—and something from which Washington could learn.

After ten years in government, I moved on to a career at health plans, big and small, focused on Medicare, Medicaid, and commercial coverage. I served in a number of roles, focusing on starting up Medicare Advantage, Medicaid, and Obamacare Exchange plans. During my Connecticut budget position, I had been named by then Health and Human Services Secretary Tommy Thompson to sit on a commission to integrate state drug assistance programs with the new Medicare Part D prescription drug program. Later, I was appointed to sit on the state of Florida's Medicaid Reform advisory panel.

One of my most life-changing jobs was serving as the chief operating officer of a nonprofit HIV/AIDS plan in south Florida, an epicenter for the AIDS epidemic. Two of our biggest constituencies could not have been more disparate—previously well-off gay white men and impoverished African American women. Here, I learned first-hand about the healthcare barriers and challenges faced by Americans with chronic conditions and how social determinants of health impact overall outcomes. It was both humbling and eye-opening. We were able to create a paradigm of private, managed care that offered great healthcare benefits and services to many in great need. The national organization that ran it, the AIDS Healthcare Foundation, continues to do tremendous work.

In 2010, two health plan IT executives founded a new healthcare technology firm, Medical House of Knowledge (MedHOK or, more recently, MHK). It was a tremendous success, creating medical and pharmacy clinical management software for health plans and pharmacy benefit managers (PBMs). It focused on ensuring that plans and PBMs meet the emerging compliance regime from the Centers for Medicare and Medicaid Services (CMS) and state Medicaid agencies. I was one of its first executives. As chief strategy and compliance officer, I oversaw strategy, compliance, product development, innovation, release management, business analysis, and quality assurance.

Over six years later, the company had grown so much that it was sold to the Hearst Corporation, a leader in healthcare technology companies such as First Data Bank (FDB), MCG Health, and now MHK. In October 2019, I was appointed executive vice president and chief operating officer of MHK and became its president in January 2020.

I am an avid blogger and podcast host on healthcare issues, some of them covering healthcare generally but often on the technical emerging Medicare compliance and quality regime. Look me up on LinkedIn, my blog site (**https://mhk.com/resources/strategic-insights-blog/**), or my podcasts, *Healthcare Revolution with MHK.*

On the personal front, I am a Roman Catholic. I have been married for over thirty years and have three children. The newest love of my life is my first grandson, Owen, to whom this book is dedicated. It actually is dedicated not only to Owen, but all children who deserve affordable access to healthcare. So that is ultimately why I am writing this book. My own personal transformation has helped me understand that if healthcare is not a right, it is darn well close to it. It is certainly not a privilege. Every developed nation provides affordable universal access—*except* America. The lack of such access has huge consequences not only for the well-being of individual Americans but for the economy as a whole. Supplying such coverage does not have to break the bank, either. Indeed, it can save money over time, if done right. I can't think of a better reason to reform healthcare but ensuring the health and well-being and economic prosperity of the next generation.

Marc S. Ryan
Tampa, Florida
June 2021

CHAPTER 2

Uncle Otto:
"All Hail Bismarckian Socialism"

> "Laws are like sausages; it is better not to see them being made."
> – *Otto von Bismarck*

I thought it might be interesting to begin our American healthcare journey with the origins of the modern social welfare state. For that, you can thank Uncle Otto, or Prince Otto Eduard Leopold von Bismarck, a German statesman in the latter-third of the 1800s in Germany.

How could a nineteenth-century German be responsible for the modern welfare state? Before we get into the details, let's give you a general background on Bismarck's life. He was born in 1815, to a modestly wealthy aristocratic family. He had a fine education, eventually studying law. He was in the Prussian civil service and helped manage his family's land holdings. In 1849, he became a member of the Prussian parliament. He held a series of diplomatic posts. In 1862, he was named prime minister and foreign minister of Prussia by King Wilhelm I.[2-1]

In 1871, Wilhelm became kaiser (emperor) of a united German Empire after a series of wars and diplomatic maneuvers engineered by Bismarck. Bismarck was named chancellor as well as prime minister of the empire, serving in the all-powerful position until 1890, when Wilhelm II unceremoniously ousted him.[2-1]

Bismarck is known for many things—here are four of them:

First, he is known for his great modernization of Germany, introducing a series of programs to expand its economy, encourage free trade, and introduce a civil and criminal code.[2-1]

Second, Bismarck, the Iron Chancellor, essentially united the weak German states of the north and south into one powerful empire.[2-1]

Third, Bismarck is best known for his realpolitik approach—the emphasis on the practical rather than the ideological, moral, or principled. The notion harkens back to the times of Machiavelli and the "end justifies the means" philosophy. Whether foreign or domestic, Bismarck was the ultimate pragmatist. His realpolitik united the empire and forged the great economic and social modernization of Germany.[2-2]

Fourth, the main reason I am talking about Bismarck in this book is his response to socialism. In the late 1800s, this philosophy was on the rise in Europe (the *Communist Manifesto* pamphlet by Karl Marx and Friedrich Engels was created in 1848). The social democratic movement began to win favor with the people, as it preached worker justice and the benefits of socialism. Bismarck and others in the new kingdom saw this as a threat. His realpolitik philosophy kicked into action. While he was by no means a democrat or socialist, the pragmatic chancellor set out to co-opt the social democratic movement by championing measures in the Reichstag (parliament) meant to protect workers. Bismarck argued that these worker protections would further grow the economy and the empire by shielding Germany from even grander socialist ideals.[2-3, 2-4, 2-5]

Little did he know how far-reaching his moves would ultimately be. His efforts led to the following:

The first modern-day national health insurance program, 1883—In this scheme, employers' and employees' contributions were tied to wages.

(Employees contributed about two-thirds of the funds.) The workers were eligible for a broad range of healthcare services. A healthcare provider fee schedule, the insured's payment schedule, and sick leave were also introduced. The system was not technically run by the government, but by quasi-public health bureaus with employer and employee representation, although workers dominated.[2-6]

The first form of modern-day workers' compensation, beginning in 1871 with a liability act and culminating with an insurance scheme in 1884— Although such programs date back to the Sumerian civilization around 2000 BC,[2-7] Uncle Otto established the first workers' compensation laws in modern Europe. Under the system, injured workers received a pension and medical care. The pension was equal to two-thirds of wages (a ratio that is still present in many places across the United States). Employers paid the freight and set up quasi-public insurance organizations to administer them.[2-8]

The first modern pension act, 1889—A pension act was passed that paid workers a pension when they reached seventy years of age (somewhat old for those times) or if they were disabled. The government ran this program, the financing for which was a mix of government, employer, and employee.[2-9]

Bismarck, through his realpolitik ideology, became an unintentional social welfare pioneer, revolutionizing many facets of the first social welfare state. His opponents defined the new vision as Bismarckian Socialism or State Socialism.[2-5] It also led to the concept of the social market economy in the mid twentieth century, where the free market forms the foundation of the economy. However, the state intervenes in two crucial areas: It safeguards fair competition to ensure the market operates correctly, and it adds social protections in the form of worker and equal opportunity rights as well as social welfare programs to fill economic voids.[2-10, 2-11, 2-12]

The social market economy is often seen as the middle ground between two other economic theories—the absolute unfettered operation of laissez faire free market economics and socialism/communism. In laissez faire, there is no government intervention. Scottish economist and philosopher Adam Smith saw laissez faire as a natural law system that would produce the greatest potential for everyone. In socialism/communism, the state or cooperative entities own the assets and means of production. Market concepts could be used in some forms of socialism to guide aspects of the economy. This can be seen, for example, in China today. Socialism/communism should not be confused with the State Socialism of Bismark.[2-12]

Bismarck's model was broadly adopted in Europe and eventually made its way to the United States. For all his aristocracy and conservatism, Bismarck is held up today by American liberals (not the classical type) as a positive example of the need for government intervention due to the inherent abuses that emerge within the free market mechanism. Those on the American Right see him as something of a traitor. They think the social welfare system, coupled with the free market, is anything but economic security.

So thus far, we have gone back to ancient Sumer and sped through almost 4,000 years of history. What have we concluded?

First, government intervention in the market and even healthcare has been around for a long time—perhaps for good reason. There have been countless failed socialist states over the years. It is also hard to find a properly functioning laissez faire free market around the world, although some would say it was never given a shot. However, history shows some of the excesses that can occur without some government controls.

So, while there are philosophical holdouts on each side of the political spectrum, we now seem to be debating not whether government should be part of the economy and everyday life, but rather how big its involvement should be and what level of interference is necessary in the free market. It is in this context that our unique American healthcare system has emerged and, truthfully, somewhat languished thus far.

Second, hero or foe, Bismarck introduced the modern-day concept of government social welfare, including healthcare benefits, that took root in our modern free-market economies.

Third, many of Bismarck's mechanisms remain. Employer-employee bureaus or organizations control various benefits and organizational practices throughout the world. In Bismarck's day, an employee-employer bureau administered the health fund. This is no longer the case in other developed nations, but this concept is still active in America, with employer-sponsored healthcare and union and employer self-insurance funds.

So, as you thank the Lord for that healthcare you have when you are sick or loathe that health insurer for denying that migraine medication that is $560 per month out-of-pocket, remember Uncle Otto, that health insurance trailblazer from the nineteenth century.

CHAPTER 3

Origins and Brief History of U.S. Healthcare

hile Bismarck's views did make their way to America and influenced its system, America did not go down the national health system route as much of Europe did. So, let's talk about the origins and history of healthcare in this country.

Early America did have doctors and certain healthcare facilities, but the system was not yet formalized. The provision of medical care was often left up to individual doctors, who had various levels of formal and informal education and training. Doctors charged little for care and often were paid in things other than currency. Sometimes groups formed on a voluntary basis to furnish care. Charitable and religious organizations also furnished a large share of medical services in the country's early years.[3-1, 3-2, 3-3, 3-4]

With the advent of technology and the Industrial Revolution, healthcare in America took on a more specific role. In the second half of the 1800s and into the early 1900s, we saw a series of medical discoveries and developments that helped usher in the modern medical era. Investment in health and medicine suddenly paid dividends in terms of recovery from accident or illness. Medical training became more formal. Medicine became a true profession.[3-5, 3-6]

The Industrial Revolution brought major changes in the way Americans lived and thrived. Entrepreneurs and industrialists of the day formed various enterprises, including railroads, lumber, mining, steel, construction firms, and shipyards. The Industrial Revolution offered average workers huge opportunities and social advancement. But with the opportunities came great risk as well. They worked under dangerous conditions, often for long hours. Accident and illness were commonplace.

The combination of medical advancement and the perils faced by workers during the Industrial Revolution sowed the first seeds of health insurance in America. While it might have been altruism on the part of some entrepreneur owners, the introduction of employer-based coverage had much to do with pure economics. Given the accidents, injuries, and illnesses of their workers, business owners looked for ways to get their workers treated and back on the job as quickly as possible. As it is today, attracting and training workers is always an expensive proposition, especially compared with the low cost of healthcare and treatment at the time.

Various early models emerged to treat workers for accidents and sickness. Sometimes companies hired local doctors to work as company doctors to treat their workers. In other cases, companies paid all or a portion of the costs of treatment at a private doctor's office in the community. Over time, businesses began entering into formal arrangements to pay physicians and other providers to care for employees. Employees then began paying a share of that cost. Unions were born and organized in the late 1800s and into the 1900s. They began creating sickness and injury funds to care for their members. In many regards, though, what was emerging could be best described as accident, sickness, or workers' compensation insurance, rather than full-fledged healthcare insurance. (Most did not initially include hospitalization.)[3-7, 3-8, 3-9]

The transformation continued. The American Medical Association and American Hospital Association became very prominent. Insurance companies began to cover costs via employer premiums. State insurance laws and agencies matured as well; the National Association of Insurance Commissioners was founded in 1871. [3-7, 3-8, 3-9]

Then, several laws were passed at the federal and state levels on the social welfare front that spurred further action. At the turn of the twentieth century, trustbuster Teddy Roosevelt seemed to embody many of Bismarck's ideas. He famously took on big business to stop monopolies and oligopolies, although the actual anti-trust act had passed in 1890. He also argued for social welfare protections. Our first workers' compensation laws passed in 1908. The muckraker journalists exposed abuses during the Progressive Era of the early 1900s and helped forge a series of worker protection acts. [3-7, 3-8, 3-9]

As the early 1900s moved on, however, there was some notable resistance to creating a national healthcare system for several reasons. Healthcare was still relatively cheap, unlike the costs today that often bankrupt families hit by a catastrophic accident, a life-threatening disease, or even chronic conditions. Further, a national system seemed anathema to America's entrepreneurial spirit. The first modern lobbying groups were also at odds regarding healthcare. While some academic groups supported national health insurance legislation at the state and federal levels, physician, hospital, business, and most labor groups saw the system as a threat to their existence and prosperity. The opponents laid waste to various initiatives over the years. [3-9]

With a national program unlikely, the private sector kept filling the void. From the 1920s to the 1940s, the U.S. healthcare system firmly took root, especially as costs began to rise. Employers wanted so-called prepaid arrangements, where hospitals and physicians accepted payments to take care of firms' employees—the precursor to what are now known as risk arrangements with providers. To meet the demand, hospitals and physicians went beyond organizing simply as groups and formed arrangements to offer healthcare benefits in an insurance-type model. Insurers continued their growth, offering accident and sickness insurance.

Some healthcare insurance firsts:

- ○ In 1910, the Western Clinic in Tacoma began offering a suite of prepaid healthcare benefits to employers, specifically lumber firms.[3-10]
- ○ Retailer Montgomery Ward is said to have offered the first health policy to its employees starting in 1910.[3-7]
- ○ In 1929, the Dallas Teachers' Union entered into a prepaid arrangement with Baylor University Hospital. Baylor offered a low fee of fifty cents a month to obtain several weeks of insurance a year (the exact number is of some debate). This was the start of the Blue Cross movement, where hospitals began offering such plans to employers. Eventually, Blue Cross Plans offering hospital-based insurance benefits popped up all over the country.[3-11]
- ○ Also, in 1929, the Los Angeles Department of Water and Power began offering its public sector employees a prepaid medical plan.[3-10]
- ○ Blue Shield, the group formed by physicians combining efforts, began initially in California in 1939, when a California physician group offered prepaid arrangements to employers. Again, these Blue Shield plans offering community physician benefits emerged throughout the country.[3-11]
- ○ At about the same time, industrialist Henry Kaiser (known for shipbuilding, steel, aluminum, and construction) participated in the creation of insurance plans for his workers and their families. This eventually became what is known as Kaiser Permanente, a mammoth integrated delivery system featuring physicians, other providers, hospitals, and health plans.[3-10, 3-12]

The Blue Cross plans, Blue Shield plans, and insurers continued their marked growth throughout the 1930s and 1940s. The Blue Cross and Blue Shield plans usually did not compete against each other and over time began cooperating to offer joint benefits in many cases. They became subject to the same insurance regulations as the other insurers and eventually merged into one entity in their regions to compete on the benefits front and gain efficiencies. The two national associations merged in 1982.[3-11, 3-13, 3-14]

Insurers initially stayed out of the healthcare market that the Blues were now in. They stuck with accident and sickness coverage due to fears of "adverse selection," a phenomenon where sicker individuals pick up coverage while healthier ones do not—as they don't usually need it. This means that an extremely sick cohort can cause premiums to skyrocket, increasing the risk of the product. As the years went on, however, insurers began to offer what we think of as healthcare coverage as well. The Blues plans were non-profits and offered rates based on community rating (the same cost per enrollee regardless of health or conditions), while traditional insurers took into consideration health risk—the process known as underwriting.[3-7, 3-9, 3-11, 3-14, 3-15]

The growth of private health insurance was propelled by two government actions during the World War II era. Given the need to allocate as many dollars in the economy as possible toward the massive war effort, and to control inflation, wages were frozen by government mandate. Benefits were not. To attract high-quality employees (in high demand because many were fighting the war), more and more employers offered healthcare benefits and continually enriched them.[3-14]

The other action was a regulatory interpretation by the Internal Revenue Service that made the costs of providing employee health coverage tax deductible for corporations. This lives on today.[3-9, 3-14]

In addition, the rise of unionism also played a role in adding people to the healthcare rolls. During collective bargaining, unions now had the ability to push for increases in both wages for the worker and health benefits for the worker and his or her family.[3-9, 3-14]

The 1940s through the 1960s saw a rapid rise in the number of Americans and dependents with health insurance. According to various sources, it appears the insured rate jumped from about 10-15% in the early 1940s to between 50-55% in 1950. By 1960, about 75% of Americans had coverage. In all decades, the vast majority had employer-based coverage. The system that emerged was what is known as the fee-for-service (FFS), indemnity, or transaction system, where each service gets a payment.[3-7, 3-15, 3-16, 3-17]

Why didn't the United States go down the same road as Germany and the rest of Europe? While there were attempts to bring national health insurance to America, the politics of the time stopped it. America adopted other reforms and initiatives instead.

Teddy Roosevelt had argued that social welfare programs were needed in order to be compassionate while also ensuring economic prosperity. Roosevelt included national sickness insurance in his 1912 platform when he attempted to regain the presidency through his alternative Progressive Party (also known as the "Bull Moose Party"). However, Roosevelt's efforts at that time were spurned by organized lobbying and a general lack of support.[3-17]

After the stock market fall of 1929, the economy crumbled and ushered in the Great Depression. Franklin Delano Roosevelt had to take concerted action. He created a series of New Deal Programs, including the Social Security Act of 1935, which brought public pensions, unemployment compensation, and care of dependent children and the disabled after death or injury of loved ones. FDR toyed with the idea of national healthcare as well, but again there was a lack of general support and fear that the entire Social Security Act would be tanked. FDR's successor, Harry Truman also wanted universal healthcare as part of his Fair Deal. But again, opponents stopped it, this time branding it as a socialist plot.[3-18, 3-19]

While we did not get national healthcare, it quickly became evident that we had a nation of "haves and have nots." Seventy-five percent of the nation or so had coverage in the 1960s, but 25% did not. For the most part, if you worked for any level of government (the federal employees health benefit program began in 1960 and the military had coverage) or had solid employment in the private sector, you had coverage. Otherwise, you were one of those who fell through the cracks. You had no nexus or connection to healthcare. You might be in and out of employment or at the lower end of the income scale and could not afford the benefits that your employer offered. You might not be part of the workforce—aged, disabled, or poor.

In 1965, in lieu of a national healthcare program, Lyndon Johnson promoted and Congress passed amendments to the Social Security Act—Titles XVIII and XIX—that created Medicare, for the elderly and later the disabled, and Medicaid, for those with low incomes. We will discuss their specifics in coming chapters. One interesting trivia side note: Johnson gave a great deal of credit for Medicare to Truman's earlier efforts and enrolled Truman, and his wife, Bess, as the first Medicare beneficiaries after signing the bill into law.[3-20]

Not to be outdone, a Republican president, Richard Nixon, advocated for something close to universal access to healthcare. He advocated an employer mandate to cover health benefits, with protections as to how much cost would be borne by the employee. The government was to help pay for coverage for small businesses and low-wage employers. He wanted to replace Medicaid with a federal program that would cover most others, with people paying premiums and other healthcare costs based on a sliding scale tied to income. If Nixon's proposals sound familiar, read on.[3-21]

Although these proposals did not pass, Nixon was instrumental in ushering through the Federal Health Maintenance Organization (HMO) Act in 1973, which sought to further ingrain the emerging managed care concept throughout the nation.[3-22] Managed care has its roots in the prepaid plans discussed earlier, but it truly came to the fore in the 1970s and later. The West Coast adopted the concept first and it quickly moved east. The HMO Act was an important catalyst to nationwide adoption. The HMO-managed care model attempted to displace the inefficient FFS model mentioned previously. It was not entirely successful, but it did redefine the healthcare system in America.

Attributes of the HMO model: [3-23, 3-24]

- The use of networks versus any available provider to obtain deep discounts on fees and costs
- Focus on wellness, prevention, and primary care, with capitation payments and other forms of incentive-based reimbursement to providers, especially assigned primary care physicians (PCPs)
- Comprehensive benefits, but with tiered cost-sharing to encourage members' appropriate use of services
- Strong utilization controls, especially prior authorization of many services

|| ○   Aggressive care coordination and case management to reduce costs
and improve quality outcomes

In 1974, Nixon's successor, Gerald Ford, signed into law the Employment Retirement Security Act. This did many things in terms of regulating employee and retiree benefits. In particular, it set up the regulations for provision of self-insured employee and retiree funds run by employers and labor unions.[3-25]

Another Republican, Ronald Reagan, signed into law in 1986 the Consolidated Omnibus Budget Reconciliation Act, known as COBRA, that allows Americans to continue healthcare coverage when they leave an employer (if they pay the full premium). The act also included the Emergency Medical Treatment and Labor Act (EMTALA), which requires provision of emergency care regardless of health insurance status.[3-26, 3-27]

Democrat Bill Clinton's wife, Hillary, spearheaded a proposal, colloquially known as "Hillarycare," that included universal access, government purchasing alliances, and a healthcare control board. It died, suffering under the weight of complexity, poor public relations, and the aggressive opposition by health insurers.[3-28]

Bill Clinton did sign into law the Health Insurance Portability and Accountability Act (HIPAA), meant to protect workers when they leave jobs, protect the confidentiality of health information, and set new standards to allow data to flow through the healthcare system to reduce costs.[3-29]

In addition, the State Children's Health Insurance Program (SCHIP), Title XXI of the Social Security Act, was passed under Clinton in 1997. This act sought to reduce the number of uninsured children through a new federal appropriation. It is not an entitlement but a set amount of spending each year, reauthorized over time. It has been used to place additional children in Medicaid as well as in new state-run insurance programs. It generally covers income groups above traditional Medicaid levels. Passage had an ancillary benefit as well. Marketing around Title XXI implementation in many states led to children who were historically eligible for Medicaid to enroll and become insured.[3-30]

While Medicare was a savior for seniors and the disabled, lack of retail drug coverage meant those in Medicare continued to see huge bills. In 2003, with George W. Bush's blessing, Congress passed an act creating a retail drug component (Part D) in Medicare. It went live in 2006. The act, known as the Medicare Modernization Act (MMA), also made other changes to Medicare.[3-31]

Finally, taking cues perhaps from both Richard Nixon and Hillary Clinton, Barack Obama and a Democratic Congress passed the Patient Protection and Affordable Care Act (PPACA, ACA, or Obamacare) in 2010. Although not a national insurance model, this was America's first foray into universal access with requirements for employers to provide and individuals to buy health insurance. It, too, expanded Medicaid and set up the insurance Exchanges, which enroll the uninsured and provide subsidies for premiums and cost-sharing for some people based on income.[3-32] The act has reduced the number of uninsured in America dramatically. However, we still have a large number of uninsured compared with other developed nations.

Leaders in both parties have championed the need to fill in the gaps of our healthcare system, most recently through single-payer national healthcare or at least universal access within the model we have today. And while Democratic leaders tend to predominate when it comes to healthcare proposals, Republicans (at least in the past) have not shied away from proposing to rationalize the system and back social welfare healthcare programs and subsidies. They have argued for this on both compassionate and economic grounds. These arguments have great financial, economic, and policy merit. Throughout this book, I will discuss the need for parties to set aside their differences and forge a compromise that rationalizes how we deliver healthcare.

Fundamentals of U.S. Health Insurance

n Part Two, I lay out the fundamentals of health coverage in America, from definitions and key terminology about health plans to coverage and things that mystify us every day. I detail the various broad types of health insurance, plan or product types, and the important players or actors in the health system. I also tell you about our leap from the old indemnity insurance system to managed healthcare.

CHAPTER 4

Lines of Business

> "No longer will older Americans be denied the healing miracle
> of modern medicine. No longer will illness crush and destroy
> the savings that they have so carefully put away over a lifetime
> so that they might enjoy dignity in their later years. No longer
> will young families see their own incomes, and their own hopes,
> eaten away simply because they are carrying out their deep moral
> obligations to their parents, and to their uncles and their aunts."
> – *President Lyndon Johnson, signing Medicare and Medicaid
> into law, July 30, 1965*

So far, I have told you about the birth of modern social welfare programs and the unique nature of healthcare in America. Before I go further, however, the next few chapters will cover some of the basics of health insurance itself. This will be an important foundation as you learn more about insurance products and how the various lines of business operate in the United States.

In general, there are three lines of business in the health insurance world:

Commercial Health Insurance—This is generally the coverage derived in the private sector of the economy, with one exception. There are three subcategories of commercial coverage:

> **Employer-based or Group Coverage**—This is the predominant coverage category in America. Employers contract with health plans and insurers to provide benefits to their employees and dependents. Later, we will discuss how some large employers essentially insure themselves through self-insurance funds and use plans just as administrators, while other large employers and all small employers use health plans and fully insure with them. The Patient Protection and Affordable Care Act (PPACA, ACA, or Obamacare) now mandates essential benefits, coverage levels, and other protections. Premiums, cost-sharing, and actual coverage can vary greatly. See additional categories under Other Coverage later in this chapter regarding other private, commercial coverage offered by federal, state, and local governments.

> **Individual and Marketplace/Exchange Coverage**—If you don't receive your healthcare through an employer plan, Americans can also purchase coverage directly from a health plan. Generally, this is governed by state insurance departments, and now by the federal government as well. An employer may provide a stipend to purchase coverage on your own or you may get coverage through the ACA Marketplace or Exchanges as an individual or through the small employer program. The ACA rules mentioned previously apply here as well. Some health plans think of the ACA Exchange as almost a fourth line of business today. Premiums, cost-sharing, and actual coverage can vary greatly in the Exchanges depending on the type of plan selected.

> **Medigap or Medicare Supplement or Medicare Wrap Policy**—This is technically a commercial product. It is federally regulated, although

governed in each state by its insurance department. These policies fill in the gaps in traditional Medicare coverage, with varying coverage depending on how much you want to pay in monthly premiums.

Medicare—This line of business is a program run by the federal government, specifically the Centers for Medicare and Medicaid Services (CMS) under the Department of Health and Human Services (HHS). It was created as Title XVIII of the Social Security Act. The program covers those sixty-five and older, certain disabled individuals, as well as people with end-stage renal disease (ESRD).

Medicare has different *parts*, which can be confusing. They are:

Part A—This is the part of the fee-for-service (FFS) program that covers hospitals, acute skilled nursing care, some home care, and hospice services.

Part B—This is the part of the FFS program that covers outpatient services, such as physician services, other outpatient care, other home health, and durable medical equipment (DME).

Part C—This is the Medicare Advantage (MA) program that combines Part A and B services. As described later, this means that your Medicare is furnished through a private plan.

Part D—This is the prescription drug program. If you are in FFS, you enroll in a free-standing private drug plan. If you are in MA, usually your plan covers Part D as well. If it doesn't, you can enroll in a free-standing drug plan.

Medicare offers comprehensive coverage, but the federal government only covers about 80% of total costs in its traditional coverage. Private plans cover more. There are pros and cons of each alternative. Today, over 43% of Medicare beneficiaries are in private MA plans (based on my estimate of Medicare beneficiaries in early 2021), while about 57% are in traditional FFS Medicare (a form of single-payer healthcare). But private estimates suggest that by 2025, about 50% of beneficiaries will be in MA plans. Between 2030 and 2040, that percentage could reach 70%.[4-1]

Medicaid—This program is a federal-state partnership for poor and lower income individuals, created as Title XIX of the Social Security Act. The program is governed by CMS federally, which sets out broad policies in terms of benefits and regulations. Each state then has a Medicaid agency that administers its program. The federal and state governments share in the cost of the program based on each state's relative wealth, with a match floor of 50% from the federal government. There are mandatory coverage and benefit requirements at the federal level. States may offer the program to optional coverage groups as well as provide optional benefits. Generally speaking, Medicaid is for lower income persons without health coverage. But since its passage in 1965, various additional populations have been added to expand coverage, including the recent ACA expansion that most states elected. Medicaid offers comprehensive coverage and has little or no premiums and cost-sharing given income levels of enrollees.

As with Medicare, there is a traditional Medicaid fee-for-service (FFS) program but states also hire private plans to cover Medicaid for most populations. Today, about 70% of beneficiaries are in comprehensive Medicaid managed care plans, with about 80% being in some form of private Medicaid managed care.[4-2, 4-3]

Another program closely related to Medicaid, the **State Children's Health Insurance Program (SCHIP or CHIP)**, can be included under this line of business. This program, Title XXI of the Social Security Act, also is a federal-state partnership. The federal government allocates a non-entitlement block grant amount to each state. States must spend a given amount in order to draw down the federal funds. Match rates are higher than Medicaid in each state. States can either use the funds to extend Medicaid eligibility to children or create separate free-standing insurance programs. These free-standing programs tend to have some premiums and cost-sharing. Children covered by

SCHIP usually come from families with higher income than Medicaid. Most of these populations are in private plans contracted with the states.

Other Coverage—There are various other federal and state programs that cover millions of Americans and don't really fall into any one group. They include:

- **Federal Employees Health Benefit Program,** which is run by the federal Office of Personnel Management (OPM), contracting with national and regional private health plans. This is generally seen as private, commercial coverage.
- **TRICARE,** which is the health insurance for active military and some retirees. This is run by the Department of Defense, contracting with private health plans across the nation. This is considered private, commercial coverage.
- **Department of Veterans Affairs Hospitals and Clinics.** This is one of the programs offered in America that constitutes government-run healthcare.
- **The Indian Health Service**
- **State employees and retiree health insurance funds**
- **Local government employees and retiree health insurance funds.** This is generally seen as private, commercial coverage.

These lines of business are probably not important to the average consumer. However, they mean something to a health plan or insurer.

Health plans usually organize divisions within the insurer around these operational lines of business. While the delivery and administration of healthcare is the same at its core, each line of business can have unique compliance, regulatory, benefits, and other rules that require some segregation of staff, operations, and expertise within a plan.

CHAPTER 5

Terminology, Part 1 (Key Plan Definitions)

L et's get into some of the terminology used by health insurers and health plans in the American system. Most of it applies to all lines of business, with some exceptions for Medicaid.

While not an exhaustive list, I think these are the most important, fundamental terms. I combed various sources to select the items, including the Medicare Evidence of Coverage, Medicaid Member Handbooks, and various Exchange and commercial policy documents from a number of health plans. The definitions are my own except where I have used an open-source listing of various code or data sets or a citation is made (where an outside source contributed to the description).

Topic Area 1: You as an Enrollee and Plan Documentation

Subscriber and Dependents—Usually found in the commercial world, the subscriber is an individual who is the employee or person contracting for the coverage. The dependents are a spouse/domestic partner and children. In Medicare, enrollees are enrolled on an individual basis. In Medicaid, some states enroll by family units and others on an individual basis.

Member Handbook, Evidence/Explanation of Coverage (EOC)—These are documents issued by your health plan explaining benefits covered as well as the policies and procedures you must follow to obtain health services. These documents run from simple for a commercial health plan to extremely complex for Medicare, which runs to almost 300 pages. In the Medicaid world, states dictate that member handbooks be written at a low-grade reading level to address significant health literacy barriers in the covered population.

Pre-existing Condition—This is a documented, individual medical condition that impacted an individual's healthcare coverage prior to the passage of the Affordable Care Act (ACA or Obamacare). In the past, and in certain lines of business, health insurers might reject coverage for an individual totally, reject coverage for a given condition or disease state for a period of time, or charge higher rates for coverage due to pre-existing conditions. In some cases, for employer-sponsored coverage, an individual could provide proof of continuous coverage in a health plan and the pre-existing condition would be covered from day one in the new plan.

Now that the ACA is in place, everything has changed. It is no longer allowable to reject coverage of individuals or not cover benefits or services related to a pre-existing disease state or condition. This is the case for most insurance products today. We will discuss in greater detail later how a new rating system has taken hold with the changes regarding treatment of pre-existing conditions.

I spent a number of years in underwriting of commercial plans, including designing an individual rate structure and underwriting approach that rejected certain individuals deemed too risky to be covered, charged those with certain illnesses higher than standard rates to cover the increased risk, and granted those who were healthy lower than standard preferred rates. Now, we ran the plan honestly based on the rules at the time and applying the approved criteria and rates. But it always bothered me that we were denying people in need of coverage. Part of my desire for true universal access stems from these actuarial prediction days of mine. As well, I do believe that America is right to ban exclusion from coverage and higher rates for those who are sick.

Topic Area 2: Benefits, Networks, Provider Reimbursement, and Claims Processes

Essential Health Benefits (EHBs)—These are benefits and services that have been deemed essential and therefore mandated for health plans in the individual and small group market under the ACA. This means that plans are obligated to offer these benefits as part of all their plan offerings.

Covered versus Non-covered Benefits/Services and Formulary— Covered services are benefits or services outlined as such in your plan's benefit handbook or explanation of coverage. Non-covered benefits or excluded benefits are those that are not listed in your plan's materials as covered or are explicitly listed as excluded. Your covered drugs are listed on a drug list or formulary. The list is divided into tiers, which usually shows you the amount you pay (either a flat dollar or percentage of the costs) for that level. You may also be entitled to ask for coverage of a drug that is not on the formulary if it is medically necessary for you and no other drug could be beneficial for your disease state or condition.

Many people end up paying out of pocket for excluded or non-covered benefits, such as cosmetic surgery. A good example from my family: my grandson, Owen, had an asymmetry to his head as an infant—a relatively common condition. He needed to wear a helmet for about three months to correct the issue. His health plan benefit package specifically excluded coverage for helmets unless needed post-surgery. The doctor did say it was medically necessary to correct the asymmetry, but after an appeal to his health plan internally and a call to the state insurance department, the result was the same and the treatment had to be paid by my son out of pocket to the tune of $2,500. The doctor gave my son a break on what would have been a $4,000 billed procedure. Good news: Owen's head has been corrected, and he is as handsome as I am.

Routine dental and vision care usually are not covered by a health plan and such benefits are sold as separate policies.

Brand and Generic Drugs—Brand drugs are those that are usually still under patent. While there may be other drugs in the same or similar therapeutic class (i.e., other drugs that can be used to treat the same disease state or condition), a given brand drug is the only one sold with that exact composition. In contrast, generic drugs are generally not subject to patent, therefore any manufacturer is free to create the drug with the same chemical composition and sell it. Generally, brand drugs are much more expensive: they are hundreds—sometimes thousands—of dollars for a thirty-day supply. The average brand cost is about $567 for a thirty-day supply. Generics are usually low-cost. Over 90% are $20 per month or less and the average price is about $30 per month. Plans encourage the use of generic drugs whenever possible unless a brand drug is absolutely needed for a disease state or condition.[5-1, 5-2]

As a side note, while plans sometimes rightfully get criticized for denying expensive brand drugs that are needed, plans are largely right to encourage generic use. Too often, expensive brand drugs are prescribed when they are not truly needed. Americans request them because they are encouraged to do so by free-wheeling direct-to-consumer advertising. It is getting so bad that drugmakers are now appealing to our emotions by advertising medications for our itchy dogs. While reforms have been made, drugmakers influence on doctors is still great. Doctors are complicit in the over-use of expensive brands—it's fun to prescribe them; it looks cutting edge. So, I always ask my doctor why he recommends a brand drug and if there is a legacy generic that can do the trick just as well. It is not always the case that a generic works as well for a given disease state, but more often than not, it can. I have slight high blood pressure and mild to moderate Type 2 diabetes. I am on a thirty-year-old drug for high blood pressure and a twenty-year-old drug for diabetes. Both of these can be obtained for no cost at one pharmacy in my area and worst case for $4 each for a thirty-day supply. They both do just fine. As Mom told us, newer isn't always better. An additional advantage: legacy generics are proven in terms of side effects and potential health impacts.

Limitations—Certain services or benefits may have limitations. This means that these services or benefits are only covered up to a certain number of units or visits, or only after certain other procedures. As an example, chiropractic, podiatry, and related services often have a visit cap on them in many policies. Thereafter, visits become uncovered benefits and individuals need to pay for them out of pocket.

Different Types of Services/Benefits—Here are some of the most important types of services covered by health plans or related insurers (it may require additional coverage beyond medical coverage). Some of these services could be subject to deductibles and others not. They could have various types of cost-sharing. (See the discussion on deductibles and cost-sharing in the next chapter.) Last, some of these services could have prior authorization requirements, while others may not. This means the plan may need to approve coverage before you obtain the services.

- Inpatient hospitalization (various levels of care, including rehabilitation)
- Non-custodial skilled nursing and rehabilitation (acute stays)
- Outpatient services, either at a hospital or free-standing surgery center
- Emergency room care and services
- Ambulance and emergency transportation
- Non-emergency transportation
- Urgent care facilities
- Telehealth
- Primary care physician and provider services
- Specialist physician and provider services
- Retail drugs
- Drugs administered at a physician's office
- Laboratory services
- Imaging and radiology
- Durable medical equipment, prosthetics, and supplies
- Behavioral health and substance abuse services
- Dental services
- Hearing services

- Optometric or eye care services
- Various therapies, such as physical therapy, speech therapy, and occupational therapy
- Home healthcare and rehabilitation services
- Hospice care

Different Places of Service—Services and benefits can be delivered at various places of service (POS). Places of service are the locations where the services are rendered. These places of service are usually captured as part of the request for payment submitted by the provider or facility to the health plan. The place of service could be used in tandem with the type of service to determine whether a benefit needs prior authorization. A place of service could also dictate whether a service is subject to a deductible or higher cost-sharing.

As an example, a routine magnetic resonance imaging (MRI) request may require a prior authorization if done at an outpatient hospital setting due to the higher expense versus at a free-standing radiology center. Even if the procedure does not require a prior authorization, the costs you pay out-of-pocket could be dramatically different. As an example, an MRI for the hospital outpatient setting could be subject to a deductible as well as significant cost-sharing (explained in detail soon). The MRI at a radiology center might have just a flat co-pay amount you pay and not be subject to a deductible.

Here are some common places of service with their applicable codes that are used for payment requests and claims payment:

- 01—Pharmacy
- 02—Telehealth
- 11—Office
- 12—Home
- 13—Assisted Living Facility
- 17—Walk-In Retail Health Clinic
- 19—Off-campus Outpatient Hospital
- 20—Urgent Care
- 21—Inpatient Hospital

- o   22—On-campus Outpatient Hospital
- o   23—Emergency Room—Hospital
- o   24—Ambulatory Surgery Center
- o   31—Skilled Nursing Facility
- o   32—Nursing Facility
- o   34—Hospice
- o   41—Ambulance—Land
- o   42—Ambulance—Air or Water
- o   49—Independent Clinic
- o   50—Federally Qualified Health Center
- o   51—Inpatient Psychiatric Facility
- o   52—Psychiatric Facility—Partial Hospitalization
- o   55—Residential Substance Abuse Treatment Facility
- o   56—Psychiatric Residential Treatment Facility
- o   57—Non-residential Substance Abuse Treatment Facility
- o   61—Comprehensive Inpatient Rehabilitation Facility
- o   62—Comprehensive Outpatient Rehabilitation Facility
- o   81—Independent Laboratory

A word of caution so you become a savvy healthcare consumer—while it is almost always true that getting services at outpatient hospital (POS 19 or 22) is far more expensive than ambulatory sites (POS 24), the following is also true:

- o   There could be dramatically different rates that providers get paid within POS 19 and 22, and for that matter inpatient rates (POS 21). This depends on how good the contract is between the plan and the hospital. This can affect how much you pay.
- o   There also could be dramatically different rates paid to providers within POS 24. Again, it is all about the strength of the contract between the plan and the provider. This can affect how much you pay.

If you have to have surgery or an expensive imaging procedure, always shop around, especially if that procedure is subject to the deductible and/or has significant cost-sharing. A good example, I should be among the wisest consumers, but my wife had a fairly advanced radiology scan at a free-standing facility. We paid over $900 because it was subject to our deductible and significant cost-sharing. It was odd because, from my days negotiating contracts with providers, I knew these scans were now going for about $300 to $400. I discovered the issue just as the IV was being put in my wife's arm. A quick call to our health plan showed two other, free-standing imaging facilities where costs were estimated at just over $300.

Primary Care Physician/Provider and Specialists—A primary care physician or provider (PCP) is usually your assigned doctor handling the coordination of your healthcare in certain health plans/products. Not all plan products require a PCP, but one is always recommended. This individual is usually the first doctor you go to who handles your overall health and may refer you to specialists, doctors, or experts in a special subject area of medicine and in the treatment of specific disease states and conditions. Good examples of a PCP may be an internist, family practitioner, general practitioner, general pediatrician, gynecologist (in some plans), and gerontologist. Good examples of specialists include a dermatologist, neurologist, cardiologist, or urologist. More and more, PCPs handle specific disease states, such as diabetes and asthma.

In-network/Contracted/Participating versus Out-of-network/Non-contracted/Non-participating Providers—Depending on your type of plan, you may be limited to seeking services within an established network of contracted or participating providers or the plan will not cover those services or benefits, even if listed in your handbook or evidence/explanation of coverage. Plans publish a provider directory to let you know if your physician, other provider, pharmacy, or facility is in their network. In some cases, plans will cover in-network providers at the standard cost-sharing (described in the next chapter) as well as out-of-network providers at higher cost-sharing.

It is important to note that plans must cover certain out-of-network services, such as emergency room services and emergency admissions in the commercial world. In Medicare, health plans must cover those two services out of network as well as a thirty-day supply of drugs, renal dialysis, and urgent care. While it is not common, it is possible to petition your health plan to receive services from an out-of-network provider at in-network cost-sharing, whether the plan has out-of-network coverage or not. For example, it may be that there are no specialists that can diagnose or perform services in network and the plan approves use of that provider who is not in network.

As plans look to gain efficiencies, improve quality, and meet consumer expectations, sometimes it is possible to have additional layers of providers that are in network. A plan may offer a much-reduced co-pay if you see a preferred network provider and a higher co-pay if you see a regular network provider. It is important to understand your plan type, your in-network and out-of-network benefits, and how many types of in-network providers you might have. While not typical, it could be this complex:

Tier 1—Center of Excellence Provider (may have quality rating or other rating that differentiates the provider even from preferred providers)

Tier 2—Preferred Provider

Tier 3—In-network Provider

Tier 4—Out-of-network Provider

Provider Reimbursement Types—There are many provider reimbursement types plans utilize to pay providers for services rendered to members. Here are some of the key forms of reimbursement. Remember that it is likely that providers receive more than one type of reimbursement. It is also true that many of these can overlap:

Fee-for-Service (FFS)—In this case, a provider is paid a fee by the plan for each service the provider renders. Generally, in this system of payment and healthcare, the physician or provider likely provides as many services as possible (e.g., visits, tests, and procedures) as the more he provides, the more he makes. The fees paid are established by the provider and may be negotiated with the plan based on a prevailing fee in the marketplace or set by a regulatory authority (e.g., Medicare or Medicaid). This is known as discounted FFS. Providers may also take into consideration the volume of members from the plan in granting a discount.

Cost of Care—This model is not very popular, but in this case a provider sets a fee it charges based on the actual cost of care. This could include some room for profit.

Capitation—This is the practice of paying providers for a set of services based on a per member/patient per month methodology. As an example, this is popular with PCPs, where they are paid X dollars each month per assigned member to render all primary care services (e.g., office visits, certain limited lab, and diagnostic testing). These providers may also render other services on a FFS basis. For example, they may be paid on a FFS basis for in-office surgery. Providers usually accept capitation from a plan only if there are a sufficient number of members assigned by the plan to that provider or group.

Global Risk and Partial Risk Capitation—This goes beyond basic capitation and puts providers at risk for a broad range of services, even though they may not be responsible for most of them. The goal is to have the provider, usually a multi-specialty or large PCP group or other type of organization, emphasize care management and to avoid the costs of higher levels of care. This comes generally in two forms. **Global Risk Capitation** is when a provider is responsible for *all* the costs of the services of the members (e.g., all inpatient and outpatient services). **Partial Risk Capitation** is when a provider is responsible for *some* large amount of the costs of services of the members (e.g., certain or all outpatient services).

To ensure that providers without financial wherewithal are not saddled with costs they cannot bear, there are various rules surrounding how much risk can be assumed by providers and groups. These are called **Physician Incentive Plans (PIPs)** and are controlled by the so-called

PIP rules for various lines of business. These are embedded in federal and some state laws and regulations. Generally, these rules require an assessment of how much risk a provider group can shoulder. Various things, including patient revenue and membership, go into this calculation. There are also requirements for stop-loss insurance or reinsurance. This can be supplied by either the provider group or the health plan.

The rules lead to plans and provider groups constructing various methods of risk capitation to encourage aggressive oversight of members and cost-containment, but through financial arrangements that meet the PIP rules.

The biggest providers have stop-loss insurance. The plan gives them a significant portion of total premiums for the members assigned to them (e.g., 75-80%), and the plan is responsible for all costs. They keep all of the gains if they control costs and accept all of the losses if costs exceed the premiums given. This is known as full upside and downside risk.

Partial upside and downside risk is more popular, where providers receive part of the savings against premiums for successfully limiting costs and pay for a part of the losses if costs run over premiums. Upside only risk (full or partial) is practiced as well, with the provider sharing in savings ("shared savings") but the plan takes on the risk of over-spending against premiums.

Pay for Performance (P4P)—This reimbursement system is often used in conjunction with other payment schemes and is based on benchmarks set by the plan or regulatory authorities (quality and performance thresholds or quadrants for both performance and quality) A good example is what are known as FFS quality "bill aboves," where doctors get paid extra per quality measurement achieved or a lump sum based on overall performance driving quality in the Medicare Advantage (MA) Star or other quality programs.

Value-Based Payments—This is called either Value-Based Payments or Reimbursement (VBP/VBR) or Quality-based Payments or Reimbursement (QBP/QBR). Related to P4P above, this is an emerging reimbursement area. In this reimbursement structure, the fees paid by the plan to the provider are not based on costs or a fee, but on the outcomes or results (e.g., did the person's health improve, is the disease state or condition gone or under control, or did certain value/quality achievements occur?). We should see this morph and flourish in the future. A great deal of discussion is focused on having drug payments linked to specific outcomes.

Episodes of Care and Bundled Payments—In this example, a facility or group of providers associated with a facility might be paid a global payment to be used by all providers for a given episode of care. A good example is an inpatient procedure (e.g., hip replacement) that may require inpatient hospitalization, skilled rehabilitation, home care, and other ancillary services. This bundled episode of care payment would be shared among the providers. This encourages holistic care for these types of events, thereby limiting readmissions, speeding recovery, and ensuring quality. Medicare is practicing this in the Medicare FFS program, as are certain commercial providers. Often, the payment is to hospitals that own all the healthcare assets needed to control costs and boost quality.

Hospital and facility payments can come in many forms, including per diem payments, episode of care (e.g., Diagnosis Related Groups or DRGs), percent of charges against set fee schedules of the facility, and percent of cost.

Drugs can be reimbursed through a variety of means. Three of the most popular are based on (1) a discount to the average wholesale price (AWP), usually for retail pharmacy brand drugs; (2) the maximum allowable cost (MAC) list, usually for retail pharmacy generic drugs; and (3) the average sales price plus a percentage, usually for medical drugs (drugs administered in a physician's office or other outpatient facility).

Healthcare Codes—Providers bill health plans using various healthcare codes. These help plans pay providers appropriately when a request for payment—called a claim—is sent to the plan or in some cases other entities that help plans fulfill clinical functions, such as a pharmacy benefit manager (PBM) (usually the servicer of the retail drug benefit). There are diagnosis codes, which quantify the disease state, condition, injury, or illness that an individual may have. The diagnosis code can often be an important element of determining whether a service needed an authorization or should be paid via a claim. There are also various procedure codes, which tell a health plan what procedure or service was rendered. The codes combine with the place of service to determine proper payment for the service.

Claims are submitted in different formats depending on the type of service. More and more, claims are submitted in what are known as the Health Insurance Portability and Accountability Act (HIPAA)-compliant formats, named for the privacy and portability act I told you about in an earlier chapter.

These codes are not only important for payment of providers, but also because plans submit encounter data to regulatory agencies. The encounter data, basically all the claims a plan collects for its members, often are used in determining the risk of individual members or of the plan.

The major types of claims that come into a plan include medical, pharmacy, dental, vision, and lab claims. The major types of codes that plans utilize to pay claims to providers include:

- ◦ International Classification of Diseases or ICD-10 *diagnosis* codes
- ◦ International Classification of Diseases or ICD-10 *procedure* codes, largely used by hospitals
- ◦ Current Procedural Terminology (CPT) codes—these codes are sent to plans by providers of professional services. These codes are owned by the American Medical Association (AMA) and are designated as Level 1 procedure codes.
- ◦ Healthcare Common Procedure Coding System (HCPCS) codes— these codes are related to CPT codes. These are known as Level 2 codes. These codes are maintained by the Centers for Medicare and Medicaid Services (CMS) and are used in Medicare and other lines of business. These are largely codes not found in CPT, such as non-physician services, products, supplies, medical equipment, and certain procedures.

○ Sometimes there are codes that are unique to certain regulatory agencies, including Medicaid agencies, that are used by health plans.

○ Various Diagnosis Related Group (DRG) codes used largely for hospital payments. This is a bundled rate for the entire hospital stay that is based on diagnosis, procedure, and severity of illness. There are various DRG systems used in the commercial, Medicaid, and Medicare worlds, including MS-DRG (maintained and used by CMS in Medicare). The DRGs can be refined based on the type of population covered in the line of business.

○ Dental codes—the American Dental Association maintains its own code sets known as the Code on Dental Procedures and Nomenclature (CDP). These generally are used universally for dental procedures not captured in the medical codes.

○ Drug codes—various drug codes are used to reimburse for retail and medically administered drugs. Every drug gets a National Drug Code (NDC), which could be used in reimbursement. Two leading drug classifications are owned by First Data Bank (FDB) and Wolters Kluwer Medi-Span. FDB uses a Generic Code Number (GCN) and Hierarchical Ingredient Code List (HICL) to classify drugs. Medi-Span uses a Generic Product Identifier (GPI). These, too, can be used to reimburse for drugs. J codes are part of the HCPCS codes and reimburse for the medically administered drugs.

HIPAA Standard Electronic Transaction Formats—As noted previously, the HIPAA act set up a series of common formats that governments, health plans, and providers could use to standardize and simplify communications. These standard transaction formats are becoming more and more common, although the healthcare world still communicates in non-standard, one-off ways, based on health plans' and providers' desires. In addition, while the transaction formats are supposedly standardized, it is also true that the formats can be customized a great deal, leading to new complexity. HIPAA transaction formats include those for enrollment/eligibility, claims, payment, and authorization.

Explanation of Benefits (EOB)—An EOB is a statement sent to you by your health plan when a request for payment comes in from your doctor or other healthcare provider for a service he provided to you. These arrive periodically in the commercial world and usually monthly in Medicare. The EOB tells you what the provider sought to charge (the billed amount), the plan discount if an in-network provider, what the plan contracted amount was if an in-network provider (the allowed amount), the amount the plan paid (this is usually net of cost-sharing), and the amount you are obligated to pay if any (cost-sharing—a deductible, co-insurance, or co-pay, which are described on the next chapter). The EOB may also have explanations as to the date of submission to the health plan, the servicing date(s), and any denial or other payment information. The EOB may also show disallowed amounts. EOBs also tend to give a summary of where each member and the family (if applicable) are in terms of progress fulfilling deductibles and maximum out-of-pocket (MOOP) costs, which are explained in the next chapter. If a product has out-of-network coverage, the EOB is similar.

CHAPTER 6

Terminology, Part 2 (Payment Issues)

N ow that we have covered you as a subscriber and benefits, claims, and networks, let's get to the important stuff—what you pay as part of your health coverage. Cost-sharing is an important component of healthcare. It helps lower premiums and overall costs in the system by hopefully making you a wiser and more prudent consumer of services.

Topic Area 3: What You Pay

Health Savings Account (HSA), Flexible Spending Account (FSA), and Health Reimbursement Account (HRA)—A health savings account (HSA) and flexible spending account (FSA) are slightly different, but what they have in common is that they allow individuals to contribute to these accounts to pay for medical expenses. An HSA is owned by the individual and is usually paired with a high-deductible health plan (HDHP), a lean coverage plan that assumes you pay out-of-pocket for most services until you reach a high deductible. But the plan is there to reduce your costs (you get the benefit of negotiated rates with network providers) and in case you have a catastrophic healthcare event, such as a car accident.

The individual contributes to the HSA on a tax-free basis and uses it for medical expenses prior to hitting the deductible. All unused dollars are rolled over year to year. An FSA is usually offered by an employer and does not have to be paired with a health plan. It simply is a tax-free vehicle for individuals to contribute to and use for qualifying medical expenses. With an FSA, rollover is more limited from year to year.

A health reimbursement account (HRA), also known as a consumer-driven health plan (CDHP) is quite different. This is an employer-sponsored health plan that reimburses employees for medical expenses. Under a 2019 rule advocated by Donald Trump, HRAs were broadened to allow employers to set aside tax-free funds to give to employees to purchase insurance individually—both for Affordable Care Act (ACA)-compliant coverage and other excepted bare bones coverage.[6-1]

Premium—This is the monthly amount you pay to obtain your healthcare coverage. If you are enrolled in employer-sponsored care, usually your employer defrays much of that monthly premium the insurer charges, so you are paying only a portion of the total premium. In the individual purchase world, unfortunately you are on the hook for the whole thing. If you are enrolled in Medicare Advantage (MA) or a standalone Medicare drug plan (PDP), you may pay a premium depending on where you live in the country. While most Medicaid beneficiaries do not pay premiums to enroll in that program, there are some states that now extend coverage to optional groups and charge these enrollees a small monthly premium.

Cost-sharing—This is an umbrella term that denotes various categories of monetary outlays you make on behalf of yourself and dependents as part of your health coverage. Cost-sharing often ties to the amount of the premium paid. The lower your overall cost-sharing, the higher your premiums will be and vice versa. A relatively healthy person might want to have higher cost-sharing, as he or she won't utilize many services and wants a lower premium. It is also true that those who are ill or are high-utilizers of healthcare might be willing to pay higher premiums for lower cost-sharing along the way. There are three major types of cost-sharing:

Deductible—A deductible is the amount of money that must be spent by you before your health coverage kicks in. After that you are covered, but you may pay one of the additional cost-sharing types below. Here is where it gets complicated. In the commercial world, plan designs can use deductibles differently. In some cases, a plan benefit may subject almost every service to a deductible before the health insurer begins paying (except, for example, mandated prevention services such as wellness visits). In other cases, deductibles are targeted at specific high-cost areas to dissuade the use of these services in favor of lower-cost ones. As an example, inpatient admissions and procedures at a hospital on an outpatient basis may be subject to a deductible. At the same time, primary care, specialist, and procedures at a free-standing ambulatory surgery center might not be subject to a deductible. In the Medicare world, there is an inpatient deductible, separate outpatient deductible, and a deductible if a beneficiary elects a drug benefit. In Medicaid, generally deductibles do not apply. In the Marketplace Exchange world, the variations in the commercial world apply.

Deductibles usually apply over a twelve-month period. In Medicare they usually begin on January 1 of each year. In the commercial plan, they apply based on your benefit year, which is the twelve-month period beginning when your employer renews its coverage.

It is also important to remember that there could be individual deductibles as well as family deductibles. This means that you either have to hit your individual deductible or your family would have to hit the entire family deductible before coverage kicks in for benefits subject to the deductible. Usually, the family deductible is a bit of a break for larger families (e.g., the family deductible might be $4,500 for a family of four, when individual deductibles might be $1,500 each).

Co-insurance—Co-insurance is usually the percentage you pay of the cost of given procedures or covered benefits. As an example, in commercial healthcare, after a deductible, an insured (that's you) might pay 20% of the cost of the hospital stay, while the plan covers 80%. In Medicare, a good example may be that you pay 20% of the cost of the durable medical equipment (DME) you need. Certain retail drugs on your plan that are more expensive or that your plan has not obtained good discounts for from the drugmaker may also have co-insurance. Again, given the low-income nature of the program, Medicaid cost-sharing, including co-insurance, is not routine.

Co-pays—Co-pays are the most popular form of cost-sharing. This is the fixed dollar amount you pay to obtain given services. A good example in the commercial and Medicare worlds is that you might pay a ten- or twenty-dollar co-pay to see your primary care physician. That co-pay may be higher—say between thirty and sixty dollars—to see a specialist physician. Generally, the rest of the cost of these visits are covered entirely by the plan. Co-pays are very common for lower cost retail drugs. Very small co-pays are now being introduced in Medicaid for medical and drug benefits for some populations.

Sometimes, when you go to a provider, you could be subject to two or three forms of cost-sharing—a co-pay, a deductible, and/or cost-sharing. So, it is always a good idea to understand your benefits and cost-sharing obligations before obtaining services.

One example is when you have a procedure in a hospital. Usually, you must meet your deductible first and then pay some percentage or co-insurance of the remaining costs. This could cost you thousands of dollars.

Another example: You need to go to a dermatologist for what your wife says are suspect areas on your bald head. You spent a lot of time out in the sun over the years, and you fear it may be some form of cancer. You arrive at the dermatologist and pay a fifty-dollar co-pay. This is the amount you pay under your plan for the professional visit. For this, your doctor gives you a complete full-body exam and rules out any issues for 90% of your body.

But wait, he does say that there are issues for that bald head of yours. There are areas that look like they are pre-cancerous and must be frozen. Others require a medical procedure to extract the suspect area and send it for a biopsy. Well, you find out that your deductible of $250 (that's very low these days, so you have a good plan) applies to physician office procedures and thereafter you have 20% co-insurance. The cost of the freezing as well as the surgery is $400. You pay the following, as it is still early in the benefit year and you have not paid any of your deductible yet:

- $50 co-pay to the doctor for that full-body scan
- $250 to the doctor because in-office surgery is subject to the deductible
- $30 additional for the 20% co-insurance for the remaining surgery cost of $150
- The lab fee for the biopsy is fully covered under your plan, so there are no additional costs here

So, you got out of there for a reasonable $330 and the good news is your deductible is covered for the year. Oh, and the biopsy came back that those certain areas were not cancerous, and the doctor got everything off that he needed.

Maximum Out-of-Pocket Costs or MOOP—This is the maximum you would pay out of pocket for your health plan. Thereafter, the plan would cover 100% of the costs for the remainder of the benefit or coverage year for you. Like your deductible, this is usually on a calendar year basis or plan year basis. MOOPs can be calculated in a few different ways, so check your policy closely. It also may differ whether you are in Medicare or commercial. This doesn't really apply to Medicaid.

Traditional Medicare FFS really doesn't operate with MOOPs. There is no protection. If these beneficiaries enroll in the free-standing Medicare drug benefit, there is a MOOP. For MA plans, there are two MOOPs—one for medical and one for the drug benefit.

MOOPs in Medicare and commercial generally include deductibles, co-insurance, and co-pays. However, they do not include premiums. You will always have to pay a premium if you have one. Out-of-network costs do not count toward a MOOP for plans that have in-network only.

In the case of plans that include both in-network and out-of-network coverage, the following could apply (this also differs between Medicare and commercial):

- Some plans don't cap out-of-network costs, and they also don't count toward the in-network MOOP.
- Other plans set a totally separate out-of-network MOOP from the in-network one.
- Still others may set a lower MOOP for in-network, then have a combined in- and out-of-network one as well. MOOPs do not include member outlays for non-covered or excluded benefits.

CHAPTER 7

Terminology, Part 3
(Balance and Surprise Billing)

Topic Area 3: What You Pay (continued)

Balance Billing or Surprise (Not the Pleasant One) Billing

What you pay for your healthcare should be fair and equitable. But there is a growing phenomenon of balanced billing or surprise billing that is seriously impacting Americans' financial status. I told you earlier that lack of health insurance or inadequate health insurance is a major reason for bankruptcies in the United States. More and more, however, these bankruptcies can be linked to balanced billing or surprise billing. Such bills can cost thousands, if not tens of thousands and sometimes hundreds of thousands of dollars. This chapter seeks to define it and give you some helpful hints to avoid it. Some surprise billing protection recently was passed by Congress and is covered later in this chapter.

Balance billing and surprise billing are a bit synonymous. They are umbrella terms for (1) billing by a network provider for the difference between his charges and the combined amount of what a health plan contractually should pay the provider and what you are obligated to pay under your insurance through cost-sharing; (2) billing by an out-of-network provider above what the health plan pays (if any) because the provider does not have a contractual relationship with your insurer; or (3) in other circumstances, billing that is unexpected, erroneous, or even illegally billed from an in-network or out-of-network provider.

Balance billing or surprise billing is quite common for emergency services (whether in-network or out-of-network) as well as with complex inpatient and outpatient procedures done at hospitals or surgery centers. These bills can also be tied to the fact that prior authorization was not sought from the plan, prior authorization was denied by the plan, or the services are for uncovered or excluded benefits.

Balance billing or surprise billing is on the rise in healthcare. There are several reasons for this. Due to the managed care backlash, beginning in the late 1990s and early 2000s, plans increasingly introduced products with more out-of-network benefits. This opens up issues with out-of-network provider payments. More recently, some plans (especially in the Exchanges) have introduced narrower networks in order to contain costs. This increases the likelihood of getting treated by an out-of-network provider.

Plans also are closely scrutinizing what they pay and how much. If plans negotiate a good deal with providers, then that is the rate they are willing to pay for out-of-network services, if applicable (perhaps somewhat more in certain circumstances). They are trying to keep costs down, and it is hard to blame them. On the flip side, providers argue that plans are unwilling to pay reasonable rates both to in-network and out-of-network providers.

As important, members often do not know who is in network and who is not, and they do a poor job of studying such issues. Add to this the complexity of the myriad providers who often take part in complex procedures. For example, in a moderate-to-complex procedure on an inpatient or outpatient basis, you may have many of the following providers: surgeon, consulting surgeon, anesthesiologist, pathologist, laboratory, hospital or surgery center fee, skilled nursing or rehab facility, home health agency, physical therapist, hospitalist, or hospital attending physician.[7-1]

Balance or surprise billing comes in many forms:[7-1, 7-2]

A simple mistake. The in-network provider billed you instead of your insurance company. This may occur because you did not present your insurance card at the time of service or the insurance was not updated.

Claim not submitted or submitted incorrectly. A provider may not have submitted a claim or did not submit it correctly, and it has been rejected. The provider turns around and bills you instead of working it out with the health plan.

Claim processed wrong or initially denied. The health plan processes a claim wrong or initially denies a claim, and providers begin billing you for the whole bill. It could be a mistake by the plan, or you won on an appeal. Providers often need to resubmit claims to have all of this straightened out.

Provider ignores no-balance-bill contractual or legal provisions. A provider is ignoring his contract or the law and bills you the difference between an allowed or contracted amount and his prevailing rate, even if you pay a co-pay or co-insurance. A provider may seek to bill amounts from certain individuals who have both Medicare and Medicaid (the poorest of the "dual eligible" enrollees) when they are not allowed to under law. Under federal law, what Medicare and Medicaid pay are deemed payment in full.

You see an out-of-network provider, but you don't have out-of-network coverage. You are seeking care from an out-of-network provider, and your plan has no out-of-network coverage. In this case, the plan won't cover anything, and you are responsible for 100% of the bill. More important, the provider can charge you whatever he wants. In most cases, members can seek emergency care out of network and be covered.

You have an indemnity plan or managed care plan with out-of-network coverage and don't know the out-of-network payment rules. You have an indemnity plan or a managed care plan that has out-of-network coverage. The provider is seeking payment above what the health plan paid for the service in question. While your indemnity or out-of-network benefit may call for the plan to pay a percentage of the costs (e.g., 50%), the plan may limit its reimbursement to a lower rate, such as a usual and customary rate (UCR or a reasonable rate) or a rate based in part on how much it may pay for such a provider. Thus, you not only pay for 50% of the plan paid amount but also 100% of the balance up to the amount billed by the provider. This can occur even if you received prior authorization from your plan beforehand. Sometimes, an out-of-network provider will agree to accept the plan's allowable amount as payment in full.

The plan does not cover or limits payment to an out-of-network provider when you sought emergency care. There are several scenarios here:

> First, you are in an accident or have another emergency and you need to seek emergency care. While emergency care usually is covered whether in-network or out-of-network, the surprise bills come flying in. You could have a major cost-sharing bill come in the mail because the plan denies payment to an out-of-network facility or other out-of-network provider rendering care at an emergency room or for an emergency inpatient admission.
>
> Second, the facility or other provider rendering emergency services is out of network and the health plan limits the amount it pays the non-network-provider to a UCR or rate it would pay in-network for such services.
>
> Third, you had to receive emergency care from an out-of-network provider at an in-network emergency room or inpatient hospital. The plan either denies those payments or limits them and the pro-

viders bill you. Sometimes an out-of-network provider will agree to accept the plan's allowable amount as payment in full. Some plans, but not all, have rules that require an in-network facility using out-of-network providers to require the out-of-network provider to accept in-network rates of payment and not balance bill. Note that ground or air ambulance to the emergency room and transport between hospitals is often one of the biggest surprise billing areas.

You followed all the rules and are at an in-network provider for a non-emergency procedure, but an out-of-network provider enters the picture. Similar to the emergency cases above, you arrange for non-emergency treatment at an in-network facility or provider, but one element of the services or procedure you receive are furnished by an out-of-network provider. You may not be aware of it or you signed an acknowledgement early that morning of the surgery or procedure. The plan may argue the cost needs to be borne 100% by you. Some plans, but not all, have rules that require a facility using out-of-network providers to require the out-of-network provider to accept in-network rates of payment and not balance bill.

A provider did not seek prior authorization for a service. An in-network provider did not seek an authorization for a service from a health plan, and the plan has denied the service after the fact through the claims process because it did require prior authorization. (Sometimes the plan may review the claim retrospectively, grant authorization, and pay the claim.) Under some contracts with health plans, a provider cannot bill you for that denied service as he did not seek authorization. Or he may be allowed to bill you only for applicable cost-sharing. Instead, the provider bills you anyway at the discounted rate or the provider's billed rate. In certain cases, a provider can bill you, and you may be responsible for the entire bill.

An authorization was denied but the service occurred anyway. An in-network provider did seek authorization for a service from a health plan and the health plan denied the service. The service took place anyway. Under some health plan contracts, the provider cannot bill you at all or the provider can bill the member for applicable cost-sharing at the negotiated discount rate but does not receive a payment for the difference from the health plan. Instead, the provider has billed you for the full amount anyway, either at the negotiated discount rate or the provider's billed rate. In certain cases, a provider can bill you and you may be responsible for the entire bill.

No authorization was obtained by you for an out-of-network service. You have an out-of-network benefit, but the services require prior authorization, and you did not request it before the services were completed. In this case, the provider will likely bill you at his full provider rate.

The health plan thinks it should be secondary coverage due to an accident or other event. Health insurance is secondary to another insurance in cases of accidents and other events. Based on diagnoses or procedures, your health plan suspects you may have been involved in an accident and denies your provider claims because you did not get back to them to substantiate that no accident occurred and therefore an automobile, homeowners, or workers' compensation insurance policy is not involved. Your provider bills you for either a plan discounted amount or the billed rate when the health plan denied his claim.

Your coverage is limited for certain services you received. In unique circumstances, plans may limit the maximum amount it pays for certain services. This could be a cap on the amount paid per visit, a cap on the number of visits per coverage year, or a maximum amount paid per coverage year. Under the Affordable Care Act (ACA), this usually can only occur for benefits that are not deemed essential health benefits (EHBs). In this case, the provider bills you for amounts over these limits. The provider should always seek your concurrence before treatment, but sometimes he does not or you have forgotten you signed acceptance some time ago. Note that this is different from a provider discount (that a provider should not bill you for). In this case, the plan places a maximum on what it will pay under your plan benefits and may or may not have negotiated a discount rate.

The service you received is non-covered. A provider performed a service that was specifically not covered by your plan or excluded. In this case, you are responsible for the entirety of the bill and the provider can charge you what he wants unless you negotiated this upfront. Usually, for in-network providers, plans require providers to disclose beforehand the fact that services are not covered or excluded and will be billed at the provider's usual and customary rate (UCR). Watch for this in many lines of business for certain laboratory or other testing. Always ask if a lab or test is covered.

Your plan specifically allows balance billing. Plans negotiate discounts with providers from their UCRs or agree on a fee schedule. In the commercial line of business, some plans allow providers to bill above such amounts if the patient agrees in writing beforehand. In addition, certain charges may be disallowed under contracts but can also be billed if the patient agreed beforehand.

You don't understand your cost-sharing and benefit structure. While this is not really a form of balanced or surprise billing, I call it out here. Many people are often surprised when they get a bill in the mail from an in-network provider because they did not scrutinize their benefits or do their homework enough before getting surgery, advanced radiology, or the like at a given in-network facility. They often think that a given service or procedure is not subject to a deductible and/or may have a flat co-pay versus co-insurance. They also may be surprised by the magnitude of a bill, having heard a procedure was low-cost but the bill says something quite different. It is important to remember that benefit designs do take into consideration places of service and provider rates can vary dramatically from facility to facility even for the same place of service. This means that consumers must always do their research before obtaining non-emergency service in network. In addition, shop around for the best deal. In Chapter 5 I told you of a scan my wife had where the difference was $600 for providers within the same place of service.

A recent study finds that over forty-two percent of patients hospitalized or treated in an emergency room received surprise bills in 2016. Another survey stated that 18% of emergency room visits, on average, resulted in at least one surprise bill. Many emergency rooms are being staffed by outside emergency room provider groups who sign very few in-network contracts.[7-3, 7-4, 7-5,]

While rules are rules for some of these events (they actually are meant to help control healthcare costs and limit premiums), some state legislatures have passed laws to rein in some of the unseemly balance billing tactics. Thirty-two states have enacted surprise billing protections, but only seventeen are deemed comprehensive in nature. These laws generally cover emergency and in-hospital services. They generally seek to set reasonable rates that providers can charge, have insurers pay usual and customary-type rates for non-network providers, bar certain balance billing from out-of-network providers if you were at an in-network facility, protect insureds by having plans only charge in-network cost-sharing for emergency services and in-patient procedures, and setting up binding dispute resolution.[7-5, 7-6, 7-7, 7-8, 7-9]

There is an existing law disallowing balance billing for Medicare patients if the provider is enrolled in Medicare fee-for-service (FFS). In this case, a provider cannot bill more than the Medicare-approved rate for services whether to a Medicare FFS patient (because they are in-network) or a Medicare Advantage (MA) member. This represents 95% of all providers who see Medicare patients. Most of the others can balance bill no more than 15% above the Medicare rate that the government pays them. This is a strong protection for members, except that balance or surprise billing may still occur in certain circumstances (such as non-covered or excluded services). There is also a blanket protection against any cost-sharing and billing for certain very low-income Medicare enrollees that are also Medicaid eligible (but higher income ones can be balanced billed if applicable).[7-2, 7-9, 7-10]

Since there is little or no cost-sharing in Medicaid, low-income patients do not have the worry of balance billing. States usually allow services only in a Medicaid FFS network or in a plan managed care network. In both cases, federal and state law disallow balance billing for covered services in network. In the case of emergencies where an out-of-network provider sees an enrollee either in Medicaid FFS or managed care plan, the provider must accept as payment in full what otherwise would have been paid by the Medicaid FFS program. Medicaid recipients still could face balance billing in other scenarios (such as using out-of-network providers and non-covered or excluded services).[7-2, 7-9, 7-11, 7-12]

The new federal law, passed in late 2020 and effective January 1, 2022, applies to commercial insurance across the nation. Here are the key elements:[7-5]

The bill prohibits balance billing in all emergency care circumstances. Thus, if an out-of-network provider (facility or physician) renders care, it will be deemed in-network and you only pay the applicable in-network deductible or cost-sharing for the services to each provider.

It also prohibits balance billing for air ambulance transportation. Thus, if an out-of-network provider renders care, it will be deemed in-network and you only pay the applicable in-network deductible or cost-sharing for the service. Ground ambulances can still balance bill.

It also prohibits most out-of-network balance billing for non-emergency care at an in-network hospital or facility if you are unknowingly treated by an out-of-network provider. Thus, if an out-of-network provider renders care, it will be deemed in-network and you only pay the applicable in-network deductible or cost-sharing for the services.

Some balance billing still is allowed. In a non-emergency situation, if a provider notifies a patient seventy-two hours before the services are rendered that he is out-of-network and furnishes potential good-faith charges, and the patient consents, balance billing can be charged. For certain services, consent only needs to be given on the day of the service. Many providers are barred from seeking consent so as not to get around the general prohibition on out-of-network providers balance billing when they render care at an in-network facility.

To get bills paid, health plans and providers will negotiate differences between in-network rates and rates charged by providers. Health plans will then pay the amount to the providers on members' behalf. If a payment is not negotiated in thirty days, then the dispute goes to an arbitrator. The arbitrator cannot consider Medicare or Medicaid FFS rates or the provider's billed charges but can look at the median in-network rates in the region for such services, among other factors.

The uninsured potentially get some breaks as well. A provider-patient bill dispute resolution process will be set up to address similar circumstances. This new federal law also applies to self-insured employer health insurance, which could not be considered by state laws due to a federal prohibition.

I am of two minds about the federal legislation that passed. On one hand, it will begin to make a huge difference on the issue of surprise billing. It should give tremendous relief on the emergency front and most non-emergency, in-network situations. At the same time, arbitration is costly, cumbersome, and time-consuming and will mean excessive payments for such bills. As this book was being written, the Biden administration was issuing regulations that offered some hope that arbitration would not be slanted toward providers and their high charges.

So, to sum up this chapter: Caveat Emptor or Buyer Beware! Remember that when it comes to out-of-network services you almost never get the advantage of the discounts that plans negotiate on your behalf with in-network providers. Even if you have out-of-network coverage, your deductible, cost-sharing, and maximum costs for out-of-network services are usually very high. And, most important, for the most part you can be charged whatever rate the provider deems appropriate, which may be well above a plan contracted rate or even a usual and customary rate (UCR). Further, your plan may adjust the charged rate to something more reasonable, pushing more of the cost to you.

Here are some best practices for you to protect yourself from surprise/balance billing, or at least limit your exposure, whether you are seeking in-network or out-of-network services:[7-1, 7-2]

> Before seeking services, check to ensure that the service or benefit in question is covered or is uncovered or excluded. Further, check to see if the provider is in network or out of network and if you have out-of-network coverage or are allowed to go out of network in isolated cases. Next, scrutinize your plan benefit design to determine what your cost-sharing (deductible, co-insurance, and co-pay) is for such services. Pay attention to places of service and shop around. Inventory all the procedures or services to be rendered and each provider. Discuss with the plan and providers what needs authorization or not and whether the plan has approved these services.

> While seeking services, scrutinize all documents signed in a provider's office for possible surprise billing areas. Seek an upfront accounting of the costs of your care from each provider that may be involved in a procedure or services.

> Negotiate upfront costs for the services with the providers or your health plan.

> If an inpatient or outpatient procedure is complex, ask if any out-of-network providers will be rendering any of the services.

As well, plan in advance what emergency room(s) and hospital(s) you would use if you could in emergencies and determine if they use out-of-network doctors in general. You have a better chance of limiting your surprise bills when in network.

Study and use the great surprise billing guide from the Healthcare Financial Management Association (HFMA) at this link (**https://www. aha.org/system/files/2018-11/Avoiding-Surprise-Bills-FINAL.pdf**). It walks you through how to approach various complex procedures and emergencies.

After the services are rendered, examine your Explanation of Benefits (EOBs) closely and ask questions of your plan for services and claims you have questions on. The EOB should tell you why a claim was rejected or paid, for what amount, and whether your provider can bill more.

Know your state laws and Medicare rules against balance billing or what is allowed under those laws and regulations. Study the provisions of the new federal law, which takes effect January 1, 2022. It will be implemented throughout 2021 and be well-publicized.

Report issues to your health plan or file a grievance, whether in network or out of network. Plans will take care of in-network issues and may intercede even on out-of-network issues, especially emergency care ones. Plans are obligated to offer out-of-network emergency services coverage.

Remember to raise holy you-know-what. Exhaust all of your internal and external appeal rights. Contact your various state and federal representatives. The Department of Insurance and your state attorney general like these types of cases. You may also hire an expert to negotiate your bill or hire an attorney to take legal action.

CHAPTER 8

Terminology, Part 4 (Clinical Practices)

N ow let's look at some of the clinical practices of plans. This is divided into two categories. The first category is utilization management (UM), where plans scrutinize the utilization of services to ensure appropriateness and reduce costs. The second category includes population health, care management (CM), and quality assurance. Through these processes plans seek to assess and promote quality outcomes in its members. Both categories have upfront and retrospective approaches.

Topic Area 4: A Plan's Clinical Oversight

Utilization Management (UM)—This is an umbrella term and a series of policies and processes used in managed care to reduce unnecessary or over-utilization of services and to ensure care is delivered in the right place, efficiently, and safely. The term covers both the medical and drug worlds. At its foundation, plans should use evidence-based criteria to determine whether a given service or benefit at a given place of service should be rendered or not. Plans generally do this in several ways. As part of the benefit structure, plans designate what services and locations need to be pre-approved. Plans then use prior authorization (PA), pre-certification processes, utilization review, and appeals processes when members or providers request them. Plans also use concurrent review of inpatient and other facility visits. These are day-by-day assessments of whether a member qualifies for continued stay in the facility.

UM features also include discharge planning or care transitions, which are the appropriate planning for services when a member leaves a hospital or other facility.

Plans may also use edits in their claims system to flag questionable services or to deny claims. Plans also perform retrospective review of high-cost services, such as inpatient visits, outpatient services, and certain drugs. These determine if processes were followed, whether additional services need to be added to prior authorization or pre-certification lists, and whether provider education needs to occur for those not following plan policies.

Plans may perform peer reviews with doctors if they are outliers in terms of practice patterns or on given cases.

Medical Necessity, Prior Authorizations (PAs), and Appeals—Medical necessity is the standard used by health plans and health insurers to determine whether a benefit or service should be rendered to a covered individual. In most cases, plans do not require members or their providers to prove this upfront. As an example, primary care services, most labs, and low-cost services largely are deemed necessary. However, expensive benefits and services, such as high-cost radiology, inpatient admissions, and many outpatient services/procedures require approval of the plan prior to the benefit being covered. This is called prior authorization or pre-certification.

Members and providers file requests for prior authorization. If the request is denied, the member or provider can appeal the denial. If the plan denies again, in most cases a member can then appeal to an external entity. Both the plan and the external entity must use evidence-based medical criteria to determine medical necessity. Regulatory agencies now often audit health plans in many lines of business to ensure prior authorizations and appeals are carried out timely and that evidence-based criteria are used consistently across the population in the plan or product.

Drug prior authorizations can get very technical. Plans publish covered drugs on the formulary or drug list. Some of these drugs may require different kinds of prior authorizations.

In the drug world, prior authorization (PA) is the required approval by the plan to use the given drug on the drug list. Step therapy is similar in that the plan must approve the use of a given drug on the drug list, and you must show that the use of a generic drug or other preferred brand on the drug list was not efficacious or there was or would be a safety issue if used. Plans also set quantity limits (QL) to ensure safety, and you may require approval by the plan to exceed such limits.

In some products or lines of business, you can seek what is known as an exception to the drug list, in which case the plan may approve the use of a drug not on the drug list if it is medically needed and no other drug would be efficacious. In addition, if a cost of a drug on the formulary is prohibitive for you, you may request what is known as a tiering exception. If the plan approves it, your cost-share would be based on a lower tier because the drug is medically necessary and the other drugs on lower tiers would not be efficacious.

If part of the covered benefit, a member may also request reimbursement for certain out-of-pocket costs if they used an out-of-network pharmacy or provider. Sometimes, these do not require a prior authorization but in certain cases they do.

If you are seeking care from an in-network provider, generally the burden is on the provider to seek authorization from the plan if needed. And, as we noted under surprise billing, usually you are protected if authorization is not sought and the service is performed. But this is not always the case. Therefore, you should always check with your health plan and the provider to determine whether a service requires prior authorization, and if the service or procedure has been authorized before it is performed. Mistakes can happen. This may save you great anxiety and potential out-of-pocket costs down the road.

In the case of out-of-network services (if available and except for emergencies), while the provider may facilitate approval, the burden usually is on you as the subscriber to ensure all prior authorizations have been made and approved.

It is very important to note that prior authorization does not always mean guaranteed payment to the provider by the health plan. There could be a variety of reasons why a payment may be rejected or reduced even with a prior authorization. In addition, just because something was authorized doesn't mean you know what your cost-sharing will absolutely be in every instance. For an out-of-network provider, it may be that the plan limits your payment as discussed in the balanced or surprise billing chapter. And as we noted, there are even instances of surprise billing when in-network services are sought.

Referral—Some types of products or plans require a member to obtain a referral from their primary care physician to receive certain specialty services. Sometimes, certain specialists do not require a referral, such as obstetrics, gynecology, and routine dermatology. Some plans require these referrals to be filed with the health plan while others simply have the referral sent to the chosen specialist by the primary care physician.

Grievances—A grievance is a complaint made by a member to a health plan. Regulatory bodies, such as a state Medicaid agency or the Centers for Medicare and Medicaid Services (CMS) as well as accreditation agencies, require plans to have a grievance process. This could relate to denial of an authorization or appeal or be a general complaint regarding the health plan or a provider. Plans are required to log each grievance, investigate, establish root causes, and notify the member of the resolution, all within a prescribed timeframe.

Quality-of-care complaints or grievances are handled in a different manner and call for investigation by the plan to ascertain if quality of care was insufficient or somehow faulty. There are external entities for Medicare and Medicaid lines that could also get involved in quality-of-care complaints at the request of a member or a state Medicaid agency.

It is also possible for a member to complain directly to a regulatory entity about the health plan. As an example, a Medicare beneficiary enrolled in a Medicare plan could complain to CMS at 1-800-MEDICARE. In this case, the plan is notified and must respond to CMS within a prescribed period of time, depending on the severity of the complaint. Plans usually use a similar system to investigate and resolve these complaints as they do for grievances.

The Prudent Layperson Standard for Emergency and Urgent Care Services—This standard applies to the utilization of emergency rooms and related emergency services (ER care). Federal and state laws generally require health plans to cover trips to the emergency room if an insured, exercising reasonable judgment, seeks ER care services believing that sickness, injury, or symptoms could place the insured's life in serious jeopardy without immediate medical attention. Under this standard, the symptoms of the patient rather than the actual diagnosis dictate whether the service will be covered. This is an important protection memorialized in law. But members must exercise good judgment when seeking ER care—as opposed to going to urgent care or calling their primary care physician. The former is obtained when your life and well-being may be at risk. Urgent care is sought when you need medical attention, but your PCP is unavailable.

Topic Area 5: Population Health and Quality

While utilization management (UM) remains a primary focus of health plans, more and more population health and care management (CM) are coming to the fore. CMS is pushing plans and providers to focus more on care management versus UM as they see this as changing the paradigm from a cost and quality perspective.

> According to the Centers for Disease Control and Prevention (CDC), 75% of all healthcare spending can be tied to treatment of chronic diseases. This percentage is higher in Medicare and Medicaid, 96% and 83%, respectively.[8-1] And as you will learn later, a great deal of that cost is due to exacerbation of these chronic conditions because they are not well maintained.

While more needs to be done to convert from a UM focus to a CM focus, most plans do dedicate significant resources to effectively manage members' care through population health and care management. In so doing, a plan seeks to reduce current and future costs of care. This happens in a number of ways:

Risk identification and stratification—Plans use clinical data and algorithms to identify and stratify members based on disease states and conditions, service utilization, and financial utilization, among others. This allows them to craft intervention strategies to lower risk and improve quality outcomes.

Care management (CM) and coordination—Plans create programs to manage and coordinate care. Discharge planning and care transitions were listed under the UM section. However, these are also functions that fall under care coordination or care management. Others include:

> *Case management*—A plan may assign a case manager to a member for a catastrophic episode (e.g., a car accident with serious injury) or for members who have multiple chronic conditions. The goal is to reduce costs and improve quality by coordinating and managing all care.

> *Disease management*—A plan may assign a disease case manager to oversee members who have chronic conditions or disease states, in order to reduce overall costs and improve outcomes by helping members better manage chronic diseases.

> *Health education, wellness, and prevention*—A plan may create programs to educate members on wellness and preventive benefits and required visits. In addition, a plan may also engage in health education. Health education also has a non-clinical component that may involve educating members on barriers to good health rooted in social determinants, including poverty, homelessness and shelter, food insecurity, and health literacy.

Ultimately both member and provider engagement are keys to successful care management, as is sharing data mined by the plan.

Quality review assurance and improvement—Plans also set up important quality review and assurance programs. These programs use analytics to periodically assess effectiveness of operations and clinical outcomes. Through periodic assessment, plans can practice continuous quality improvement by adjusting policies, processes, and programs to improve outcomes and quality.

Quality review and improvement programs can impact many areas of the health plan enterprise and include quality and safety of member care, provider performance, health delivery performance, specific clinical outcomes (including performance under various external quality measures and member satisfaction surveys), ensuring the plan abides by the various requirements of accreditation organizations' standards of care, and addressing racial and other disparities to quality-of-care attainment.

Health Enhancement Programs (HEPs)—HEPs are a generic term and can go by a variety of names. In general, these are programs set up by health plans to promote members taking an active role in their own healthcare and disease management, thereby reducing current and future outlays by the plan. In return, plans may offer a variety of incentives or rewards. Such incentives might include reduction of premiums and cost-sharing (including deductibles, co-insurance, and co-pays), additional health and non-health benefits, and cash outlays or credits against future healthcare costs.

Requirements of HEPs can differ across plans, but often include requirements to complete recommended preventive wellness visits and screenings (e.g., vision screening, dental cleanings, colonoscopies, and mammograms). Those with underlying disease states would have to complete various disease-specific testing (e.g., glucose and HbA1c tests). Some plans may give those with disease states extra rewards if test results are within recommended levels for that disease state.

Last, members might have requirements to participate in disease education and management programs if they have certain disease states (e.g., diabetes, asthma/chronic obstructive pulmonary disease, hypertension and various heart diseases, and high cholesterol).

These programs are most common in commercial plans but will grow in public programs over time. For example, some states have Healthy Behaviors programs in Medicaid, where incentives are paid for completion of preventive and wellness visits and hitting disease management benchmarks. This is also coming to Medicare Advantage.

CHAPTER 9

Fee-for-Service (FFS) versus Managed Care

n Chapter 3, we discussed briefly the concept of fee-for-service (FFS) and managed care. To refresh on the history, health insurance in America firmly took root in the first half of the twentieth century. The Blues Plans began in the 1920s and 1930s, as health insurers began to move from accident and sickness insurance to full-scale health insurance. By the end of the 1950s, about 75% of Americans had health insurance, mostly through their employers.

The system that emerged goes by several names. First, it is the fee-for-service (FFS) system. Second, it is also known as the transaction model because a fee is paid for every healthcare transaction or service. Third, insurers built a product around this system called the indemnity policy, where the insurance company pays a portion of each bill for each service and you pay the rest. Generally speaking, an insurer would pay 80% of the bill and the insured 20%, but those ratios have changed over time. In the commercial world, an insurer offered this type of plan to an employer or directly to an individual. As you will learn, this indemnity product is near extinct.

Because health insurance was so new and it was still relatively cheap, few worried about whether the emerging system was a good one. But over time, it became clear that FFS has three glaring faults. It is very costly, it is inefficient, and it does not promote quality. This is true for several reasons.

First, physicians and other providers are encouraged to provide as many services as possible. There are few, if any, cost constraints. High utilization is encouraged because the more the provider sees you or tests you, the more he gets paid. It does not mean that those services are even necessary or appropriate. Providers could be recommending expensive services when cheaper ones would be sufficient for most people. The system encourages over-utilization and high costs because the system is essentially unmanaged. It is a free-for-all.

Second, in a transaction-based system, providers have much greater incentive to increase fees continuously. Since there are no networks, there are few if any discounts in the form of negotiated rates. Health plans may not know how often or by how much providers raise rates. The only way for them to limit increased costs is to limit the amount they will reimburse, which transfers the price hikes to the insured.

Third, there is little or no attention to rewarding health outcomes, short of having a really caring doctor. Providers have no incentive to treat patients holistically and there is no care coordination or management of the member. Quality in the system is poor because physicians and providers are transaction- or service-focused and not patient-outcome oriented.

Finally, while healthier, well-educated people may not suffer under this system, and may even prefer the freedom it offers, those who are sicker or less health literate tend to have very poor health outcomes in a FFS system. They are very much on their own and have to navigate the complex system alone. This increases costs as these consumers access healthcare late and often during catastrophic circumstances.

As costs increased in the 1950s and 1960s, it became apparent to both government and businesses that the system had to change. Average Americans even recognized that their premiums, deductibles, and cost-sharing were increasing as healthcare costs crept up.

That is where managed care came in. As discussed in Chapter 3, managed care has its roots in the prepaid plans created between 1900 and the 1930s. But managed care as we know it today began as an idea from Dr. Paul Ellwood, an adviser to then-President Nixon's Administration, who conceptualized health plans and insurers morphing into entities that compete on price and quality. The idea was to refocus plans on contracting with providers not on a per-transaction basis, but on new prepaid reimbursement arrangements that promoted holistic care—wellness, prevention, primary care, and care management. He also coined the term, "Health Maintenance Organization or HMO."[9-1]

The theory is that costs would drop because plans would be monitoring for unnecessary services. Over time, outcomes would improve as prevention and member health were emphasized, which would also reduce costs.

The Nixon Administration's work with Ellwood and others led to the passage of the Federal HMO Act in 1973, which created grants and loans for entities to start up these new HMOs. It also pre-empted some state laws to encourage HMOs' growth. The act also required employers with twenty-five or more employees to begin offering federally qualified HMOs if they offered FFS insurance. HMOs had to prove they had comprehensive benefits, adequate networks, quality assurance, grievance processes, and financial solvency.[9-1]

The act was a defining moment for the growth of managed care. It forced employers to think about healthcare differently and helped HMOs and managed care grow in the employer sector. In addition, the act also laid the foundation for the adoption of a new type of managed care regulation in state insurance departments.

From the early 1970s to the end of the century, HMOs and managed care displaced indemnity policies in the private sector. Growth was especially great in the late 1980s and into the 1990s. By the mid-1990s, the vast majority of plan offerings were managed-care oriented. By the early 2000s, FFS or indemnity was very small.[9-1]

The state of California was among the first states to endorse Medicaid-managed care approaches in the early 1970s.[9-2] They began modestly. Most states have now endorsed private HMOs as their delivery model, with between 70% to 80% of Medicaid recipients in some form of managed care for an element of their benefits.[9-3, 9-4]

Medicare managed care was introduced as demonstration projects in the 1960s through 1990s. In 1997, the program became formalized. Today, over 43% of Medicare beneficiaries are in private, managed care plans.[9-5]

So, let's go a little deeper on the philosophy of managed care and HMOs specifically. As noted, these were formed to correct the inefficiency, high costs, and poor quality exemplified by the FFS system. Most of the managed care entities seek to redefine the relationship with the insured and with the provider. In this case, managed care tries to tie health plans, providers, and members together and give each one responsibility and reward.

On the insured side or what became known as the member side, managed care sought to change the behavior of the member through varying cost-sharing and enhancing benefits. Theoretically, members would be deliberate in how they thought about accessing services and would prioritize preventive health. Their responsibility was taking an active role in health. Their reward was lower costs and some enhanced benefits.

On the provider side, managed care sought to change the behavior of providers by changing reimbursement approaches by linking it to quality and cost-effectiveness. Their responsibility was a greater role in managing their patients. Their reward was increased compensation, at least for the providers focused on prevention and primary care.

The following are the broad features of managed care.[9-1, 9-6, 9-7] In general, most of these apply to HMOs and managed care entities closest to them, such as open access HMOs and point of services (POS) plans.

Use of networks. Managed care plans credential providers as to their quality and fitness to serve members. Plans prefer networks for a number of reasons:

- First, they can obtain discounts from various providers by theoretically generating greater volume to the practices or facilities. This can be the case whether the provider is paid a fee-for-service (FFS) rate or a prepaid amount for assigned members, known as capitation or a capitated amount. The term "capitation" has its roots in Latin: *caput* meaning "head." In this case, the health plan is counting heads to pay the provider, who is assigned a number of health plan members to take care of.

- Second, they can negotiate withhold arrangements, penalties, and bonuses for achieving cost-savings and quality targets. They also may enter into risk arrangements, where providers share upside profit and some downside loss on their assigned members.

- Third, they can aggressively negotiate rates with facilities, including hospitals. Hospitals that do not offer significantly discounted rates can be excluded from the network.

- Fourth, they create a bond between the health plan and the provider. Often, contracts require providers to perform care management and other functions with or on behalf of the plan. Data-sharing is also prioritized. This relationship does not exist in a FFS model, where all the provider wants is to get paid.

- Fifth, they can ensure that members of the health plan pick a provider to be their primary care physician (PCP), whether formally or not. This creates a better nexus between the plan, the member, and the provider.

- Sixth, they can have the network steer members to the lowest cost providers or to the places of service that are most appropriate.

- Seventh, to save costs, pure HMOs do not allow out-of-network services except in emergency cases, while other forms may allow it.

Required or encouraged designation of a PCP by each member.
This ensures a single point of contact for each member's healthcare
needs. It also creates a gathering point for all that goes on with the
patient. Members are asked to tell other providers who their PCP is so
that records and results can be sent there. HMOs began with so-called
gatekeeper PCPs. Some still have them. Members had to see their PCP
before they visited a specialist or sought other services.

**Managed care has comprehensive benefits that usually go beyond
traditional indemnity policies.** These include upfront prevention
services and wellness visits, drug coverage, physician and outpatient coverage, mental health and substance abuse coverage, and hospital coverage.

Strong utilization management (UM) controls. High-cost and often
over-utilized services, benefits, or drugs require prior authorization before
a member can receive them. In addition to the importance of reviewing
authorization requests for evidence-based medical necessity—does the
member need the given service, drug, or benefit?—managed care considers two other important factors: Is the provider in network or out
of network? Except for emergency-related services, HMOs usually do
not approve requests for providers that are not in network. Is the place
of service (POS) appropriate for medical treatment? As an example,
managed care favors the appropriate use of ambulatory service centers
and even physicians' offices for surgeries as opposed to more expensive
inpatient services or outpatient surgery at a hospital setting. Plans will
evaluate whether the disease states of a given member or the current condition of that member dictates approval of surgery on an inpatient basis
or at a hospital on an outpatient basis. The vast majority can utilize the
more cost-effective places of service. Plans, too, drive people to the lowest
cost place of service by applying deductibles and higher cost-sharing to
the more expensive places of service.

Managed care usually has drug lists or formularies. These lists show what drugs are covered or should be tried first. Authorizations may be needed.

Managed care usually stratifies cost-sharing to encourage the use of the earliest, most cost-effective, and appropriate treatment option or place of service. This is true in HMOs and stricter managed care plans. This means that PCP visits, preventive services, and routine labs may have little or no cost-sharing to encourage their use. For example, a free-standing, ambulatory surgery center may have a flat dollar co-pay to encourage members to choose the lower-cost option. An expensive, hospital-based outpatient procedure, as well as inpatient stays, may have a deductible and costs-sharing. The stratification of cost-sharing is meant to reduce the overall cost burden on Americans by introducing more modest co-pays and reduced co-insurance compared with the high-percentage cost-sharing in most FFS plans. Managed care had a major impact on consumer out-of-pocket costs, at least initially. In some part, this was due to lower cost-sharing of the product compared with FFS. At the same time, a good portion of the reduction was tied to restrictions on what services members could obtain due to prior authorization (including high-cost hospitalizations). Despite some over-zealousness on the prior authorization front, my view is that both were perhaps positive developments.

Managed care focuses on wellness, prevention, and primary care. This encourages doctors and members to work together to utilize the lowest cost services and avoid high-cost places of services, such as the emergency room. Primary care is incentivized by generous upfront capitation payments. In return, providers are asked to ensure their assigned panel of members receive regular visits according to published wellness and prevention guidelines, including well care visits, screenings, and testing. It encourages early-intervention outreach to them in concert with health plans. Incentive-based reimbursement to providers, especially assigned PCPs, often exists to drive health outcomes and quality.

Managed care practices care coordination and case management to reduce costs and improve quality outcomes. This coordination and management can be for a relatively healthy member that might have suffered a catastrophic event and needs help in his or her recovery. More often, the coordination and management services are for those who have multiple co-morbidities and need constant attention. It could also include health education for the entire population, especially those with documented disease states or those that need reminders on wellness and prevention exams or drug refills. Case managers or care managers are often assigned to individuals with high healthcare needs.

Managed care performs a great deal of retrospective review of claims and utilization. This scrutiny helps reduce future costs as well. It might entail provider education as to whether a provider's practice pattern is outside of norms based on his panel's demographics or risks. Plans focus extensively on reducing the use of inpatient care, high-cost outpatient care at a hospital setting, and emergency room use. As part of this effort, plans today also invest heavily in technology to reduce fraud, waste, and abuse. In addition, plans like to analyze claims to ensure the correct site of care (another definition for place of service) is used and help change practice patterns over time.

Managed care puts in place quality review, assurance, and improvement programs. These are mandated by regulatory agencies and outside groups that accredit the plan. These programs aim to improve the performance of the plan and providers as well as boost health outcomes of members. Managed care may pay providers bonus reimbursement if they achieve high marks on the quality front or boost member outcomes.

Next, let's discuss different forms of HMOs. HMOs have come in a few different models over the years. Often, HMOs combine the different models below.[9-8]

The early days saw the creation of **the staff model HMO.** In this form, the HMO plan, physicians (primary and specialists) and sometimes facilities, including hospitals, are all owned by one entity. The staff model has huge advantages over other forms. Because the doctors and sometimes facilities are owned by the same entity as the plan, they often have integrated care management technology to share clinical information. In addition, providers are compelled to follow the plan rules and care management protocols. In the staff model HMO, members usually gravitate to the HMO because the doctors and facilities are known to them. In return, for the most part, they must stay in the captive or closed panel of doctors.

The group model HMO is similar to the staff model except that the HMO plan or a common entity does not own the providers (primary physicians and specialists and facilities). It contracts with them, sometimes on an exclusive basis. **If the group is exclusive to the HMO plan, it is a closed group model.** The HMO may actually create the physician group, or it might simply have just a very strong contractual relationship. **If the group serves other HMOs, it is an independent group model.**

The group model can have many of the same advantages as the staff model. A closed group could work with the HMO plan on technology and data sharing as well as ensure the physicians and providers follow the HMO plan practices. This may be possible with independent groups but could be more difficult. Provider availability may also be more limited as with the staff model.

The network model HMO is where the HMO contracts with multiple provider groups. These provider groups may also contract with other HMOs. Here it is harder to coordinate care given the multiple provider organizations, but greater provider access is a benefit to members.

The Independent Practice Association (IPA) model is where the HMO contracts with an IPA entity. In this case the IPA is a group of physicians that have gotten together to negotiate with health plans. They generally contract with multiple health plans as well. The IPA model is the most popular form of an HMO today and usually is a hybrid with the direct contract model below. Coordination with these providers is more challenging and takes a great deal of investment in provider relations to achieve strong managed care costs-savings. On the flip side, provider choice is usually greater.

The direct contract model is where an HMO directly contracts with a physician. More and more, physicians join IPAs to have bargaining power, but some providers continue to negotiate on their own. The providers may contract with many HMOs. The pros and cons of this model are similar to the IPA model.

Historic healthcare spending data shows that managed care's adoption helped bend the cost curve for a period of time. Earlier, I noted that managed care's greatest growth was from the mid-1980s to the mid-1990s. As managed care's adoption peaked, the impact on spending was felt. Various assessments and studies say that healthcare spending growth moderated rather dramatically roughly between 1993 and 2000, with the lowest annual increases from 1994 to 1996. Healthcare spending as a percentage of gross domestic product (GDP) held flat in the 1993 to 2000 period. In addition, studies show that the more managed care penetrated a market, the more healthcare spending reacted and moderated. It also had a positive impact on growth in the remaining FFS products. Studies also show downward trends in service utilization, especially admission rates and lengths of stays in hospitals.[9-9, 9-10, 9-11]

To validate what sources are saying, I like to check the math. The best source for doing that is mining the Centers for Medicare and Medicaid Services (CMS) National Health Expenditure Data (NHED) website. It has a wealth of information on trends. I looked at healthcare expenditures as a percentage of GDP over time. Clearly, as managed care penetration reached its peak in the 1990s, the moderation in healthcare costs kicked in.[9-12]

- 1960: 5.0%
- 1970: 6.9%
- 1980: 8.9%
- 1990 12.1%
- 2000: 13.4%

Despite HMOs' and managed care's growth from the 1970s and into the 1990s, Americans became disenchanted with the strict form of managed care. Americans felt the pendulum swung too far from the freedom of FFS. They wanted something more in the middle for the following reasons:[9-1, 9-9, 9-10, 9-11, 9-13, 9-14]

First, Americans hated the lack of flexibility they had in choosing providers that they were used to with FFS/indemnity plans. To control costs, plans set up tight networks and often enrollees had no idea who was in or not.

Second, Americans disliked the tight control HMOs had over their healthcare, especially in the area of utilization management (UM) and prior authorization. There was a perception, perhaps real, that managed care was over-zealous on UM.

Third, some felt that they should not have to go through a gatekeeper PCP to access other parts of the network, especially specialists. My wife reminded me as she edited this that she was one of the critics of gatekeepers back before our first child was born. She complained that she had to go to the PCP to get referred to her gynecologist to be told she was pregnant. This was something she had already figured out by taking a home pregnancy test. Imagine!

Fourth, Americans complained that managed care plans were infringing on the doctor-patient relationship by dictating what should or should not be covered. Long-established relationships with primary care doctors and specialists had to be severed and transitioned as many doctors were not in network. Doctors were no fans at all, complaining about reduced rates as well as administrative burdens that impacted the time they could spend with patients. Too, they complained of plans' contractual provisions that served as gag rules related to what they could say or not say to their patients.

Fifth, the HMO Act wanted to see choice between FFS/indemnity and potentially multiple managed care HMOs. Many businesses, seeking savings, restricted choice or offered just one tight network HMO product. Businesses failed to explain what managed care was and essentially took away too many choices.

In summary, while Americans wanted relief from high costs, they felt managed care as they knew it just went too far. HMOs bungled their rollout and got black eyes. They concentrated on the negative aspects to drive cost reduction and not the positive aspects of the other benefits of managed care, such as wellness, prevention, care management, and quality. In fact, the combination of prior authorization, tight networks, and lack of seeing the positives of managed care led Americans to conclude that quality was actually suffering under the model.

To respond to the criticism, several things occurred to move what was a strict form of managed care into something less onerous and restrictive. Plans began creating and businesses adopted lighter forms of managed care. We will review these different managed care products in the next chapter, but they include exclusive provider organizations (EPOs) or open access HMOs, preferred provider organizations (PPOs), and point of service (POS) plans. All of these alternatives to strict HMOs offered Americans some relief from the onerous restrictions, but at the same time preserved certain cost-savings capabilities. As an example, plans with both in-network and out-of-network coverage were created. Plans that did not require seeing a PCP before seeking certain services were introduced.[9-1]

States also passed various reforms, including prohibiting those gag rules mentioned above, strengthening grievance and appeal rights, passing prudent layperson laws regarding emergency care, and putting in place benefit protections given HMO's perceived over-zealousness on the UM front.[9-1] As an example, so-called "drive-through births" (where mothers were ushered out of the hospital too quickly after giving birth) were reined in by requiring a minimum number of in-hospital days for a regular birth and additional days for C-sections.

More recently, CMS has introduced a fairly strict compliance and quality regime in Medicare, Medicaid, and the Affordable Care Act (ACA/Obamacare) Exchanges. The Medicare regime is the most mature, and the other lines of business programs are just now being rolled out. These regimes force plans to be accountable on many fronts, which will be discussed in great detail later in the book. Plans must spend a set amount of money on medical expenses. This ensures most of the premium that an insured or employer pays goes to actual medical care. In addition, it limits the amount a plan can spend on administrative costs and reduces profit margins.

Plans must follow compliance dictates to ensure that requests for authorizations and appeals are considered on a timely basis. Plans are required to follow evidenced-based practice and criteria in their analysis of whether a benefit, service, or drug is deemed medically necessary for the member. Various appeal levels are also dictated to ensure fairness to the member. In addition, they must process grievances timely.

Plans must meet vigorous quality standards or face enrollment freezes or cancelation of their contracts. In addition, the best plans receive added revenue and in most cases it is directed to be used to further augment member benefits.

Now, the backlash and realignment performed by plans clearly had an impact. Beginning in the early 2000s, there was a notable increase in health-care trends, indeed a reversal in the moderation seen in the 1990s. Annual inflation began to surge in the late 1990s and early 2000s. This was largely due to the looser UM and network frameworks of the alternative managed care plans. HMO and similar product enrollment declined markedly in favor of the much-less-restrained Preferred Provider Organization (PPO) product. The regulatory response clearly contributed a great deal to the inflation trends as well.[9-1, 9-9, 9-10, 9-11]

If we go back to CMS's National Health Expenditure Data (NHED) website to validate the increase in healthcare expenditures as a percentage of GDP, I found that by 2010 healthcare as a percentage of GDP increased to 17.3%. This is a 29% increase in a decade—a clear return to the high inflation prior to managed care.[9-12]

Today, things have seemed to right themselves when it comes to managed care. There are various offerings that go from the tightest HMOs to more flexible managed care products. There has been a moderation of inflation once again for a variety of reasons. Today, almost all commercial providers offer some form of managed care, and most of the tiny percentage of indemnity plans have adopted some managed care principles. Many Americans are able to choose between low-cost, high-deductible HMOs versus higher cost, managed care alternatives. They can weigh the pros and cons of paying more. It is a budgetary decision. In some sectors, especially small businesses, choice may still be limited.

Of course, it is not the perfect system. People still complain that health plans have too much control and deny care. However, the compliance regime will continue to mature and provide better accountability. Complaints still exist about tight networks, but people now often have the ability to opt for more open plans or use a piece of their plan for out-of-network coverage at higher out-of-pocket costs. Promises on wellness, prevention, care management, and quality are still evolving and should get there over time, especially with the role technology can play in the future.

People are offered comprehensive benefits at a cost (premium and cost-sharing) that is well below what it would have been in the FFS system. We see this because the Medicare and Medicaid FFS systems still exist. While affordability is a big issue in the United States, managed care has brought greater affordability to tens of millions. It also provides a mechanism to control costs and is bringing quality.

Managed care is not a panacea. But we seem to have a much better model today. It, too, should be the lynchpin for moving reform forward. Coupling private health plans and managed care principles with affordable universal access and value-based care is the right recipe for the future.

CHAPTER 10

Types of Plans/Products/Coverage

Now let's discuss the various types of plans. This is a general overview that applies to most lines of businesses. But it is important to note that plan and product types can differ a little by line of business based on regulatory rules. I will be going into greater detail on some of these issues in subsequent chapters. Terminology could be slightly different for each state and even within a health plan's offerings.

Most products fit into these six broad product areas, with some consumer-directed health plans (CDHPs) or health reimbursement accounts (HRAs) mentioned in Chapter 6 taking hold over the last several years. It is important to note that health plans may mix and match some of the following products to create their own new plan or product type.

Except where cited, the descriptions are my own, derived from designing various insurance products over the years in my work at health plans as well as studying plan websites.

1—Fee-for-Service (FFS) or Indemnity—The last chapter covered how the FFS model got started and its many problems. It is also called the indemnity model or product. As you know from Chapter 4, this system lives on in the Medicare and Medicaid worlds, which will be discussed shortly. FFS and indemnity policies are dying out in the commercial world and have become very rare (a percentage point or two in the commercial world); their last bastion as a true insurance vehicle are heavily unionized employers and government employee plans. Some of these remaining products have incorporated a few managed care principles and have become what is known as managed indemnity.

From a commercial product design perspective, networks are not a key component of the model, but products can sometimes have network or payment arrangements with providers. This may be because the plan offers other products where networks are established and they "piggyback" off of the other product.

An insured usually is free to see whatever primary care physician or specialist he or she wants and most facilities as well. A small minority of plans may pre-certify or prior authorize certain services, but overall there are few utilization controls on services laid out by the plan.

Depending on whether the insurer has payment arrangements with the provider (which creates the semblance of a network), you may have to pay upfront and get reimbursed by the plan. If there are payment arrangements, the plan's payment for the service might get paid by the plan directly to the provider and the provider would bill you for the remainder.

Because the product type is extremely inefficient and very costly, these plans have high deductibles and individuals also pay at least 20-30% (if not higher) for each service.

As well, because there may not be payment arrangements in all cases, the plan may calculate what it pays based on what is known as the "usual and customary rate (UCR)" or prevailing or reasonable rate for that service in your area. If the plan has arrangements with the provider to accept a certain fee or this UCR payment, you simply owe the cost-sharing amount on that arranged payment; if not, you could be on the hook for paying 100% of anything above that rate. There are no guarantees here. This is a form of balance billing discussed earlier. Note that UCR may also apply to out-of-network benefits for some managed care plans explained later.[10-1]

But if you can afford the expense and put up with the reimbursement paperwork, you get the freedom to go anywhere!

In Medicare, the federal government contracts with almost two million providers nationwide (from my calculations on the Centers for Medicare and Medicaid Services (CMS) Medicare website) to form a very broad network of Medicare FFS providers. In Medicare FFS, the government acts as the insurer and covers about 80%, with seniors and disabled paying 20%. As noted, some Medicare recipients will get Medigap policies to fill the gaps.

Similarly, states contract with tens of thousands of providers in most cases to form a very broad Medicaid network in each state as well. Because enrollees are largely poor, the states (supported by the federal government) pay 100% of the bill to providers for Medicaid.

Forms of Managed Care:

2—**Preferred Provider Organization (PPO)**—This product is based in part on the FFS model. In the PPO world, there are large but established networks contracted by the health plan. But in return for being in the plan's network and theoretically getting members fed to them by the plan, providers pass on a FFS discount from their usual rate to bring the cost of overall healthcare down from the FFS product cost.

This is a very popular product today although it can be on the expensive side. Primary care physicians (PCPs) are not required. Referral requirements are limited or non-existent. Plans prior authorize certain services (especially high-cost ones), but generally there are fewer cost controls than HMO or similar managed care products. There is little care coordination. There is out-of-network coverage at higher costs (usually at a percentage co-insurance). As noted in Chapter 5, there may be a separate maximum out-of-pocket (MOOP) cost for out-of-network services or no limit at all. Cost-sharing, deductibles, and premiums are higher than in more restrictive products.

The Medicare Advantage (MA) world has added PPOs as a product with slightly different rules. The out-of-network component is based on the Medicare FFS network. The advantage here is that out-of-network fees are based on the established Medicare FFS rates, which insulates members from exceedingly high bills for such services.

3—Health Maintenance Organization (HMO)—This is the most restrictive type of managed care product that was outlined a great deal in Chapter 6. As discussed, the HMO limits you from making your own decisions but usually is the cheapest in terms of premiums, deductibles, and cost-sharing. You must have a PCP, who may act as your gatekeeper to higher levels of care. In many cases, they must refer you to specialty care. Many services require prior authorization. You have an established network and cannot leave it, or you are on your own in terms of paying that provider whatever rate he dictates.

Health plans sometimes liberalize certain rules to attract people wary of HMOs. As an example, you may be allowed to see certain providers without a referral—you may visit providers specializing in dermatology, gynecology, chiropractic, podiatry, etc. for a certain number of visits per year without referral.

Both MA and Medicaid managed care have network products that follow most of the principles.

4—Exclusive Provider Organization (EPO) or Open Access Health Maintenance Organization (OA-HMO)—These entities are basically the same. They have all the restrictions of an HMO with one exception: you don't have to have a PCP and do not need referrals within the network. Prior authorizations and other restrictions will apply and you do not have out-of-network coverage. This is one of the most popular HMO-type products today as it saves consumers a lot, but the hassle of having a PCP as a gatekeeper and the PCP referring you to other doctors is gone.

MA and some Medicaid managed care also have this type of product.

5—Point of Service (POS)—This product is somewhat unique and seeks to combine the Health Maintenance Organization (HMO) or exclusive provider organization (EPO) with the ability to access care outside of a network at higher deductibles and cost-sharing. Think about it this way: if you stay in network, your costs are low because you are agreeing to abide by referral rules, prior authorization rules, and networks. But if you see an out-of-network provider (or in some cases a broader network than the basic

HMO type one), you are paying a very large percentage of the bill out of pocket as a cost-share (you may have to pay up front and get reimbursed as well). Depending on the POS plan, you may or may not have to have a PCP. POS designs can vary, so read the fine print. As with the out-of-network coverage for the PPO, there may be a separate MOOP for out-of-network services or no limit at all.

MA has POS plans. MA rules are somewhat different in design than commercial ones.

6—High-Deductible Health Plans (HDHPs) or Catastrophic Plans— HDHPs are increasingly popular in the commercial world given ever-increasing costs. These plans have high deductibles and may be tied to one or more of the insurance types above. Under law, certain preventive services and some primary care visits are extended to the member upfront; virtually all other services are subject to the initial very high deductible. After the deductible, you receive 100% coverage.

These plans are often paired with health savings accounts (HSAs) so employees can set aside money tax-free to cover their medical expenses before the health plan payment kicks in after the deductible.

A catastrophic plan is similar in nature and is an option in the Marketplace Exchanges. Individuals under thirty years old can purchase catastrophic plans that act much like high deductible plans but HSAs may or may not be paired with them.

In 2019, the Trump Administration expanded the types of preventive services that can be covered pre-deductible, including certain low-cost tests, medical devices, and drugs.

One trend of late has been companies offering HDHPs, sometimes as the only option. This is due to the sheer costs in the system. Many businesses have no choice. Before you pass on insurance because it is the only option your employer offers, remember that some coverage is better than no coverage. In Chapter 16, I go into detail about why health insurance is very important from a consumer perspective. The good news is that it appears the percentage of companies offering only HDHPs is coming down. The National Business Group on Health's annual survey of employers' healthcare strategies predicts that just 25% of employers will offer only HDHPs in 2020, down from 30% in 2019 and 39% in 2018.[10-2]

Summary

Here is a quick cheat sheet summary for health plan product types. They are in order from the most cost-effective/most managed care elements to the least/none:

- HMO (strictest) and EPO (slightly less strict)—tight network; stringent requirements on you; no out-of-network coverage except emergencies
- POS—in network, it looks exactly like an HMO; has out-of-network flexibility
- PPO—broader network with looser requirements on you; has out-of-network coverage
- FFS/Indemnity (no managed care elements, unless a managed indemnity plan where elements are few)—very loose requirements; by and large no network constraints

Suffice it to say, all this is confusing even for experts. Every plan is different and nuanced. No two insurers or products are the same. It is always important to study your coverage closely as well as ask many questions of your plan when you access services and benefits.

CHAPTER 11

Players in the U.S. Health Insurance System, Part 1

B y now you should have a firm foundation in the history of the U.S. health insurance system and the various terminology, including lines of business and products. You also know that managed care, in its various forms, is the basis for our health insurance system today. The next two chapters are devoted to the various players in the health insurance system.

Except where cited, the descriptions of the players are derived from my work over the years at health plans and a healthcare software technology firm, review of various government and regulatory websites, and review of various state health insurance laws.

Government Regulators

This group includes various federal and state government agencies, beginning with the **Centers for Medicare and Medicaid Services** (CMS, www.cms.gov), **within the Department of Health and Human Services (HHS).** CMS formerly was known as the Healthcare Financing Administration or HCFA and HHS was formerly known as the Department of Health, Education, and Welfare.

In general, we can call HHS/CMS the overall policymaker for all things healthcare. They directly or indirectly do the following:

CMS sets policy for and runs the Medicare program. This includes the traditional Medicare fee-for-service (FFS) program and the private plan options, Medicare Advantage (MA) and the standalone Part D drug plans.

CMS sets national policy for Medicaid and finances the federal portion of the Medicaid system. CMS oversees the Medicaid program nationally by implementing congressionally mandated basic eligibility, benefit, and other rules in the program that states must follow. It is then up to the states to file plans and waivers with CMS as to how their state-specific Medicaid programs will operate, maintaining the minimum requirements and sometimes by adding additional eligibility groups and benefits.

CMS sets policy and oversees the Obamacare Marketplaces or Exchanges under the Affordable Care Act (ACA) of 2010. It does so along with the federal Labor and Treasury Departments. CMS is the lead on most healthcare policy issues. It sets benefits, coverage rates, actuarial, and policy rules for how the Exchanges are run. It also runs the federal Exchange and collaborates with states for the state-specific Exchanges.

Given its wide breadth of responsibility, it is clear that CMS is the pivotal player in future healthcare reform. We will see CMS driving all lines of business to a common compliance, accountability, and quality standard. I am a huge fan of the strides the agency has made in Medicare and it should have similar success in Medicaid and the Exchanges. While plans and individuals complain about the rigor that has been put in place at times, there is little doubt that it is the only way to bring accountability to the system, root out waste and inefficiency, and improve quality. Building a national program based on quality is the only way to truly bend the cost curve and begin seeing national healthcare expenditures as a percentage of gross domestic product (GDP) that are more in line with other developed countries.

This is perhaps one of the most important developments in our healthcare systems and needs to be understood and championed. In Chapter 29, I have a detailed analysis of the new accountability regime being built by CMS.

| For more information, go to **www.cms.gov**

Another government player involved in healthcare is the **U.S. Department of Labor** (DOL, **www.dol.gov**). The agency's role in overseeing health policy is primarily in administering the healthcare insurance provisions of the Employee Retirement Security Act (ERISA) of 1974. This set out standards for certain employee and retiree health plans in the private sector that preempt most state laws. ERISA rules also form the backbone of the ACA. Labor, HHS, and Treasury basically copied ERISA and augmented it for the regulation of Exchanges.

The ERISA regulations specify rules regarding healthcare provision for employers, unions, and other entities that self-fund healthcare. Such entities do so by setting up their own health funds and taking on the risk of the cost of care. In this case, an insurance company is not at risk—even if it helps administer the plan for the employer group. In an insurance risk arrangement, the health plan or insurance entity is entering into a risk contract with the employer group and is responsible for the employer group's health costs. It would not be covered under ERISA and state insurance laws would apply.

ERISA was amended by several other acts, including the Consolidated Omnibus Budget Reconciliation Act (COBRA) in 1985, the Health Insurance Portability and Accountability Act (HIPAA) in 1996, and the ACA of 2010. These acts added certain provisions applicable to these self-insured plans. The ACA had a major impact on ERISA, although it did not apply all rules (e.g., essential health benefits [EHBs]).

ERISA plans are a majority of employer-based coverage. As the size of a business increases, the more they elect to set up self-insurance funds rather than contract with an insurance company on a traditional risk basis. In addition, there is retiree coverage under ERISA. At last count, about 60% of all employee-coverage is tied to ERISA.[11-1] The regulations outline employee rights and the need to supply plan information, including benefits, cost-sharing, participation, funding, grievances and appeal rights, and other features.

The regulations also lay out the fiduciary responsibilities of the sponsoring group (usually a union or employer) in running the welfare and benefit funds.[11-2]

For more information, go to https://www.dol.gov as well as www.dol.gov/agencies/ebsa/laws-and-regulations/laws/erisa.

State Medicaid agencies are an essential part of Medicaid's state-federal partnership, since the program is governed at the national level and administered at the state level. A state Medicaid agency is the state government department designated under federal law to administer the Medicaid program in that state. Such an agency could be a free-standing department dedicated just to Medicaid, but more often is part of another master state agency, such Healthcare Administration, a Department of Health, a Department of Social Services, or a Department of Human Services. A state Medicaid agency sets all state policies related to the discretionary portions (eligibility, benefits, and other policies) of the Medicaid program in the given state. States must file, amend, and negotiate the state Medicaid plan or waivers with CMS for the state-specific program. States must also send appropriate financial data to receive the appropriate percentage reimbursement from the federal government for outlays in the state Medicaid program.

The state Medicaid agency also carries out the day-to-day policy and operations of the program. It usually administers both a fee-for-service (FFS) program as well as a private managed care program.

For more information, go to https://www.medicaid.gov/. In addition, visit state Medicaid agency websites, especially California and New York. Individual state contacts can be found at www.medicaid.gov/about-us/contact-us/contact-state-page.html.

State departments of insurance (DOIs) and other state agencies play a fiscal and regulatory role in all lines of business, with the exception of Medicaid in some states. A DOI is the chief regulatory agency for licensure and solvency of insurers and managed care plans. Sometimes the insurance department can be an office within a broader financial regulation or services department. In addition, some states have now merged their departments of insurance (DOIs) and banking into one entity.

The National Association of Insurance Commissioners (NAIC, www.naic. org) is an important, non-profit group of insurance commissioners that sets important global insurance standards and fiscal solvency policies nationally, which states generally adopt. In addition, CMS and state Medicaid agencies look to it for important guidance and may adopt its guidance in regulation.

It is important to note that while federal law preempts state law in many healthcare programs, state DOIs play an important role in almost every case. The power to license a plan alone gives the agency great sway over the insurer. Here are some good examples of the power of state insurance regulators:

Medicare—CMS has authority over all aspects of the benefits and policy and generally pre-empts state laws. However, CMS does require that Medicare Advantage (MA) and standalone Part D plans be licensed in each state that they are doing business as a condition of award of an MA or Part D contract.

Medicaid—While federal laws may pre-empt certain state laws, generally the state Medicaid agency and DOI are given cognizance over Medicaid in that state. DOIs generally cover largely the licensure and financial solvency areas unless the state Medicaid agency is given cognizance over this for Medicaid-only plans.

ACA Exchanges—Plans must have state licensure. In addition, state DOIs review rates along with CMS in certain circumstances.

Self-insured ERISA—Although employers are self-insured, health plans often administer these plans and usually have a third-party administrator (TPA) license or full insurance licensure in the state.

Commercial—Plans must have state insurance licensure to offer other commercial plans in a state.

A state insurance agency's main responsibilities include accepting applications for licensure of new insurers, HMO entities, or other entities operating in the insurance world. A good example is delegated entities of a health plan, as they may be required to obtain a TPA license in order to process claims, provide services, and to show financial stability. State insurance regulators also may license other players, such as brokers and agents selling health insurance or life products.

Insurance regulators also periodically audit or examine insurers, HMOs, and other entities for solvency and compliance with insurance regulations (e.g., network, consumer protection, grievance, claims processing timeliness, and quality assurance). They also investigate consumer complaints against an insurer or HMO and set fiscal solvency standards for regulated entities. In general, a risk-based capital standard is used to ensure that plans have sufficient reserves to cover claims for insureds.

State insurance agencies also must approve health insurance rates. Given the passage of the ACA and Exchanges, this duty is done in concert with CMS for individual and small groups. State insurance agencies generally do not approve rates for large group risk arrangements (this is based on each employer's unique experience). There really is no rate-setting for self-insured large groups. State insurer entities do not generally play a role in setting Medicare or Medicaid rates.

Sometimes states have multiple agencies involved in insurance regulation. In some states, while licensure may be in the hands of the DOIs, the state Medicaid agency may have cognizance over most other policies related to provision of managed Medicaid. In some states, regulation of certain plans may be outside of a DOI and be under a state Medicaid agency or other department.

For example, these plans may serve Medicaid or government-program eligibles exclusively and only be partially at-risk or partially capitated. They can also be considered pilot healthcare programs or unlicensed provider networks or organizations. In some states, other agencies (e.g., Health, Human Services, Social Services, or Healthcare Administration) may have joint responsibility with a DOI or explicit cognizance over certain regulatory areas, including network adequacy, benefit provision, quality assurance, complaints, and certification of managed care plans, among others. Therefore, plans are answerable to these agencies as well as the DOIs. A good example here is the expansive role of the New York Department of Health over managed care plans.

In California, managed care plans are actually overseen by the distinct Department of Managed Healthcare (DMHC). So, plans may have to follow rules and be accountable to both DMHC and the state Department of Insurance, depending on the types of products they sell. More on this in the next chapter.

> For more information, go to the NAIC website (**www.naic.org**). To find state department of insurance websites, especially California and New York, use the websites, **https://www.naic.org/state_web_map.htm** or **www.medicaid.gov/about-us/contact-us/contact-state-page.html**. The New York State Department of Health website is **www.health.ny.gov**. The California Department of Managed Healthcare website is **www.dmhc.ca.gov/?referral=hmohelp.ca.gov.**

Non-profit and Non-government Regulatory Entities

There are a number of **non-profit and non-governmental regulatory** entities that help regulate the provision of healthcare. These include accreditors, quality assurers, and policy decision administrators. In some cases, this is through explicit contract by government regulators. In other cases, it is because government regulators have designated that these outside entities' standards or programs be used by health plans to document how they meet quality and other standards.

These outside regulators matter because they have developed the expertise and metrics in areas that help CMS and other government regulators assess how well health plans are serving their members. They make sure that plans have the right operational processes to ensure cost-effective and quality care. Their metrics include gauging outcomes in critical clinical and process areas. These groups also serve as impartial arbiters to validate that plans are using evidence-based criteria in their prior authorization processes.

The **National Committee for Quality Assurance** (NCQA, <u>www.ncqa.org</u>) is known generally as the national quality governing entity for U.S. healthcare. This non-profit 501(c)(3) plays a number of roles. It accredits health plans to ensure they operate under quality policies, processes, and governance. It publishes the Healthcare Effectiveness Data and Information Sets (HEDIS) of quality measures. These measures are updated each year. They seek to assess clinical and quality outcomes on the medical and pharmacy front as well as have consumer assessment survey components. Various regulatory agencies recognize HEDIS in their Star or quality programs to rate plans. Plans submit data to NCQA and regulatory agencies each year to get rated for quality in all lines of business. These measures in part are used to reward high-performing plans with bonus revenue.

NCQA also is partnered with CMS to oversee the special needs plan (SNP) model of care (MOC) program in Medicare. NCQA certifies and recertifies models of care based on regulations spelled out by both CMS and NCQA.

NCQA also accredits or certifies other entities in the healthcare arena, including technology software, case and disease management entities, and accountable care organizations (ACOs, which operate as quasi-health plans in the Medicare FFS system).

The **Pharmacy Quality Alliance** (PQA, <u>www.pqaalliance.org</u>) is a bit like NCQA when it comes to quality measurement. While HEDIS has pharmacy quality measures, which are still used in Medicaid and commercial, CMS has basically chosen PQA as its quality measurement arm for pharmacy measures in Medicare. PQA measures calculate overall drug adherence. PQA measures are updated each year and incorporated into the Star program much like HEDIS measures are on the medical side.

There are several other health plan accreditation entities that review plans to certify that they meet quality standards of operation and performance. These include the **Accreditation Association for Ambulatory Health Care** (AAAHC, www.aaahc.org), which accredits ambulatory centers, surgery centers, and health plans and **URAC** (originally the Utilization Review Accreditation Commission), which accredits various utilization review entities, pharmacy benefit managers (PBMs), ACOs, health plans, and more. **The Joint Commission** mainly accredits hospitals and other facilities, but it also accredits health plans (usually associated with larger provider entities).

Other Outside Contracted Entities

There are a series of **other outside contracted entities** that contract with Medicare and Medicaid states as well as serve critical purposes in the commercial world. Following are some of the most notable that impact health plan operations or policy and regulation. We will be discussing other contractors and entities in the detailed discussion of the various lines of business.

Independent review entities (IREs), **external review/appeals entities** (EREs or EAEs), or **independent review organizations** (IROs) review authorization denials of health plans to assure an independent assessment of whether a service, benefit, or drug is needed. In Medicare, they are called the IRE. In Medicaid, there are several models, including outside review entities and sometimes state agency boards. A Medicaid beneficiary could both receive an external appeal as well as what is known in Medicaid as a State Fair Hearing.

In the Exchanges and at-risk commercial products subject to the ACA (so-called non-grandfathered plans), plans use one of the following[11-3, 11-4, 11-5]:

- A state external appeal process that meets or exceeds federal guidelines. The vast majority of states—forty-six—have qualifying external appeals processes.
- Use the HHS process set up for the ACA.
- Hire their own external appeals entity if it meets federal guidelines.

In other commercial products, state DOIs dictate the hiring of entities by plans or contract with them.

In ERISA plans that are non-grandfathered (essentially governed by most of the ACA regulations), similar rules to the Exchanges apply. External actions in court also apply. A complaint with DOL can be filed if a plan did not follow ERISA processes.

In the Federal Employees Health Benefit Plans (FEHBP), you can usually appeal to the Office of Personnel Management (OPM), which uses outside review entities.

It is important to note that members may engage directly with these outside review/appeal entities at points. Members may have to submit their external appeals to these organizations in some cases and the outside organization may communicate directly to the member and the plan with any findings and if they overturn a plan's decision to deny an authorization request.

For more, go to the following:

Medicare:

www.medicare.gov/claims-appeals/file-an-appeal/medicare-health-plan-appeals-level-2-independent-review-entity-ire
www.medicare.gov/claims-appeals/file-an-appeal/medicare-prescription-drug-coverage-appeals/appeals-level-2-reconsideration-by-independent-review-entity
https://www.medicareappeal.com/
maximus.com/capability/appeals-imr
https://www.c2cinc.com/

Medicaid:

Go to the Medicaid agency website for the applicable state and search for outside or independent review or State Fair Hearing.

Exchange/Non-grandfathered Plans:

Check your plan's documents to see if your state uses its external review entity, the plan has hired its own external appeals entity, or the plan uses the HHS process. HHS process: **www.cms.gov/CCIIO/Programs-and-Initiatives/ Consumer-Support-and-Information/csg-ext-appeals-facts.html**

External quality review organizations (EQROs) assist state Medicaid agencies in assessing the performance and quality of Medicaid managed care plans. EQROs perform audits in the areas of compliance with state contracts and Medicaid rules; assess performance and quality measures; assess performance improvement plans; validate encounter data submissions; and perform member and provider surveys of plans.[11-6]

Quality improvement organizations (QIOs) serve CMS for Medicare and are an independent entity that reviews complaints about quality of care in the Medicare FFS system and in Medicare Advantage. In addition, they also review termination of coverage and hospital stays. Similar QIO entities also work to improve patient safety, clinical quality, and coordination of care post-discharge. A member may also engage directly with the QIO. A member may file a QIO review directly and the QIO may communicate to the member and the plan with any findings or a reversal regarding termination of coverage.[11-7, 11-8]

Medicare Administrative Contractors (MACs), formerly fiscal intermediaries (FIs) handle claim payment in the Medicare FFS program. They also make policy determinations about what is covered in the program in each of their respective regions. These are called local coverage determinations (LCDs). Over time CMS assesses these LCDs and may adopt them as national coverage determinations (NCDs). MA plans are obligated to follow NCD rules nationally and LCD rules where they serve members.

CHAPTER 12

Players in the U.S.
Health Insurance System, Part 2

N ow let's look at health plans themselves and various managed care and
provider support entities that help deliver your care.

Health Plans, Managed Care Plans, and Insurers

Since Chapter 2, the terms health plan, managed care plan, and insurer have
been used often. But what do they really mean? People often use these terms
interchangeably and that is probably okay. We think of ourselves as being in a
health plan, generically. Most of us are in one of the managed care plans listed in
this chapter. And the term *insurer* refers to the fact that we have health insurance.
But let's talk a little more specifically about the actual differences in the terms.

A **health plan** is a generic term covering entities we enroll in for the provision of our healthcare benefits. Technically speaking, as you learned in

Chapter 10, a **managed care plan** would refer only to one of these types of products: health maintenance organization (HMO), exclusive provider organizations (EPO) or open access health maintenance organizations (OA-HMO), preferred provider organizations (PPO), point of service (POS) plans, and high-deductible health plans (HDHP)

Explaining truly what an **insurer** is becomes more complicated. With the advent of HMOs and managed care products, state departments of insurance (DOIs) have begun looking at regulation of the various products differently. In many states, insurance regulation may be divided into two groups: (1) HMOs/managed care plans and (2) traditional insurers.

An HMO and related managed care products generally have stricter regulation to ensure that the plan is meeting network access, adequacy, credentialing, and other rules. At the same time, capital reserve requirements (to ensure there is enough money to serve members and pay claims) could be less for managed care, given its tight networks, network discounts, and lower risk.

On the other hand, traditional insurers may have less onerous regulatory requirements but higher capital reserve requirements. This is because their networks may be looser or non-existent and therefore cost and risk is higher. Insurers, too, may be licensed in multiple states, while HMOs and related managed care plans usually are contained as an entity in a given state.

Let's think about this a little more in terms of products. While treatment in states may differ based on specific state law, an HMO or related managed care licensure might apply to the following products (acronyms and products defined in Chapter 10): HMO, EPO/OA-HMO, POS, HDHP, and PPO. A traditional insurer licensure may apply to the following: Indemnity, PPO, standalone Medicare Part D (Prescription Drug Plan or PDP) product.

As you can see, a PPO may be regulated differently by states. It is also the case that health plans may hold both an HMO/managed care license as well as an insurer license as the products they sell fall in both categories.

States generally apply certain requirements to both insurers and HMO/managed care plans, such as what benefits are mandatory, eligibility, renewal and payments, authorization, appeal and grievance procedures, quality standards, member rights and protections, and now guaranteed issue and pre-existing condition protections due to the ACA. Then, the statutes may deviate to lay out requirements specific to insurers and differently for HMOs/managed care plans. For example, on the HMO/managed care side, state law may discuss where plans operate (known as service areas) and provider networks and credentialing. And as discussed previously, capital requirements may be laid out differently.[12-1]

Plan-Delegated Entities

These entities are responsible for certain functions that support health plans in their provision of healthcare services to members. Sometimes plans subcontract these services or benefits because they want to offer comprehensive services but do not have the expertise or technology systems to do so. They are also known as delegated or downstream entities.

These delegated entities or subcontractors look like health plans in many ways. They have to follow all the same compliance and other rules of the health plan and should be closely monitored and integrated with other plan activities. However, under federal and state laws, the health plan is ultimately responsible for the services that are rendered by these entities. Plans may contract with the entities below in one of three ways:

Administrative Services Only (ASO)—In this arrangement, the plan pays a set fee for the entity to deliver the services. In this case, the plan retains the financial risk related to the provision of the service.

Capitation—In this arrangement, the plan may pay the entity a capitation amount for each person per month. The subcontractor then has the financial risk related to providing the service.

Hybrid—In some cases a plan may pay an ASO fee but also negotiate a shared savings or penalty depending on the outcome of the projected costs of the services or benefits.

Plans should oversee and ensure coordination between all these downstream entities and the clinical staff at the plan, but they don't always do so. One major problem is that data should flow from the downstream vendor to the health plan and vice versa. Sometimes, members and providers need to ensure that vital information with a delegated entity is known to the health plan and other providers. This is often the case when pharmacy benefits managers (PBMs) and behavioral health vendors conduct clinical reviews on behalf of plans.

These delegated entities may communicate directly with members at certain points. For example, a delegated entity may handle prior authorizations on behalf of plans and the member or provider may have to communicate to that entity instead of the plan. The entity will communicate back with decisions. In some cases, grievances also may be handled by delegated entities.

A provider may submit claims directly to a delegated entity and may have to work with it on any problems. In fact, a delegated entity may have its own network of providers. While this should be included in the plan's provider directory, a member may have to work with the delegated entity to identify providers that serve the member. A delegated entity also may perform care management functions and engage with members.

It is true that you should be able to rely on your plan's member services or customer relations department to work with delegated entities on authorization and network issues. However, that does not always work out, necessitating your direct discussions with them.

Various delegated entities include:

A pharmacy benefits manager (PBM) is one example of a plan-delegated entity. Most health plans contract with PBMs to help them provide pharmacy benefits. While health plans are increasingly taking over some PBM functions due to compliance and quality concerns, they typically provide a number of services to health plans:

> **Claims adjudication/processing**—This is due to the uniqueness of paying for so-called retail drugs based on specific drug codes and classifications.

Network administration and pharmacy provider relations— Usually, PBMs create networks and administer them for health plans. Some plans, though, create their own pharmacy networks or use outside entities to build them for them as well. PBMs also negotiate prices with network pharmacies.

Quality assurance—PBMs usually credential and monitor pharmacies to ensure compliance and quality. Health plans or outside entities may also perform quality assurance and credentialing for pharmacy networks.

Drug rebate negotiation and administration—PBMs often administer drug rebates for plans. If plans are smaller, PBMs can use the aggregate buying power of their clients to gain more rebates from drugmakers. At the same time, PBMs may keep some of the rebate or fees paid by drugmakers. Increasingly, large plans are negotiating on their own. PBMs also may work with drug aggregators on rebates. Sometimes drug aggregators may work directly with health plans.

Clinical operations—This includes benefit design, formulary creation and administration, prior authorizations, appeals, external appeals and grievances/complaints. Plans may delegate to PBMs to perform these services. But many plans perform their own clinical functions using their own or purchased technology and integrate with the PBM's claim system to ensure drug claims pay once authorized. PBMs may also handle all or some aspects of member services.

Patient drug quality programs—Often, PBMs perform medication therapy management, medication reconciliation, and monitoring for drug adherence, safety issues (such as drug interactions) and opioid and other abuse. But again, many plans are in-sourcing these services and performing them on their own.

Utilization and Care/Disease Management Organizations (CMOs, DMOs)—Some plans may outsource some or all of their prior authorization and case and disease management to third parties. This could be for pharmacy and/or medical services. In these cases, the delegated entity must ensure it follows all compliance and quality requirements on behalf of the plan.

Behavioral Health Managed Care Organizations (MCOs, HMOs)—Some plans will delegate behavioral health and substance abuse services to a downstream entity that is expert in these areas. These entities will set up specialized networks and programs to ensure service needs are met on behalf of the plan. In these cases, the delegated entity must ensure it follows all compliance and quality requirements on behalf of the plan.

Behavioral health organizations usually have their own networks and are delegated for utilization management (UM)/prior authorization and care management. Members and providers often communicate directly with these entities.

Dental, Vision, and Hearing HMOs or Managed Care Entities—These are similar to the behavioral health and substance abuse entities. Plans may contract for and delegate provision of dental, vision, and hearing benefits. Such entities will set up specialized networks and programs to ensure service needs are met on behalf of the plan. In these cases, the delegated entity must ensure it follows all compliance and quality requirements on behalf of the plan.

These entities usually have their own networks and usually are delegated for prior authorization if it applies. Members and providers may engage with them.

Third-Party Administrators (TPAs)—These may administer comprehensive health plan services or a subset of services. Good examples of things TPAs perform for plans include enrollment and member services, network management, and claims processing. They can also administer clinical services, such as prior authorization and appeals, as well as case and disease management.

It is not uncommon for plans, large and small, to administer one line of business within the organization while delegating vast pieces of other lines of businesses to TPAs. It is also quite common for members and providers to directly engage with TPA entities if they are delegated whole lines of business or significant member-facing services, such as enrollment and member services.

Note that many of the delegated entities listed before TPAs are actually TPAs that specialize in specific clinical or benefit areas.

Provider Entities

While this book is about health plans, it is important to outline some of the major provider entities that either compete with health plans for membership in a given line of business or enter into contractual agreements with plans. Provider entities below can go by different names, depending on the state or region of the country.

It is important to understand the function of these provider entities and their relationships with plans. Some provider entities are functioning in between the actual healthcare provider and the health plan. This can sometimes lead to complications.

These provider entities may also be providing critical services on behalf of the health plans, so you may encounter them via mail or phone. They also may act as extensions of the provider and the health plan. This is not terribly common right now but will grow in the future. Important provider entities impacting health plans include several types of organizations:

Accountable Care Organizations (ACOs)—These are provider entities that have been created as demonstration projects within the Medicare fee-for-service (FFS) program. The goal was to reduce costs and improve quality in what I have deemed as a terribly antiquated, inefficient, and poor-quality system. The program began in 2011 with a set of pioneer ACOs. The program was expanded and has a number of types of ACOs now. As of early 2021, there were about 500 ACOs participating with about 12 million members. This is less than half of the enrollment in Medicare Advantage. The number of ACOs has been shrinking in recent years.[12-2, 12-3]

ACOs usually are composed of hospitals, physicians, and facilities. They are assigned Medicare beneficiaries based on claims data that show members who regularly visit doctors who have joined a given ACO. They are encouraged to focus on avoidance of inappropriate services, monitoring care transitions from hospitals, providing care management and care coordination, and boosting quality metrics.

Initially, most ACOs continued to receive all of their provider FFS payments. At the end of a year cycle, ACOs were then given a portion of any shared savings, or penalized for losses in some cases, against the expected spending. They were only paid the shared savings bonus if they also achieved certain quality improvement results. The Centers for Medicare and Medicaid Services (CMS) now is moving ACOs toward an upfront payment model and increasing the amount of risk the organizations will take on.

I am generally a proponent of experimentation to encourage new ways of thinking and to usher in reform. But the truth is the program has shown minimal savings achievement thus far. Where savings did appear, it was largely with experienced provider entities and those with integrated delivery systems.

There are a variety of other provider-based pilots in the Medicare FFS system aimed at reducing costs and improving quality. There are also some ACOs in the commercial and Medicaid world serving millions more members.[12-3]

Provider Sponsored Networks (PSNs)—Similar to ACOs, a PSN is a provider network set up to serve the Medicaid population. Generally speaking, where PSNs operate they do so in direct competition with health plans in the Medicaid managed care program. Depending on the state, these provider entities may need state insurance licensure or be deemed solvent and qualified by the state Medicaid agency. As with ACOs, doctors, hospitals, and other facilities band together to look like a plan and contract with the state Medicaid agency to deliver full or partial Medicaid services. Sometimes, these entities are paid up front, or they get paid by the FFS system and then earn an incentive payment if they save money and improve quality.

Similar provider organizations consisting of physician groups and hospitals are working together through pilots in the Medicaid FFS systems in various states. The aim is to reduce spending and improve quality.

Integrated Systems and Networks—These go by several names: Integrated Delivery Systems (IDS), Integrated Delivery Networks (IDN), or Integrated Health Systems (IHS). This terminology signifies hospitals, physicians, and other facilities that are usually under common ownership and have formed an integrated system to deliver healthcare. These systems may or may not be interested in forming ACOs or PSNs. They may simply want to act as sophisticated providers in the health system and contract with plans.

These systems often have a great advantage in controlling costs because they are their own care continuum and work closely together across the various provider types. Various medical systems and data may be integrated across these provider types as well.

Physician-Hospital Organizations (PHOs)—Similar to Integrated Systems and Networks, physicians and hospitals may get together to form a contracting entity to negotiate with plans. The entity is usually governed by a board composed of both hospital and physician members. In addition, the PHO may provide various services to the health plan or the individual providers. PHOs may perform health plan negotiation, payment administration (billing, correct procedure, and diagnosis coding and capitation payment collection), and other back-office operations (accounting, financial management, human resources, technology, and risk management). It may also perform clinical services, such as prior authorization and care management.

The PHO should be able to demand higher rates given the integration of the providers and hospital and commitments the PHO can make in terms of operating more like an integrated delivery system. It also reduces risk to the individual provider given volume and the backing of usually well-heeled hospitals.

PHOs can also sell themselves as networks or portions of a network to plans and directly credential their providers. While PHOs often negotiate with plans, they, too, now are going directly to self-funded Employee Retirement Security Act (ERISA) employer plans. PHOs are often precursors to ACOs.

Independent practice associations (IPAs), **medical groups**, and **management service organizations** (MSOs)—In this case, physicians band together to create a contracting entity known as an IPA. This gives individual physicians and other providers a great deal of additional fire power to negotiate with plans. They aim for the best rates possible based on the fact that the IPA can help bring members to a plan and work together to control costs. In some cases, physicians and providers could also come under common ownership in a large-scale medical group to obtain better rates from health plans.

IPAs can limit themselves simply to negotiating rates with plans or may provide additional services, in which case they take on the functions of an MSO as well. As with PHOs, MSOs can provide myriad back-office services to serve physicians and providers but also to further boost revenue from plans. Medical groups can be their own MSO as well. MSO activities include negotiating and managing various health plan contracts administering billing and capitation collection, and accounting, financial management, human resources, and risk management. Sometimes the MSO performs clinical services (including prior authorization and care management). MSOs will also ensure correct diagnosis and procedure coding of billing submissions, operate electronic health/medical record systems, and credential providers within the IPA/MSO/Medical Group.

Sophisticated Provider Entities Acceptance of Downstream Risk

In the most mature healthcare markets, the most sophisticated PHOs, IPAs, medical groups, and MSOs may also enter into downstream risk arrangements with health plans. A portion of each assigned member's premium (premium set aside) is placed in a risk pool and the entity is put at risk for the provision of services. These arrangements occur in all lines of business but are especially popular for MA, given high premiums throughout the country. The MA risk-sharing arrangements are governed by the physician incentive plan (PIP) regulations laid out by CMS.

These arrangements cannot be formed to limit necessary care. Plans also must ensure that the downstream entities have stop-loss reinsurance. The provider entity can buy this on the open market, purchase it from the plan, or the plan may craft other ways to insulate downstream entities from a level of risk that triggers the need for the stop-loss insurance.[12-4]

The risk pools can take on many forms, including upside risk only (where providers are rewarded if costs come in under the premium set aside), full upside and partial downside risk (where providers get reward fully for savings against the premium set aside and only partially penalized for expenses above the premium set aside) and full upside and downside risk.

Plans and providers may also negotiate what services are in or out of the risk pool. For example, physician and outpatient services could be in the pool, but inpatient services and perhaps drugs carved out.[12-4]

In many cases, entities that accept such risk arrangements look almost like plans. They have very sophisticated prior authorization and care management departments. They set up their own quality monitoring shops to drive Star bonus revenue to increase their premium set aside and the amount they ultimately gain. They also set up risk adjustment coding shops. These sophisticated providers are seeking to ensure that all diagnoses on each member are documented and submitted to the plan as this drives the amount plans receive for each member (and therefore adds to the premium set aside they receive).

The last two chapters show a complex interchange between plans, providers and groups, delegated entities, and regulators. All of these entities must work together to help redefine healthcare in America if quality and cost savings are to be achieved.

PART THREE

Where We Are Today

In Part Three, I tell you all about how big our health system is, where we spend our money, and why you need coverage. I also outline how a health plan operates, in hopes you can better maneuver the insurance system. I give you details about the various broad types of health insurance, what is better known as lines of business. I begin to outline why I think Medicaid is good for the country and why private alternatives, like Medicare Advantage, make the most sense.

CHAPTER 13

Healthcare Statistics

For me, the best source of information on statistics in U.S. healthcare is the Centers for Medicare and Medicaid Services' (CMS) National Health Expenditure Data (NHED), published annually by the CMS Actuary. Most of the detailed statistical analysis out there can be tied back to this main source of information. I am writing in early 2021, so the latest information available is for 2019. Most of the information in this chapter, unless otherwise cited, can be found at CMS' NHED website.[13-1, 13-2]

In 2019, national healthcare expenditures hit roughly $3.8 trillion, or $11,582 per person. In 2018, expenditures were $3.63 trillion, or $11,129 per person. The costs are so large that if our healthcare system were its own country, it would be the fifth largest in the world—behind only the United States, China, Japan, and Germany. Total national healthcare spending in 2019 grew 4.6%. Growth in 2018 was 4.7%. The average annual growth since 2016 has been 4.5%.

A good measure of the efficiency of the healthcare system is to compare the percentage of the so-called healthcare pie against the nation's gross domestic product (GDP). GDP is the productivity of a nation, measured by the value of all the final goods and services produced in a given time period.

In 2019, national healthcare expenditures accounted for 17.7% of GDP, about the same as in 2018, which was 17.6%. As you will learn, our healthcare spending, both as a percentage of GDP and per capita, is markedly above that of other developed nations.

As discussed in earlier chapters, healthcare spending in America as a percentage of GDP has rapidly risen throughout our modern history. Let's repeat what we showed earlier:

> 1960: 5.0%
> 1970: 6.9%
> 1980: 8.9%
> 1990: 12.1%
> 2000: 13.4%
> 2010: 17.3%
> 2018: 17.6%
> 2019: 17.7%

The growth from 1960 to 1990 was tied to the widescale adoption of health insurance in America and the general rise in the cost of healthcare. The relative moderation in the increase seen from 1990 to 2000 was attributed to the advent of managed care in the private employer sector in the 1980s and 1990s. From 2000 to 2010, costs trends took off again given the managed care backlash and the adoption of looser managed care models.

Since 2010, we have seen a moderation in cost increases in healthcare. Inflationary pressures have been relatively moderate in key areas, including drug prices. The Affordable Care Act's (ACA's) expansion of coverage also reduced cost pressures. This is not to say that costs are under control or that our crisis has been averted. Businesses struggle with affordability and continue to reduce or eliminate healthcare coverage today. Many of those who would have become uninsured have moved over to Medicaid or the Exchanges.

Let's review some key facts from CMS' national healthcare expenditures breakout and parse this out a little more.

Who pays the healthcare bills (again in 2019)?
    Federal government—29%
    Households—28%
    Employers—19%
    State and local governments—16%
    Other—7%

The federal spending is for government healthcare programs and the direct costs of providing coverage to employees. The employer spending is for self-insured costs of operating their own healthcare funds or risk payments to insurers for health coverage for employees. State and local government spending is for healthcare programs and employee costs.

So, what is the household cost? It is a mixture of premiums paid for healthcare insurance, out-of-pocket costs for healthcare services (whether covered by a health insurance plan or not), and the costs that the uninsured pay for treatment on their own.

What is the allocation of spending by the three major coverage programs in the United States? Private health insurance consumes 31%, Medicare consumes 21%, and Medicaid/State Children's Health Insurance Program (SCHIP) consumes 16%.

Looked at another way, there was about $1.2 trillion spent on private health insurance in 2019, but about $1.4 billion spent on Medicare/Medicaid/SCHIP. So, government spending on the big programs alone now exceeds private health insurance. All federal, state, and local government expenditures on healthcare total almost 50% of national healthcare expenditures. So, who says we don't have government healthcare already?

There were an estimated 328 million Americans in 2019. There was reported coverage totaling about 384 million because people can have more than one form of coverage. As examples, they can have two employer-sponsored coverages, Medicare and employer-sponsored coverage, and Medicare and Medigap.

How does coverage breakout?
    Private employer-sponsored coverage—176.4 million

Other Private health insurance coverage—31.3 million

Marketplace—9.8 million

Medigap (companion to Medicare for those on the traditional fee-for-service [FFS] system and sold privately)—12.3 million

Medicare—60.2 million

Medicaid—72.3 million

SCHIP—7.1 million

Other Public Coverage—14.4 million

TOTAL—383.8 million

There were about 31.8 million Americans who were uninsured as of 2019 statistics, or about 9.7% of the population.

Employer-sponsored coverage is about 46%, but private coverage (excluding Marketplace) is about 57% of all coverage. This is down from the peak of about 75-80%. Medicare, Medicaid, and SCHIP coverage, at 36%, has seen huge growth in the past thirty years. (It was just 22%, or 52 million, in 1987.) The reasons include aging as well as the many Medicaid expansions over the years, including under the ACA in 2010.

As a side note, the ACA helped reduce the rate of the uninsured dramatically, although the rate has inched up again since 2016. Prior to implementation of the ACA, which expanded Medicaid in many states and introduced the Exchanges, the uninsured rate was 14-15% according to NHED. In 2016, it had fallen to below 9%.

The Census Bureau has some interesting additional statistics before the ACA's implementation and after. Note that the NHED statistics generally comport with the census data, but numbers may vary for several reasons (timeframe, methodology, etc.).[13-3]

From 2013 to 2017, the number of people with either employer or directly purchased private coverage increased from 201 million to 217 million. Most of this was in the direct purchase arena due to the introduction of the Exchanges—with 36 million enrollees in 2013 and 52 million now. But strict employer coverage did increase from 174 million to 181 million. (The sub counts don't equal the full count due to duplication or overlap in the subcategories.) This employer trend is a good sign. The economy had been doing well prior to the COVID-19 pandemic, which added jobs and insureds. In addition, employers seemed to be able to better afford insurance given the moderate spending growth.

From 2013 to 2017, enrollment in government programs increased as well, from 108 million to 122 million. Medicare enrollment increased due to aging and normal growth from 49 million to 56 million. Medicaid grew from 55 million to 62 million in large measure due to the expansion of Medicaid under the ACA. The actual number of people covered under the Medicaid eligibility expansion is greater (it is offset here by other reductions).

The uninsured number in this timeframe went down from about 42 million to about 29 million.

An Urban Institute study reports that the ACA led to a surge in coverage for young adults. The uninsured rate for people aged 19 to 25 declined from 30% to 16% between 2011 and 2018. Medicaid enrollment for this age group increased from 11% to 15% in the same time span. We know that getting young adults covered is still a struggle and the lack of this relatively healthy pool has played a role in overall high Exchange costs and premiums.[13-4]

What is important, too, is that ethnic and racial disparities were reduced tremendously with the adoption of the ACA. One source, the Kaiser Family Foundation (KFF), relying on data from the Census Bureau's American Community Survey, found the following:[13-5]

As of 2013, prior to the ACA implementation, the rates of uninsured for these racial and ethnic groups were as described in the graph. (This is for non-elderly adults and children, regardless of citizenship status.) As of 2017, all categories recorded huge gains in coverage, but blacks and Hispanics the most. Thus, the ethnic and racial disparities related to healthcare coverage are closing.

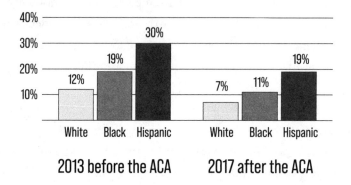

2013 before the ACA   2017 after the ACA

A second source, the Commonwealth Fund, performed a similar study using the same data. Even though Hispanics have a disproportionate share of people who lack citizenship status and therefore are not eligible for premium and cost-sharing subsidies under the ACA, Commonwealth concluded that racial and ethnic disparities in insurance coverage were reduced with the introduction of the ACA. The biggest declines were in states that expanded Medicaid. In the nation as a whole, the coverage gap between non-elderly adult blacks and whites went down from 11 percentage points in 2013 to 5.3% in 2017. Similar trends were seen for non-elderly Hispanic adult citizens versus whites: 13.2% to 6.8%.[13-6]

So, what has happened during the COVID-19 pandemic of 2020 with regard to the uninsured rate? It is hard to say as of this writing in early 2021. Various studies estimate that up to 15 million may have lost employer coverage during the initial COVID-19 outbreak in the first half of 2020. The Economic Policy Institute (EPI) suggests that as many as 12 million Americans lost employer-based coverage at the time due to the COVID-19 pandemic, with about 6 million employees and 6 million dependents.[13-7] Some who lost coverage have regained jobs and coverage and others have found their way to Medicaid, the State Children's Health Insurance Program (SCHIP), and the Marketplace

Exchanges. Enrollment in these programs has gone up dramatically. The best guess at the time of this book's writing is that the uninsured count has remained about the same.

How could the COVID-19 pandemic and other recent forces impact costs in healthcare and the percentage of the economy it will take up? The COVID-19 pandemic will materially impact previous estimates as to costs in 2020. While final numbers were not out as of this writing in early 2021, utilization was dramatically down in 2020 for a number of quarters. Even in the second half of 2020 and into 2021, there was still lower utilization compared with the pre-COVID-19 history. Thus, we will see a drop in overall healthcare costs in 2020, and we should see a return to rising costs and inflation in 2021, 2022, and beyond. However, the COVID-19 pandemic alone likely will not fundamentally impact overall long-term predictions. The NHED projects that healthcare spending will be $6.2 trillion by 2028 and take up just short of one-fifth of the overall economy.[13-1] There could be some lower re-estimates coming out, but the upward trajectory will not stop just due to the pandemic.

One research firm, however, is predicting that other forces could begin to change projections. Deloitte is now predicting that healthcare spending will be markedly lower than estimates by CMS actuaries. Deloitte actuaries are predicting that the positive trends in the healthcare system—I outline them in Chapter 29—will actually create an annual "well-being dividend" of $3.5 trillion due to new business models, emerging life-saving technologies (in part driven by the pandemic), and highly engaged consumers. Thus, they say our spending will be $3.5 trillion less annually by 2040 than previous estimates. Deloitte says CMS' estimate of healthcare spending by 2040 was projected to be $11.8 trillion annually and might only be $8.3 trillion. Deloitte says that in 2019 about 80% of health spending went toward care and treatment. By 2040, it says 60% of spending will go toward improving health and well-being.[13-8, 13-9]

We don't know for sure if this will occur, but it should be celebrated if it does. It means critical reforms will take hold. At the same time, if it does come true, Deloitte notes that healthcare spending as a percentage of GDP will still be 18.4% (as opposed to 26.1%). So, America's healthcare spending will still be out of control and far above what other developed nations spend per capita and as a percentage of GDP.[13-8, 13-9]

So, we have learned a few things in this chapter. Healthcare is a huge part of our economy and GDP. Everyone contributes a great deal to our system, from the average American, to employers, to the government. Despite what many believe, government is a big part of the healthcare system even though we have one of the few employer-based insurance systems in the world. The ACA had a positive impact in reducing the number of uninsured, especially among ethnic and racial minorities.

CHAPTER 14

Pieces of the Healthcare Pie

So, we have covered some of the current healthcare statistics of the times, including how much of our economy is devoted to healthcare, who pays for it, where people get coverage, and uninsured statistics. Let's now turn to understanding how much of the healthcare pie, so to speak, is consumed by the various service categories.

Some words of warning. Data in this area are a bit "all over the place," in part related to the fact that statisticians and healthcare economists do things differently, the scarcity of data in some cases, and the inability to reliably parse the data.

Where are the pieces of the healthcare pie and how big are each?

Again, looking at the Centers for Medicare and Medicaid Services' (CMS) National Health Expenditure Data (NHED),[14-1] the CMS data is not broken out as you and I might like. The terminology is a bit arcane, too. But here is my best effort to explain the pieces of the healthcare pie. The percentages are rounded to the nearest percentage point in each category.

Hospital Care

This seems fairly straightforward, but it is not. The category covers all services furnished by hospitals, both inpatient and outpatient services. It also includes various other services furnished as part of those inpatient or outpatient visits. So, in this category are the following depending on the type of visit: the inpatient clinical care charges, room and board at the hospital, the outpatient clinical care charges, services of resident physicians at the hospital, any pharmacy or drugs provided on an inpatient basis, hospital-based nursing home and home healthcare, and other ancillary charges.

In 2019, hospital charges were about 31% of total healthcare expenditures.

Physician and Clinical Services

This includes all healthcare services provided by physicians in facilities operated by them, such as those provided in offices, outpatient care centers or ambulatory surgery centers, as well as any medical laboratory services billed independently by laboratory providers. Included here, too, is the cost of surgery or other services that are billed separately by doctors for hospital care above.

It is important to note that what we think of as outpatient surgery is split between hospital care and physician and clinical services. In general, we think of outpatient care as care provided in an outpatient hospital setting, an ambulatory surgery center, or in a physician's office (whether a visit or a surgery). But for CMS' purposes, outpatient hospital is in hospital care and the other two are in this category.

Health plans increasingly push to have surgery and routine procedures done in a physician's office or ambulatory surgery center rather than through an outpatient hospital visit. This is because costs at the outpatient hospital setting (place of service or POS 22) are far greater than at ambulatory surgery centers (place of service or POS 24) or physicians' offices (place of service or POS 11). Given the trend, many hospitals are allying with physicians or setting up their own ambulatory service centers to compete, sometimes in the backyards of their competitor hospitals. In this case, the ambulatory surgery centers partially or fully owned by the hospitals shows up in this bucket.

In 2019, physician and other clinical services were about 20% of total healthcare expenditures.

Prescription Drugs

This includes the so-called retail side of prescription drugs (i.e., those obtained at a pharmacy). It does not include over-the-counter drugs that do not need a prescription but does include certain diagnostic equipment and supplies that need a prescription (e.g., diabetic supplies and test strips). In addition, it does not include the so-called medical drugs that are administered in inpatient, outpatient, or in physician office settings. These are captured in other categories.

In 2019, prescription drugs were about 10% of total healthcare expenditures.

Other Health, Residential, and Personal Care

This includes spending for Medicaid home and community-based waivers, care provided in residential care facilities, ambulance services, school health, and worksite healthcare. In 2019, these services were about 5% of total healthcare expenditures.

Nursing Care Facilities and Continuing Care Retirement Communities

This includes spending for nursing and rehabilitative services provided in freestanding nursing home facilities. In 2019, nursing care and related facilities were about 5% of total healthcare expenditures. This is expected to jump considerably with the aging of America.

Dental Services

These are services provided by various doctors of dentistry in their facilities. In 2019, dental services were about 4% of total healthcare expenditures.

Other Services and Products

In total, these other services and products accounted for about 10% of total healthcare expenditures in 2019.

Other Professional Services are namely those provided by health practitioners in their facilities other than physicians and dentists. CMS includes private-duty nurses; chiropractors; podiatrists; optometrists; and physical, occupational, and speech therapists, among others. In 2019, other professional services were about 3% of total healthcare expenditures.

Home Health, includes spending for medical care provided in the home by freestanding home health agencies, accounting for about 3% of total healthcare expenditures in 2019.

Durable Medical Equipment (DME) includes items such as contact lenses, eyeglasses, and other ophthalmic products; surgical and orthopedic products; wheelchairs; medical equipment rental; oxygen; and hearing aids. In 2019, it was about 2% of total healthcare expenditures.

Other, Non-Durable Medical Products includes non-durable medical products, such as non-prescription drugs and medical sundries. This accounted for about 2% of total healthcare expenditures in 2019.

Summary

That adds up to 85%, rounded up. Where is the rest?

Well, there is about 8% that is tied to administration by states, the federal government, and private insurers as well as insurers' profits. Over 80% of that is private insurer administration and profits. (You will learn my view later on why the amount of administrative spending in private healthcare is not a bad thing and that profits are reasonable.) The remaining 8% includes public health expenditures, government research, and other investments.

In looking at spending in other nations, the percentage we spend in these categories is not really the issue. The issue is that our overall spending is too high, and we have little focus on prevention, management, and quality.

Employer Coverage Spending by Category

Several groups break out healthcare expenditures and statistics within a given line of business in a different way, which can be quite informative. Let's look at employer-sponsored insurance (ESI). The best source for this is the Health Care Cost Institute (HCCI), a non-partisan group dedicated to analyzing the rise in U.S. healthcare costs. It published an annual Health Care Cost and Utilization Report. The 2017 report examines spending, utilization, and average prices. It is based on healthcare claims data from 2013 through 2017 for Americans under the age of sixty-five with ESI. The report relies on de-identified claims data from Aetna, Humana, Kaiser Permanente, and UnitedHealthcare. I encourage you to review the report and available data. It has a wealth of information. The 2017 HCCI report includes some key findings, which I summarize below:[14-2]

I mentioned previously that, although spending increases moderated in the 2000s, that did not mean prices or spending stopped climbing. HCCI reports that in 2017 per-person spending for ESI reached a new high of $5,641.

The spending increase from 2016 to 2017 was 4.2%, down from 4.9% from 2015 to 2016. The fact that per person spending grew 16.7% over the claims period is concerning. While this is relatively moderate, the growth continues to outpace growth in personal income, overall inflation, GDP growth, and per capita GDP growth (growth per person).

From 2013 to 2017, utilization declined 0.2%. In 2017, utilization grew 0.5% over 2016 levels. Therefore, price increases drove overall spending. Average prices increased 3.6% in 2017. This is down from 4.8% earlier in the claims period. This is in part due to lower overall increases in drug costs.

Out-of-pocket spending per person increased 2.6% in 2017. This is a sign that businesses overall (not all of them) are able to absorb moderate increases from year to year and not transfer them to employees.

Here is a better breakout of price (unit cost), utilization (how much the service use increased), and spending increases in ESI over the 2013 to 2017 claims period: [14-2]

Category	Price Increase	Utilization Increase	Spending Increase
Pres. Drugs:	25.0%	3.1%	28.9%
Outpatient:	18.9%	0.3%	19.3%
Inpatient:	15.6%	-5.0%	9.8%
Professional:	12.4%	0.3%	12.7%
Total:	17.1%	-0.2%	16.7%

Let's now look at how spending areas stack up for ESI, according to 2017 statistics from HCCI, which I summarize below. [14-2]

Inpatient spending accounted for 19.4% of ESI spending. In this case, HCCI counts only inpatient admissions in the inpatient spending category. The breakout of admissions is below, with the percentage of spending that each represents in the inpatient category. Mental health/ substance abuse saw a major increase in spending over the claims period (with substance abuse driving this).

- Surgical admissions: 49%
- Medical admissions (a stay for other than surgery): 28%
- Labor/delivery/newborn: 19%
- Mental health/substance abuse: 4%

Outpatient spending accounted for 28.0% of ESI spending. In this case, HCCI includes the broad categories below in the outpatient category. The percentage of spending in the list below represents that category's amount against the outpatient total. HCCI does note that ER spending increases over the claims period were high compared with other categories.

- Outpatient surgery (hospital and non-hospital facility based): 36%
- Emergency room: 24%
- Radiology: 13%
- Laboratory: 5%
- Durable Medical Equipment: 3%
- Observation (usually in a hospital or ER): 3%
- Ambulance: 3%
- Other 13%

Professional spending accounted for 33.6% of ESI spending. In this case, HCCI includes the broad categories below in the professional category. The percentages of spending below represent that category's amount against the professional total. This spending would be related to the physician's professional charges and the fees for a given service, such as drugs, radiology, or anesthesia, at a physician's office or when the physician visits the patient in an inpatient or outpatient setting. HCCI notes that office visits and administered drugs accounted for more than half of the cumulative increase over the claims period. Further, administered drugs grew at a faster rate than any other professional services subcategory in each year of the claims period.

- ○ Office visits: 21%
- ○ Surgery: 15%
- ○ Administered drugs (chemotherapy and other infusibles/inject-ables): 13%
- ○ Lab/pathology: 8%
- ○ Radiology: 8%
- ○ Anesthesia: 6%
- ○ ER visit: 5%
- ○ Other: 26%

Retail prescription drug spending accounted for 18.9% of ESI spending. In this case, HCCI includes drugs and devices (e.g., glucometers and supplies) obtained at pharmacies. HCCI notes that the costs here include negotiated discounts at the pharmacy level but do not count the impact of rebates from drugmakers.

There are some key facts to note here about retail prescription drug spending. Over 75% of spending was for brand drugs. As we discussed in Chapter 5, plans drive utilization of generic drugs, but the average price point of a generic is about 5% of that of the average for brand drugs—$30 versus $567. Thus, even with high utilization rates for generics, brand drug spending will dominate costs in this category. HCCI notes several sources indicating that rebates can offset between 10-20% of drug costs, depending on the line of business. Rebates in the commercial world are toward the lower end, with Medicare rebates at the higher end.

Medicare Coverage Spending by Category

We will go into a great level of detail about the various parts of Medicare in Chapter 19. In the meantime, let's investigate Medicare spending, based on various category breakouts, which are somewhat different than those of the NHED or HCCI.

In terms of overall spending, the NHED reports that gross spending for Medicare was about $799 billion in 2019.[14-1] NHED reports Medicare enrollment was 60.2 million in 2019, compared with 61.5 million for the year on another CMS site,[14-1, 14-3] giving us a per capita annual cost of between $13,000 and $13,300 for all Medicare spending. This compares with $5,641 annually for ESI, which is well less than half the per capita spending. Note that this calculation is based on 60.2 to 61.5 million total Medicare beneficiaries having Part D drug benefits, although I calculate from CMS membership data that only about 49 million actually do so through a standalone Part D plan or their Medicare Advantage (MA) plan in early 2021. (For example, some may have drug coverage under a retiree health plan). However, it does represent a reasonable allocation of total costs against the total eligible population.

A good source on public programs spending is always the Kaiser Family Foundation (KFF). It reports that in 2014, per capita costs were just under $11,000, with costs ranging from roughly $8,200 per year in the lowest state to $12,600 in the highest state. So, per capita costs range from 34% *below* the national average to 15% *above* the national average.[14-4]

In another report, KFF indicated that federal fiscal year 2017 Medicare benefit payments were about $688 billion (numbers can differ slightly depending on how it is calculated). KFF reports the following breakout for that year[14-5]:

- Medicare Advantage medical payments (not Part D drug payments): 30%
- Traditional Medicare fee-for-service (FFS) inpatient services: 21%
- Part D payments for both Medicare Advantage (MA) and traditional FFS: 14%
- Traditional Medicare FFS physician payments: 10%
- Traditional Medicare FFS hospital outpatient services 7%
- Traditional Medicare FFS skilled nursing facilities: 4%
- Traditional Medicare FFS home health: 3%
- Traditional Medicare FFS other services: 11%

Based on membership percentage, I have allocated Part D spending between Medicare FFS and MA (I assumed the same costs between the two populations). I then computed out just Medicare FFS costs and found these rough percentages for major categories of spending:

- ○ Inpatient: 33%
- ○ Physician services: 16%
- ○ Retail drugs: 12%
- ○ Outpatient: 11%
- ○ Skilled nursing: 6%
- ○ Home health: 5%
- ○ Other: 17%

If you compare the Medicare breakout to that of employer-sponsored coverage, the following is clear. Inpatient is a much greater share of the healthcare pie cost due to the age and disabilities of enrollees in Medicare. Medicare also has a high utilization of skilled nursing and home health services. The other categories' percentages tend to be skewed by the utilization noted previously. It is also true that spending in Medicare is generally higher in any category compared with commercial because per capita costs are much higher.

Medicaid Coverage Spending by Category

Getting a good breakout for Medicaid is difficult because each state runs its own system. In addition, managed care is the majority of acute medical care now in Medicaid. As a result, data from plans are challenging to gather and collate. In addition, FFS program data for acute care are unreliable, given the small population base. Showing it here would skew your understanding, although the largest category is inpatient spending and related hospital payments.[14-6]

According to KFF, the 2017 breakout of the total $577 billion in Medicaid spending nationally was as follows:[14-7]

- ○ Spending in the traditional, acute FFS system of each state: $142 billion
- ○ Spending in the traditional, long-term care FFS system of each state: $119 billion

- ○ Managed care spending: $282 billion
- ○ Medicare premium and cost-sharing payments for dual eligibles (see Chapter 18): $19 billion
- ○ Payments to hospitals for underfunding and uncompensated care: $15 billion

The NHED reports that gross spending for Medicaid was about $613 billion in 2019.[14-1] This is the state and federal spending in the partnership program. Enrollment from CMS for that year was about 75 million beneficiaries,[14-3] giving us a per capita annual cost of about $8,200 annually for all Medicaid spending. This compares with $5,641 annually for ESI and about $13,000 for Medicare. Note, though, that the Medicaid figure includes both acute and long-term care costs so comparison is not entirely valid.

Given the challenging data collection efforts, the best source is 2013 data in a recent KFF report, which says that in 2013, rough Medicaid costs were as follows:[14-8]

Acute Care (annually):

- ○ Children: $2,400
- ○ Adults: $3,100
- ○ Elderly: $4,300
- ○ Persons with disabilities: $10,700

Long-Term Care (annually):

- ○ Children: $100
- ○ Adults: $50
- ○ Elderly: $9,000
- ○ Persons with disabilities: $6,300

CMS published the following in January 2020, and it combines acute and long-term care Medicaid services costs for 2017:[14-9]

- ○ Children: $3,555
- ○ Adults: $5,159
- ○ Medicaid Expansion adults: $5,965
- ○ Elderly: $14,700
- ○ Persons with disabilities: $19,754

Thus, the Medicaid acute care spending profile would actually appear more like the commercial profile than the Medicare one for most categories of enrollees. The $5,641 annual average cost for ESI has a range of ages, from child dependents, to younger and middle-aged employees and dependents, to older members of the workforce nearing retirement. While the ESI cost per capita would appear to be higher than in Medicaid, it is tied in great measure to the fact that Medicaid rates are extremely low, whereas commercial rates are artificially high to make up for underpayments in Medicaid and to some extent Medicare. It is also true that the disabled with acute Medicaid coverage look a lot like Medicare. The elderly category cost for Medicaid is low because Medicare is primary, and Medicaid is secondary coverage.

CHAPTER 15

How a Health Plan Operates

Before we get started on our chapter about health plans operations, let's dispel the notion that somehow health insurers or health plans are reaping huge profits these days. We will go into greater detail on this in succeeding chapters. But the fact is that the days of health plans earning double-digit percentage earnings are gone. As you will learn, various regulations now impose new requirements. Certain amounts of a premium must be spent on medical expenses. Administrative costs are implicitly limited, which limits margins in the industry. Excess premium dollars must be directed to member benefits. Rebates to member or government entities are required if not enough is spent on medical expense.

Looking at 2018 earnings of top health plans compared with other leading healthcare entities, the facts are clear[15-1]:

Percentage earnings:

- o Brand drugmakers—19.4%
- o For-profit health systems—6.1%

- ○   Health plans—4.3%
- ○   Not-for-profit health systems—3.0%

In an earlier chapter, we discussed the difference between a health plan and an insurer, although these terms are often used interchangeably. But how does a health plan operate and deliver healthcare services to ensure efficiency and quality? Like any business, it has its various departments with defined scopes and duties.

In this chapter, we will review these various departments and what role they play in the delivery of healthcare. The explanations and definitions are my own and are based on my time running various health plans in all lines of business.

The most important thing to know is that, except for a plan that is provider-owned (such as the staff model HMO), health plans generally do not furnish direct healthcare. A health plan arranges healthcare services and pays for a portion of it, minus your cost-sharing. Health plans do help coordinate care that may be furnished across many providers. In addition, they are tasked by state and federal law to ensure its efficiency and quality.

Health Plan Board of Directors and Key Executives

Generally speaking, a health plan is led by a **board of directors.** Most states require a board to be formed to oversee the licensed insurance or managed care entity. States also may require those on the board to have expertise in some form of plan operations and clinical affairs or experience with regulated insurance entities. Even if the state does not have such rigor, health plans today look for board members with varied backgrounds and experience in the health field to ensure that the plan is successful and delivers quality care.

The board is a pivotal part of the governance of the health plan. Along with other high-level executives, most state insurance regulators require board members to undergo extensive background checks to ensure they have no criminal backgrounds and are not barred from overseeing an insurance entity.

The board of directors is required to ensure the health plan is run in a fiscally sound manner and that the plan has enough assets or reserves to cover members' care. The board is the fiduciary agent of the licensed insurance entity.

Most state laws, as well as Medicare and Medicaid regulations, require boards to be actively involved in the delivery and quality of care. A quality committee is usually set up and includes board members as well as key executives of the health plan. The quality committee governs the overall delivery of care and constantly strives to improve quality through a continuous quality improvement analysis process.

Under state and federal laws, the board is also the main overseer of compliance with various security, regulatory, and fraud requirements. The Health Insurance Portability and Accountability Act (HIPAA), along with related laws, require health plans to ensure the privacy and security of protected health information (PHI). This includes data related to enrolled members as well as their clinical information. Ultimately, the chief compliance officer of the company must have direct access to the board as a safeguard against fraudulent or non-compliant activities within the health plan.

As with most businesses, a **president and chief executive officer (CEO)** often leads the company in association with the board. The president and CEO is the ultimate executive authority of the business and leads day-to-day affairs of the plan. State and federal regulators like to see the president, along with the board, participate actively in the operations of the plan and quality planning and tracking. The president should be an active member of standing committees of the board and involved day-to-day in other clinical and operational aspects of the plan.

Health plans also have a **chief medical officer (CMO).** The CMO usually is a licensed physician who generally oversees all aspects of the clinical functioning of the health plan but may also assume additional responsibilities. The CMO usually chairs the committees governing quality, provider credentialing, pharmacy and therapeutics (which sets the plan's drug list and prior authorization requirements), and grievances and appeals. The CMO also oversees (with the quality committee) any delegated entities that carry out plan functions, such as pharmacy benefits managers (PBMs) and behavioral health vendors.

A **chief operating officer (COO)** may serve one of two types of roles. In some cases, he may be an executive layer between the CEO and other primary executives of the company. In other cases, the COO may oversee aspects of the health plan that are non-clinical in nature, such as sales, member services, claims, and IT operations.

The **chief financial officer (CFO)** is the person responsible for ensuring fiscal soundness of the health plan, including auditing, accounting, and consistency with all financial regulations. Sometimes a CFO may also oversee claims and other functions.

The **chief information or technology officer (CIO/CTO)** may oversee all aspects of the technology systems in the company and information flow.

And as noted, the **chief compliance officer (CCO) or compliance officer (CO)** oversees the required regulatory compliance and security program. The CCO/CO usually reports to the president, the compliance committee, and the board simultaneously.

Sales and Marketing/Product Design Department

The sales and marketing department is responsible for attracting members to the health plan through various marketing and direct sales initiatives. Voluntary enrollment, and therefore the need for sales activities, is key in the following lines of business:

> **Medicare**—Medicare has direct, voluntary enrollment by individual members in Medicare Advantage (MA) and standalone prescription drug plans (PDPs). It also has group sales for employer wrap-around benefits for MA and PDP. "Wrap-arounds" are where retiree health benefits are more generous than the Medicare program and businesses wrap or add their benefits to the standard Medicare medical and retail drug benefits.

> **Exchange**—While members generally enroll via the healthcare.gov or state websites, sales activities include promoting the various plan offerings to independent sales agents who then urge members to enroll in a given plan online.

Commercial—There is a sales and marketing process to sell group insurance in the small and large group markets as well as for Employee Retirement Security Act (ERISA) self-funded businesses.

Medicaid—Sales and marketing is limited. Some states bar it and enroll members through choice counselors and/or through auto-assignment to health plans based on previous use of a plan's providers and other variables. Some states do allow direct marketing to beneficiaries.

Product design may have its own department, or it may exist within sales and marketing. This is the group responsible for creating and designing various products to sell in the marketplace. A great deal of market intelligence and internal analysis goes into designing products for a health plan.

This group is responsible for entering new counties or service areas and designing new plans or products; updating, making more competitive, or diminishing benefits, plans, or products in existing service areas due to current costs or market activities; and exiting existing counties or services areas due to costs or risks.

This group also works closely with the finance actuary to ensure development of rates, benefits, premiums, and cost-sharing for each product or plan. Each line of business usually has defined rules on what benefits must be covered, what maximum cost-sharing might be, and what the actuarial value (the percentage of expected benefit costs versus the premium) of the plan/product must be.

Enrollment Department

Once a prospective member goes through the sales process, the enrollment department takes over. Enrollment is responsible for actually enrolling the member in the health plan and setting up premium billing, if any, for the member.

The enrollment processes can vary significantly by line of business. Enrollment in MA or PDP can be very complex. The enrollment department forwards the member information to Medicare and resolves any issues in that process. Medicaid enrollment may be done by the state Medicaid agency sending an electronic enrollment file to the health plan or the plan sending information to the state and awaiting a response. The Exchange world largely involves receiving an electronic file from the federal or state Exchange. Other commercial enrollment is achieved by employers sending information to the health plan usually through online portals.

In each of these lines of business, including Medicaid in some cases, the enrollment department also sets up premium billing, sends it to the members each month, and resolves any disputes.

Member Services Department

I think of the member services department as the lifeblood of health plan operations. A good department, with well-trained employees, can drive customer and provider satisfaction, reduce grievances and appeals, and ensure retention of members. A poor one can prove disastrous to a health plan.

Generally, the member services department will field calls from members as well as providers. Sometimes the provider relations department also is involved in fielding provider calls. Member services deals with numerous matters, including enrollment questions and matters, welcome calls to new members, non-clinical health risk assessments or education programs, fielding member calls on benefits and covered drugs, resolving complaints or taking grievances, taking prior authorization or appeal requests, helping members find providers for certain covered services, and conducting satisfaction surveys.

Provider Relations Department

The provider relations department serves several functions.

First, it will create various networks for the health plan or various products. To do so, it must follow various rules by state and federal regulators, including ensuring that the network is robust enough to serve the number of members to be enrolled. This usually includes measuring various provider specialty types against time and distance requirements to ensure reasonable member access and maintain a sufficient overall number of providers in each category. This includes all of those types covered earlier in the book, including primary care physicians (PCPs), specialists, hospitals, other facilities, and ancillary services.

The department will then contract with individual providers or through the independent practice associations (IPAs) or related entities, as discussed earlier. The contracts include federal, state, and other plan contractual language and, most importantly, outlines how a provider is paid.

Negotiated payments can be in many forms. Some of the most popular are the following:

Fee-for-service (FFS) payments for each service rendered. This can be a flat fee, based on a government fee schedule, or based on a percentage of charges from the provider.

Capitation, where a set amount is given to the provider for each member for certain covered services each month.

Risk pools, where providers are held responsible for some or all of the costs of the member whether or not they provide the services. The provider or group shares in upside and/or downside risk for the cost of assigned members. This is most often practiced with PCPs.

Per diems—global daily payments to facilities covering all services rendered. Sometimes, expensive services are paid a separate FFS payment.

Case rates—a set amount paid for a given procedure or episode of care for certain providers and facilities.

Second, the department collects information from providers and credentials each one. This ensures the competency of providers and quality in delivery of the plan's healthcare services. Credentialing essentially means that the health plan has reviewed the provider and is attesting that the provider furnishes quality services.

Credentialing includes looking at the provider's educational background, licensure status, society, and board specialties; continuing medical education requirements; malpractice insurance and record; lawsuits; stop-loss insurance (if participating in a risk payment arrangement); and any complaints against the provider through state and federal regulatory agencies. There are various service providers today that perform the background screenings and searches required for credentialing.

Credentialing is ultimately decided by the plan's credentialing committee, usually chaired by the CMO and composed of other providers in the community. A health plan may also delegate credentialing to an IPA, related entity, hospital, or delegated service entity. In this case, the provider relations department, supervised by the quality committee, will periodically audit these entities to ensure a quality credentialing process and one that follows plan and regulatory requirements.

Third, together with member services, the department fields calls and complaints from providers and seeks to address issues over claims payment, authorizations, appeals, and other aspects of health plan functions.

Fourth, the provider relations department also engages in the education of providers on plan responsibilities and mandatory activities passed down to the provider via the contract. Some of this involves the need to submit encounter and claims data, to ensure that the plan can file them with the state or federal government. This directly impacts the amount of revenue a plan receives. Provider representatives also review utilization management (UM) practices, referral patterns, and costs with providers. This is meant to ensure that each provider furnishes cost-effective and quality care.

In most lines of business, governmental agencies are measuring quality attainment and providing bonuses to plans that score well on quality or Star measures. Thus, plans also spend a great deal of time educating providers on quality attainment. Plans may also share such revenue with high-performing providers.

Fifth, along with the CMO and the quality committee, provider relations will play a role in overseeing the provider and network aspects of any delegated services (pharmacy, behavioral health, dental, vision, hearing, etc.).

Last, more and more, plans are capitating providers for certain basic services or delegating risk to providers for some or all services. The provider relations department may also handle overseeing the capitation and premium risk pools and addressing any questions.

Clinical and Quality Management Department(s)

Usually reporting to the CMO or another high-level clinical executive, the clinical department or departments directly oversee the clinical operations of the health plan. Various units or departments include:

UM or medical prior authorization—This department will review requests for services requiring prior approval on the medical benefit side. Certain services may be delegated to outside entities under contract with the plan to provide certain benefits or services. Nurses and medical directors are usually required to review requests prior to denial. Evidence-based criteria must be used. The UM department or care management department may also perform concurrent review daily within facilities to ensure cost effectiveness and care transitions planning.

Pharmacy prior authorizations and quality—This department will review requests for services requiring prior approval on the pharmacy side and sometimes on the medical side. Pharmacy technicians, pharmacists, and medical directors will review such requests for consistency with the formulary or drug list and render decisions on whether certain drugs will be covered if they require prior authorization or step therapy or have quantity limits. Some plans perform these functions internally, while others delegate this function to their pharmacy benefits manager (PBM). Evidence-based criteria must be used. The pharmacy department may also carry out various pharmacy quality functions if not delegated to the PBM, including medication therapy management, drug utilization review and safety assessment, and opioid monitoring.

Medical and pharmacy appeals—When requests for services or drugs are denied, the initial denial may end up being appealed by the member or provider. Generally speaking, appeals must be considered by the same types of clinical professionals, but the same persons cannot not render the decision on the appeal. Evidence-based criteria must be used. If denied at the appeals level, a member can ask for an independent outside appeal.

Grievances—Members have the right to file complaints or grievances against the health plan on almost any matter—benefit denials, provider, or plan behavior, etc. In this case, grievance coordinators will receive the complaint or grievance from a member and seek to resolve the issue within a prescribed regulatory timeframe. The coordinator will gather additional information from the member, providers, or others involved in the complaint. Grievances or complaints not resolved with the member on the first call go to a grievance committee to ensure fair resolution to the member as well as to ensure that root causes are established at the aggregate level and any remedial activities are undertaken.

Care management—the care management department will engage in case and disease management on behalf of members. Care managers may work with members, caregivers, providers, and facilities to coordinate care. The goal is to ensure that disease states are adequately controlled, care transitions from facilities and to home occur seamlessly and with adequate service supports, readmissions are reduced, and that quality of care is ensured. Care managers may also participate in population health activities (perhaps with the quality department), seeking to identify risks and gaps in care of members and address them. This could include basic health education programs for the vast majority of members and intensive case management for those most in need.

Quality department—The quality department oversees reviewing and improving quality of healthcare services and their delivery. This will involve assessing operational effectiveness and clinical outcomes.

Through periodic assessment, plans can practice continuous quality improvement by adjusting policies, processes, and programs to improve outcomes and quality. Plans may also create quality improvement programs when deficiencies and areas in need of improvement are identified. The quality department also oversees population health initiatives. In addition, it supervises the annual filing of the National Committee on Quality Assurance (NCQA) Healthcare Effectiveness and Data Information Set (HEDIS) with NCQA and state regulators as well as other quality and Star attainment filings.

As a side note, while I am not a clinician, some of my fondest memories in healthcare tie to my engagement with clinicians at a health plan. Contrary to the conventional wisdom, these folks are among the most caring individuals I have ever met. While they do oversee whether given procedures will or will not be covered, in my experience they also were most concerned about ensuring members received the right care at the right time. I remember sitting with care managers overseeing some of the sickest individuals when I was operating an HIV/AIDS health plan. Hearing members' stories, understanding their healthcare challenges, and witnessing the engagement of our care managers was humbling and changed me for the better.

Claims Department

The claims department is responsible for reimbursing any claims coming from providers on behalf of members that were served. This is usually on the medical side only, as a PBM pays all retail drug claims on behalf of a plan. The claims department employs claims analysts as well as stands up sophisticated software that receives, analyzes, and pays such claims. The claims system stores provider-specific information, including specific contracted rates by line of business, in order to pay claims accurately. Various software technology used in prior authorizations and appeals will send information to the claims system to ensure that a service requiring prior approval is paid. The claims department is required to process claims within specific timeframes based on regulatory and contractual requirements.

The processing of a claim is a complex undertaking that considers numerous factors, including the following:

- Is the member eligible for the date of service?
- Is the provider in network or out of network?
- Is the submitted benefit a covered benefit or service?
- Did the service or benefit require prior authorization and was it sought and approved?
- What is the cost-sharing for the service—is it subject to the deductible, co-insurance, or a co-pay?
- If applicable, has the deductible been fulfilled?
- Has the member hit any maximum of out-of-pocket cost (MOOP)?
- Is the claim "clean"—does it include all the information and medical documentation needed to properly adjudicate the claim?
- Was the claim submitted timely based on regulatory or contractual timeframes?
- Does the member have out-of-network coverage if it is covered?
- If it is out of network and coverage is available, what is the prevailing or usual and customary rate (UCR) that would be used to determine payment?
- Is there other primary coverage (e.g., automobile, homeowner's, workers' compensation, or other liability coverage) that the claim should be submitted to?

The claims department also works with the information technology department to furnish explanations of benefits (EOBs) to providers and members.

Information Technology (IT) Department

This is a key department within the health plan. It is responsible for ensuring that the health plan can communicate with health plan customers (state and federal programs and employers), providers furnishing services and seeking payment, and, of course, members. While this list is not exhaustive, here are the major technology systems the IT department will need to procure and maintain:

- Sales tracking system
- Eligibility system, including the ability to accept HIPAA-compliant transactions
- Premium billing system
- Member services and call center platform
- Medical claims system, including the ability to accept HIPAA-compliant transactions, an encounter submission system, and a risk adjustment processing and submission system
- Pharmacy claims system (usually through a PBM)
- Provider credentialing and network database
- Accounting and financial services system
- Pharmacy prior authorization system
- Medical prior authorization system
- Care management system
- Appeals, grievance, and complaints system
- Various pharmacy quality intervention systems
- Quality tracking and filing system
- Provider complaints resolution system

The Information a Health Plan Collects

Here is a review of the types of information a plan may have related to you, which is protected under the Health Insurance Portability and Accountability Act (HIPAA) as protected health information (PHI) or personally identifiable information (PII):

- Member eligibility information and demographics
- Information about your providers
- Medical claims

- ○   Pharmacy claims
- ○   Laboratory claims and results
- ○   Disease states and conditions
- ○   Prior authorization history
- ○   Appeals history
- ○   Grievance and complaints history
- ○   Case and care management history
- ○   Results of health risk assessments and medication reviews
- ○   Various risks and care gaps

Finance Department

We covered a great deal about the finance department under the CFO earlier. The finance department carries out various functions, including state insurance department reporting, which includes financial and solvency reporting; other federal regulatory reporting; accounting and calculation of revenue, medical expense, and administrative costs, based on various service categories; assessing the health of the products based on the medical loss ratio (MLR) (usually around 85% of premium revenue); sales and administrative costs (usually about 10%), and margin (usually about 5%); revenue collection and reconciliation with government payors and members; participating in product and benefit design based on financial information available, including calculating per-member-per-month (PMPM) revenue and expenses; annual budgeting for the organization; and procuring stop-loss and other insurance to mitigate financial risk.

A finance department may also include an actuary (internally or as an outside consultant) to work with the product department to design benefits and calculate premiums, medical expenses, and other costs filed with state and federal regulators for premium bids.

Compliance, Security, and Risk Department

This department has a number of key duties in a health plan. Broadly speaking, it ensures that all federal and state laws and regulations related to the delivery of healthcare are met by the various plan departments. The department serves in an oversight capacity over each department to ensure this compliance. The department ensures healthcare delivery laws and regulations are met, including ongoing assessment of changes. This can include accreditation standard requirements. The department maintains an effective compliance plan to ensure laws and regulations are met. This will include the flow of information to departments to ensure they understand rules and regulations as well as the changes they are required to meet. The department creates policies and procedures with other departments that show how laws and regulations are enforced. It also carries out and oversees mandatory training of all associates on laws and regulations and ethical behavior.

The department audits each department periodically to ensure compliance. This broadly includes laws and regulations, but also specific requirements related to timeliness of cases, use of evidence-based criteria, and regulatory communications to members and providers. If violations or risk areas are found, it creates, carries out, and monitors corrective actions put in place.

When a government regulator audits the plan, it usually leads and supports such activities in conjunction with other health plan officials. It also oversees the operations and compliance of downstream subcontractors that have been delegated certain functions, activities, or delivery of care by the plan. These downstream subcontractors act in the role of the plan and thus must follow all the same rules mandated by state and federal authorities.

Last, the department also conducts investigations related to fraud and other activities that are inconsistent with laws and regulations. A hotline and other disclosure mechanisms are maintained, which allows associates as well as associates of downstream subcontractors to contact the health plan on fraud or compliance issues. This can always be done anonymously. It reports suspected or actual violations of laws and regulations to appropriate state and federal authorities as warranted.

From a security perspective, the department ensures that the health plan meets various security laws, including HIPAA, which mandates that plans safeguard members' protected health information (PHI) and personally identifiable information (PII). Further, in this security role, assessments must be conducted related to data flow and informational technology infrastructure to ensure they meet prescribed security protocols in HIPAA.

Often, the compliance officer or the department is also in charge of risk management. The risk officer is trained to identify risks and creating mitigation or corrective action plans to ensure the ongoing delivery of services and consistency with laws and regulations.

The department may also be involved with the information technology department in developing and maintaining business continuity and disaster recovery plans.

CHAPTER 16

Why Do I Need Health Insurance?

All right, we have completed a good part of our healthcare journey. You now are proficient in terminology, products, healthcare players, and how a health plan operates. But before we go further, there's one compelling question that I haven't addressed, principally, "Why do I need health insurance, anyway?"

This question is one most often asked by the younger generation. So as not to offend anyone, I won't say what constitutes this grouping, except to say that it no longer includes someone of advanced age—like me.

First, younger generations have little connection to the healthcare system. Other than seeing their parents present a health insurance card and sometimes pay very little when they needed to see a provider, most younger citizens have little or no attachment to or insight into the system. The importance and security of consistent coverage is lost on them.

Second, younger people are relatively healthy; insurance coverage usually is not on their short list of priorities—landing roughly in the same place on the list as saving for retirement. Why would the younger generation, often saddled with college debt, pay hundreds of dollars a month for one or two trips to the doctor a year?

Third, the younger generation has a bit of a superman complex or syndrome. What's that? It's all about the idea that nothing could possibly happen to someone. He or she is invincible. He or she has no Kryptonite.

Fourth, health benefits for many in entry-level jobs militate against the desirability of coverage. Premium costs are high and there may not be first-dollar coverage plans. Instead, they may be offered high-deductible or catastrophic plans.

Fifth, since the passage of the Affordable Care Act (ACA), many young people are not forced to make a decision—for or against obtaining coverage—at least until age twenty-six. Under the ACA, children are now allowed to stay on their parent's coverage as a dependent up until that age if they do not have access to group coverage of their own through employment.

Finally, overall health literacy in our nation is low. There is little knowledge of health insurance in general and the available options, including coverage under the ACA.

Overall, it is not hard to see why someone from the younger generation chooses to skip coverage prior to age twenty-six or even afterwards, when they drop off of Mom's or Dad's coverage. But here are the reasons everyone should choose to get coverage when they can—no matter how bare bones coverage may seem.

Reason 1: "Stuff Happens!"

No matter how young or healthy you are, an automobile accident or other catastrophic health event could hit. Any single major medical event could devastate you financially and cause bankruptcy. One can hope that a hospital or provider would write off the bill in favor of asking the state to consider it bad debt and eligible for grant reimbursement. However, the more likely scenario is that a single accident could have you paying bills for a lifetime. Even minor accidents today cost thousands of dollars. A short stay in the hospital could run $10,000 a day. Larger accidents could run hundreds of thousands of dollars. It could mean tens or hundreds of thousands of dollars out of your pocket because you declined or did not seek coverage.

While health insurance premiums, deductibles, and cost-sharing may not be entirely affordable, coverage is a hedge against a catastrophic event. No more dice rolling. Think of it as *insurance*: it shields you from monster bills. While paying a deductible and cost-sharing up to maximum out-of-pocket (MOOP) costs might take time, it will amount to just thousands of dollars. There is certainty. And the younger generation is allowed to obtain so-called barer or catastrophic coverage, which may better meet their needs.

Reason 2: A Health Plan's Buying Power

This advantage saves you thousands, tens of thousands, if not hundreds of thousands. Admittedly, as has been discussed, health insurance can leave you with big surprise medical bills, but more often than not, you are well protected compared with someone without insurance. With most insurance, you automatically get the advantage of the price discounts your health plan has negotiated with providers. In addition, you have the protection of having your plan cover emergency care and limits on your total outlays.

Exact numbers are hard to come by, but plan discounts are huge! One study of inpatient costs in the employer-sponsored coverage world says health plan discounts are at least 50% from provider billed charges.[16-1] Even with a high deductible and co-insurance, the savings are enormous—again in thousands or tens of thousands for a major accident or inpatient stay. Another study indicated that discounts in managed care, high penetration states could be 50-65%.[16-2]

In the case of Medicare, we know that rates are well below commercial rates. A 2018 Congressional Budget Office (CBO) assessment substantiates that commercial rates appear to be well above Medicare fee-for-service (FFS) rates across service categories (11-139% higher for twenty services studied). It also notes that Medicare Advantage plans can lower their provider costs and thus members' costs by targeting their payment rates to roughly Medicare FFS rates. This applies to both in-network and out-of-network rates given statutory limits.[16-3]

In round numbers, this means that MA costs against provider billed rates are substantially below even the 50% discount noted for commercial in the first study. Medicaid rates are a fraction of Medicare rates.

Remember, in most products, plan-negotiated discounts apply to any covered medical service you need and seek—whether you have met your deductible or not. That same discount applies whether you have a benefit-rich plan with a low deductible or a catastrophic plan with a high one. Thus, depending on what you can afford, you may go for a higher deductible plan, knowing you have the plan discount on medical costs for routine care and to hedge against a catastrophic event.

Reason 3: Free Benefits

As an added inducement to becoming covered, there are many benefits you can take advantage of, including services that incur no upfront costs or deductibles. These were dictated under the ACA and include a schedule of certain preventive services and screenings. And as a bonus, preventive care can make you healthier along the way.

Reason 4: Federal Subsidies

If you are not eligible for insurance through an employer, or if that insurance is not affordable under the law, you could get a subsidy from the federal government through the Exchange. Most people don't realize that individuals and families earning up to 400% of the federal poverty limit (FPL) are eligible for premium assistance subsidies under the ACA, with the biggest subsidies going to those with lower incomes (the FPL cap was lifted for 2021 and 2022 due to the COVID-19 pandemic). In addition, individuals and families under 250% of FPL also get support to help make their cost-sharing more affordable.

Those with incomes below 133% may also be eligible for Medicaid, if you are in an expansion state. As well, children may be eligible for coverage under a state's Children's Health Insurance Program (CHIP).

Reason 5: We Are in This Together

If the first four didn't convince you, think of it from an altruistic perspective, combined with a little economic theory. ***Getting covered lowers the cost for everyone over time.***

At the most basic level, coverage for everyone will create a healthier nation and bend the cost curve considerably over time. Getting covered now is your part in reducing overall costs in the future.

Also, at least in some parts of the commercial world, the health insurance system has now moved from one that was predicated on risk underwriting (where healthy people got coverage and those that were not healthy were either rejected or paid much higher rates), to community rating (where people of a given age and sex pay the same rate regardless of overall health). In addition, the current system has young people paying more to subsidize older people as well.

If younger and healthier people abandon coverage, the overall health pool becomes much more adverse (i.e., sicker). The greater number of healthy people we have in the healthcare system, the lower overall rates will be. You are also paying it forward as you will be subsidized by your children and grandchildren when you reach my age and need coverage.

Reason 6: Don't Be a Moocher!

As a corollary to the last point, if you did get in an accident and couldn't afford to pay your bills or declared bankruptcy, guess what? We are all paying for you! That so-called bad medical debt gets rolled into the cost of the healthcare system anyway. Unpaid bills mean providers must demand higher prices from health plans, which then must increase premiums from year to year. Businesses and employees pay more when that happens.

So there are personal reasons—financial security and health—as well as broader economic and equity reasons to get covered. Admittedly, our lack of commitment as a nation to affordable universal access dilutes the effectiveness of these arguments. But Americans should still consider all of this and get covered.

CHAPTER 17

Commercial Line of Business

The next several chapters take a deep dive into the lines of business introduced in Chapter 4. The first I will detail is the commercial line of business, known generally as private or employer coverage.

With a few exceptions, the commercial line of business is specified as insurance that is largely funded by non-governmental revenue. By far the largest is employer-sponsored coverage. Indeed, this is the largest type of health insurance in the nation. As was outlined in Chapter 3, employer-sponsored coverage is somewhat unique in the developed world. It evolved in large measure because a socialized or single-payer system did not come about in the United States as it did in many other countries.

As noted in Chapter 13, where we featured National Healthcare Expenditures, there were an estimated 328 million Americans in 2019, but coverage totaled about 384 million because people can have more than one form of coverage. There are a few categories of commercial coverage. Private employer-sponsored coverage, which includes public and private employers, had 176 million enrollees. [17-1]

Other private health insurance coverage amounted to 31 million. The Health Exchanges or Marketplaces accounted for about 10 million. While the government does subsidize this through tax credits and other subsidies, this is considered private commercial coverage by most health plans, as they are the vehicle for delivery. Medigap, the private coverage that fills the gaps in the traditional Medicare fee-for-service (FFS) system amounted to 12 million. This is paid by seniors or the disabled, not government subsidies, and is furnished in the private plan sector.[17-1]

In summary, commercial or private coverage is about 60% of all health insurance in America.[17-1]

Let's now give you details about employer-sponsored coverage. We will detail Exchange or Marketplace coverage in Chapter 27. For details on Medicare Supplement (Medigap) coverage, go back to Chapter 4 and later in Chapter 19.

Employer-sponsored coverage can take several forms: self-insured plans, fully-insured, large-group risk plans, and fully-insured, small-group risk plans. In most cases, plans usually contract with health plans to carry out the provision of healthcare services, whether they self-insure or are fully-insured.

It is also important to remember that in all these cases of employer coverage, the health insurance contract is not between you and the health plan. In fully-insured scenarios, it is between the health plan and employer, with employees as beneficiaries. In the case of self-insured plans, the employer is technically the health plan and offers coverage to the employees.

Self-Insured, Employer-Based Coverage and Plans

In this case, employers of sufficient size essentially insure themselves through self-insurance funds. These employers assess that they can pay less overall for healthcare if they take on the risk by seeding a self-insurance fund. Premiums are paid to this fund by employers and employees and the fund is tapped for healthcare claims from employees. This fund lives over time and might end up with a healthy balance if funded correctly. The employer may self-insure both employees and retirees of the company. They hire a health plan or similar entity to administer the plan. This is largely all aspects of the plan, including member services, premium and benefit management, provider network, claims payment, and clinical management. The administrator is paid what is known as an administrative services only (ASO) fee for the services it provides.

Like health plans, an employer that is self-funding may enter into several types of insurance relationships known as stop-loss or reinsurance to insulate itself from catastrophic claims.

In the self-insured scenario, the member or employee sees almost no difference. Employers are on the hook if claims exceed premium costs in this case. In the end, the employer is banking on the fact that the actual costs of claims and the ASO fee is less than what the health plan would have charged year to year through a risk arrangement.

Another big benefit is that under the Affordable Care Act (ACA) not all of the mandates (e.g., the minimum essential benefits mandate), are levied on self-insured plans. Further, state benefit mandates do not apply. Except specific ACA provisions, such as certain restrictions on benefit limits, coverage of dependents to age twenty-six, and the requirement to cover pre-existing conditions, employers have a bit of a blank slate when it comes to designing benefits. Within the rubric of self-insurance, employers can design a number of plans, including those with network only as well as network and out-of-network benefits. They may offer traditional plans as well as consumer-directed health plans (CDHPs) and high-deductible health plans (HDHPs).

Employers may contract directly with providers, use the networks and fee structure that plans have with these providers, or both. Health plans and employers may also work together to determine premiums that are paid into the self-insurance fund. The employer determines the mix of employer and employee premiums. The employer negotiates only the ASO fee with the health plan.

Self-insured plans are governed by the healthcare insurance provisions of the Employee Retirement Security Act (ERISA) of 1974. The federal Department of Labor (DOL) is the policymaker and enforcement agency for these rules. ERISA regulations govern healthcare provision for employers and certain other entities, such as unions that are allowed to maintain their own health insurance and retirement funds in lieu of the employer, and for employee and retiree healthcare benefits. As noted, for the most part, state benefit and other insurance laws are set aside or pre-empted for self-insured plans.

ERISA was amended by several other acts, including the Consolidated Omnibus Budget Reconciliation Act (COBRA) in 1985, the Health Insurance Portability and Accountability Act (HIPAA) in 1996, and the ACA of 2010. These acts added certain provisions applicable to these self-insured plans. As noted as well, the ACA had a major impact on ERISA, although it did not apply all rules.

ERISA plans are a majority of employer-based coverage. At last count, about 61% of all employee coverage was tied to ERISA. As the size of a business increases, the more they elect to set up self-insurance funds rather than contract with an insurance company on a traditional risk basis. About 84% of workers in large firms (those with 200 or more employees) are in a self-funded plan versus 23% for small firms.[17-2]

Why ERISA?

The crux of the argument for establishing ERISA to govern big employer plans nationwide was that the federal government had to step in because this is interstate commerce.

Further, large employers spanned multiple states and therefore it was difficult to have multiple states and multiple rules applying to these big employers. This is by far the biggest class of the insured in America and uniformity of regulation was important.

ERISA did bring standards to these big employer offerings, which otherwise did not exist, or enforcement might have been complicated and lax.

ERISA also reduces costs by streamlining administration for big employers. There is one set of rules to follow and administer.

And very importantly, retiree benefits are involved, and people tend to retire in states that are different than where they may have worked. The federal government has a role here to regulate these retiree benefits as a state's reach is limited if someone moves to a sunnier locale.

Oversight has become much more sophisticated since ERISA's passage in 1974. In terms of protections, while they might not appear as robust as risk-regulated plans, the DOL does have a robust regulatory regime and consumer protection focus. Large employers also tend to be fairly sophisticated and intervene when there is discrimination or errant practices by plans hired to administer benefits. In addition, various healthcare laws have been extended even to ERISA self-insured plans, including COBRA, HIPAA, and parts of the ACA.

Insured, Risk-Based Employer Coverage

Instead of self-insuring, some employers choose to contract with health plans to provide all benefits and services. These are also known as *insured plans*. What does this mean? In return for the premiums paid by the employer, the health plan is at risk if the claims exceed premium costs. At the same time, the health plan can also keep any additional profit if claims are lower than expected. This follows a new rule, known as the minimum medical loss ratio (MLR) mandate. This rule requires plans to rebate money to an employer if medical costs come in too low, usually between 80-85% of premium.

Risk-based employer coverage has to meet more of the requirements of the ACA than self-insured plans. State regulations also apply. The standard plan type offerings would apply in this category as well.

Within risk-based employer coverage, there are two groups—large and small. In the majority of states, if you have one to fifty full-time-equivalent employees, an employer is a small group. If you have more employees, an employer is a large group. In California, Colorado, New York, and Vermont, the cutoff point is 100.[17-3] For the purposes of certain ACA rules, a small group cutoff is 100. To become eligible to buy small business insurance on the Marketplace Exchange, the cutoff is fifty (more on this in a subsequent chapter).

Small Group Coverage

Small group coverage is generally regulated from a rate and benefit perspective by the ACA and states insurance laws. Small groups in each state or region receive the same rates as filed annually by each of the health plans offering such coverage in a given jurisdiction. Health plans file rates based on the experience of all of the small group individuals enrolled with their company in each state or in some cases region, as opposed to determining this per employer.

As with individual rates now, the ACA prescribes how rates are calculated and generally only allow differences for region/geography, age, and tobacco use. Health plans must accept small groups that apply to them. The ACA also mandates essential benefits, offering the so-called metal plans (platinum, gold, silver, and bronze) based on actuarial ranges and other requirements. Under the ACA, there is no mandate to provide health insurance if you are an employer, but there are small employer tax credits under the ACA as well as the ability to buy on the Exchanges.[17-4] Generally, small group plans are able to offer a range of health plans, although some stick with cheaper options, including HDHPs and HMOs.

Large Group Coverage

Large groups mostly are self-insured, but some choose to contract with health plans on a risk basis. Large groups are less hobbled by ACA mandates, although many apply. Large groups must offer insurance meeting a minimum threshold (60% of total cost of benefits) and limit how much employee's pay for self-only coverage (less than 9.78% of household income in 2020). If they do not meet these mandates, they face penalties. Unlike small groups, full-risk large group rates are not filed with the federal or state governments. They are negotiated between employers and health plans. Plans can bid for employer business and calculate rates based on history (if the employer is a current client) or based on what the employer discloses to the health plan.[17-5]

Grandfathered versus Non-Grandfathered Plans

As explained earlier, self-insured ERISA plans follow some but not all of the ACA rules regarding benefits. But there is a small subset of plans that also benefit from loosening of the ACA rules as long as they maintain their coverage and abide by some of the mandates that ACA says do apply. These are called grandfathered plans; their previous benefits and rules are included retroactively. These are opposed to non-grandfathered plans that must follow all ACA rules, mostly in the risk or insured world. Grandfathered plans can include individual coverage, although this is less the case as the years move on. They can also include employer plans—both insured and self-insured ERISA.

Grandfathered plans do not have to follow all the benefit rules of the ACA. At the same time, they cannot markedly change their benefits or they do lose their grandfather status and then would have to abide by all ACA requirements. Examples of changes that are disallowed include significant cost-sharing increases, including deductibles, cost-sharing, and out-of-pocket maximums; eliminating benefits or reducing them to a major degree; and a significant change in the level of the employer portion of premiums.[17-6, 17-7]

Late in its tenure, the Trump Administration finalized a rule that would allow grandfathered group health plans more flexibility to maintain their status. The changes include allowing high-deductible plans to have more leeway to change cost-sharing amounts and giving plans more flexibility for measuring allowable increases in cost-sharing.[17-8]

In summary, the ACA provides some so-called loopholes from following all rules. ERISA plans have some latitude regardless of whether they are grandfathered or not, especially freedom from state rules.

Grandfathered plans get to ignore certain rules as long as they follow some ACA rules and do not radically change their benefits and offerings.

The Changing Employer-Coverage Paradigm

In the past, employers looked to health plans simply to offer various traditional benefits. For self-insured employers, plans may have offered what they did in the risk world. But employers became frustrated with how health plans were performing. Commercial premiums increased dramatically year-over-year in the past, and still do, whether the employer was self-insured or contracted on an at-risk basis. Here are a few key facts from the 2020 Employer Health Benefits survey from the Kaiser Family Foundation (KFF):[17-2]

While premium increases have been tempered a bit of late, in 2020 the average annual premiums were $7,470 for single coverage and $21,342 for family coverage. The average family premium has increased 55% since 2010 and 22% since 2015. Average premiums for single coverage have grown 20% since 2015.

In 2020, 78% of eligible workers enrolled in coverage when it is offered to them. But enrollment among low-paid workers is less. Both show an affordability crisis here.

In 2020, 74% of firms offering health benefits offered only one type of health plan. 58% of larger firms (versus 25% of small firms) offered more than one plan type. (Large firms in the study were those with 200 or more employees.)

In 2020, premium contributions by covered workers averaged 17% for single coverage and 27% for family coverage. The average monthly worker contributions were $104 for single coverage and $466 for family coverage.

In 2020, 83% of covered workers were enrolled in a plan with an annual deductible for single coverage. This is up from 70% ten years ago. The average annual deductible for single coverage for all covered workers in 2020 was $1,644, about the same as last year. This amount has increased by about 25% over the past five years. The average stood at $917 in 2010. The percentage of workers with an annual deductible of $1,000 or more for single coverage was 57% in 2020, compared with 46% in 2015.

In 2019, 65% of covered workers have co-insurance and 11% have a copayment for hospital admissions.

Why did employers feel like health plans were serving them so poorly? Health plans were treating the commercial world as a cost-plus proposition, not finding efficiencies or controlling costs. They simply added increased costs to premiums year to year, with very little innovation. The cost of healthcare as a percentage of employee wages increased dramatically.

Health plans also were paying little attention to driving quality outcomes. It simply was not a focus. Employers were worried about employee illnesses and disability. This had a huge impact on productivity and turnover.

As well, the commercial market became a huge cost shift from Medicaid and, to some degree, the Medicare lines of business. Providers drove this, but health plans did little to solve for this. The cost shift noted previously as well as the high per capita cost of healthcare in America versus other developed worlds is putting U.S. companies at a competitive disadvantage.

Employers also believed that health plans were not innovating on the provider front, either. Further, employees saw their burden increase dramatically over time in the form of increased premiums, increased cost-sharing, and reduced plan options and benefits.

Given their frustration, and their need to reduce costs and drive quality, many employers have begun taking healthcare decisions into their own hands. With cooperation from some health plans, they have tackled some major reforms.[17-2, 17-9]

They are designing benefits to encourage wellness and monitoring outcomes.

They are frequently bidding healthcare, whether self-insured or at risk.

They also are separately acquiring medical and pharmacy benefit administrators or plans. This gives them the ability to leverage the strengths of different partners in the healthcare industry.

Employers, too, are creating wellness programs, rewards, and incentives for their employees to seek out primary care and preventive services and take care of chronic disease. Among large firms in the Kaiser 2020 employer study, 60% offered workers the opportunity to complete a health risk assessment, 50% offered workers the opportunity to complete a biometric screening, and 81% offered workers wellness programs such as smoking cessation, weight loss, and coaching.

Some employers are operating wellness clinics and pharmacies onsite.

Prior to 2020, about one-third of large employers had onsite clinics. By the end of 2019, about half were expected to do so. Half of employers report a 50% return on investment already.

Businesses are expanding HSAs and FSAs to help employees deal with rising costs.

They also are requiring health plans to increase transparency related to pricing at providers, including online price calculators, and encouraging the use of proven quality providers.

CHAPTER 18

What Are Dual Eligibles?

B efore moving on to government programs—Medicare, Medicaid, and the State Children's Health Insurance Program (SCHIP)—we must introduce a term of art in the U.S. healthcare world: the "dual eligible."

As described in Chapter 4, Medicare is a program run by the federal government for those sixty-five and older, certain disabled individuals, as well as people with end-stage renal disease (ESRD) and Lou Gehrig's disease. Medicaid is a federal-state partnership program largely for poor and lower-income uninsured Americans. *A dual eligible is someone who meets both Medicare **and** Medicaid criteria* and who is entitled to enroll in both programs. This is most often the case when a person qualifies for Medicare because they are over age sixty-five or have a qualifying disability **and** also has a low income.

Here are a few facts about dual eligibles. They numbered about 12 million in 2018, or 20% of the Medicare population and 15% of the Medicaid population. However, they represented 34% of Medicare spending and 33% of Medicaid spending.[18-1]

Dual eligibles tend to be much sicker than most others in both Medicaid and

Medicare. In Medicaid, most enrollees are children and mothers. While the Medicare profile is much sicker because of the age and disability of enrollees, dual eligibles usually are far more medically fragile than even Medicare's overall cohort. They tend to have multiple co-morbidities or complex conditions.

They also tend to be impacted by social determinants of health. These are socio-economic factors, such as low income, low health literacy and educational achievement, and issues related to reliable housing, food security, and transportation. If their underlying conditions serve as barriers, these social barriers or determinants create additional complications to achieving stable or quality health.

There are full dual eligibles, who receive all Medicaid benefits, and partial dual eligibles, who only receive some benefits under Medicaid. People qualify for these special dual eligible statuses largely based on income. These categories are also known as the Medicare Savings Program (MSP). Here are the major categories of dual eligibles. (To refresh yourself on the various Parts of Medicare, go back to Chapter 4.)[18-2]

Full Benefit Dual Eligibles (FBDEs)—These individuals receive full Medicare and Medicaid benefits. Medicaid pays all Medicare premiums for them as well as all deductibles and cost-sharing. The individual also receives full Medicaid benefits for services not covered by Medicare.

Full Dual Eligible: Qualified Medicare Beneficiary (QMB) Plus— These individuals receive full Medicare and Medicaid benefits. Medicaid pays all Medicare premiums for them as well as all deductibles and cost-sharing. The individual also receives full Medicaid benefits for services not covered by Medicare. This individual looks very much like an FBDE but is qualified in a different way.

Full Dual Eligible: Specified Low-Income Medicare Beneficiary (SLMB) Plus—These individuals receive full Medicare and Medicaid benefits. Medicaid pays all Medicare premiums for them as well as all deductibles and cost-sharing. The individual also receives full Medicaid benefits for services not covered by Medicare. This individual may only be temporarily receiving full Medicaid benefits due to high healthcare costs at a given time.

Partial Dual Eligible: Qualified Medicare Beneficiary (QMB) Only—These individuals receive full Medicare and have all of their premiums, deductibles and cost-sharing in Medicare covered by the Medicaid program. They do not otherwise receive full Medicaid benefits, but they receive the most benefits of any partial dual eligible.

Partial Dual Eligible: Specified Low-Income Medicare Beneficiary (SLMB) Only—This person has full Medicare, but only receives help paying Medicare Part B premiums from Medicaid.

Partial Dual Eligible: Qualifying Individual (QI)—This person has full Medicare and receives partial help from Medicaid paying for Part B premiums.

Partial Dual Eligible: Qualified Disabled Working Individual (QDWI) Program—This person pays the Part A premium for certain disabled and working beneficiaries. Medicare pays covered medical services first for dual eligible beneficiaries because Medicaid is generally the payer of last resort. Medicaid may cover medical costs that Medicare may not cover or partially covers (such as nursing home care, personal care, and home- and community-based services). Medicare and Medicaid dual eligible benefits vary by state. Some states offer Medicaid through Medicaid managed care plans, while other states provide fee-for-service (FFS) Medicaid coverage. Some states provide certain dual eligible beneficiary plans that include all Medicare and Medicaid benefits.

Because dual eligibles are in two different programs that are usually not integrated, coordinating care and funding is difficult. By and large, dual eligibles receive their prescription drugs just from the Medicare Part D program.

There may be a few drugs not covered by Medicare that are furnished by the Medicaid benefit.

For full duals, Medicare becomes primary coverage for the individual for acute medical services and Medicaid becomes secondary for these services. But often, for the full dual eligible, Medicaid can be primary, too, when Medicare does not cover a service, such as chronic long-term care services.

In the acute medical world, Medicare pays the lion's share of the costs of the full dual eligible. Medicaid acts as a wrap around the Medicare benefit and the state Medicaid agency generally pays any remaining deductibles and cost-sharing amount due to providers. Medicare covers the rough 80% as the primary insurance. The Medicaid program covers the balance (the 20% that includes deductibles and cost-sharing) as well as any premiums.

But Medicaid is allowed to cap its secondary payment or pay nothing at all. If the Medicare payment is at or above what Medicaid pays that provider, most state Medicaid agencies don't pay any secondary payment to providers. The provider must take the amount paid by Medicare as payment in full. Federal law bars a provider from asking most full dual eligibles for any cost-sharing balance.

It is clear that the MSP program helps shelter dual eligibles from burdensome premiums and cost-sharing (deductibles, co-insurance, and co-pays) in the Part A and Part B Medicare system. But with the move of prescription drugs to Part D, how are dual eligibles protected from premiums and cost-sharing they cannot afford? I will be detailing something called the Extra Help or Low-Income Subsidy (LIS) program in Part D later. Suffice it to say, the Extra Help/LIS program parallels the MSP program and offers premium and cost-sharing subsidies/protection. Indeed, many of the MSP categories are deemed as qualified into a certain LIS category.

The future costs of dual eligibles are a major concern of the Centers for Medicare and Medicaid Services (CMS). As noted previously, they already are a disproportionate share of Medicare and Medicaid costs, which will only rise with the aging of America. CMS sees it as imperative to coordinate Medicare and Medicaid acute care spending, coordinate acute spending in Medicare and Medicaid with chronic long-term care spending in Medicaid, and improve quality of outcomes for dual eligibles in both programs.

As a result of these concerns, CMS and state Medicaid agencies have undertaken some initiatives. For example, CMS has reformed how Medicare Advantage (MA) dual eligible special needs plans (MA D-SNPs) operate. These plans can only accept those that meet various dual eligible statuses. In addition, there are other special needs plans, including chronic care SNPs (disease-focused plans or MA C-SNPs) and institutional SNPs (MA I-SNPs), serving those in institutions or at risk of institutionalization. These other SNPs also serve large numbers of dual eligibles.

CMS reforms in this area include overhauling the model of care (MOC) required for all SNPs, overhauling the program audit protocols to evaluate SNPs, and requiring MA D-SNPs plans to coordinate or integrate the Medicare and Medicaid funding streams and care.

The Affordable Care Act (ACA) also created the Medicare-Medicaid Coordination Office within CMS. One such program includes three-party contracts between CMS, a given state Medicaid agency, and a health plan to fully integrate the Medicare and Medicaid acute care funding. In some states, Medicaid long-term care is being included as well.

These initiatives should help CMS and state Medicaid better grapple with the lack of coordination of dual eligibles' healthcare and the huge cost that this will continue to represent if reforms are not made.

CHAPTER 19

The Medicare Line of Business

These next five chapters are dedicated to the specifics of Medicare. This includes an overview of the Medicare program and how one qualifies for it. It also covers the Medicare Advantage (MA) program, why MA has such a great value proposition, and why it is growing. It also describes the details of special needs plans and the specifics of the Medicare Part D prescription drug program.

The program was initially founded in 1965 to provide healthcare coverage for people in old age. In 1972, it was expanded to cover those under age sixty-five with significant mental or physical disabilities. Given the significance of the diseases' cost and need for ongoing treatment, it also covers anyone, regardless of age, who has end-stage renal disease (ESRD) or amyotrophic lateral sclerosis (ALS or Lou Gehrig's Disease).

Medicare has four parts, which will be covered in detail later in the chapter.

Medicare participants either enroll in the traditional fee-for-service (FFS) program or enroll in an MA program. In the case of MA, private health plans contract with the government to stand in the shoes of CMS and provide the same coverage that a beneficiary would get in the FFS program. Over 43% of Medicare beneficiaries (based on estimates of total Medicare beneficiaries in mid-2021) are in private MA plans, while under 57% now are in traditional Medicare. Private estimates suggest that by 2025 about 50% of beneficiaries will be in MA plans. Between 2030 and 2040, that percentage could reach 70%.[19-1] We will go into depth in the next chapter about MA.

CMS says there were over 63 million people on Medicare in calendar year 2021 (full-year equivalent or average monthly enrollment). In 2017, Medicare was about 15% of total federal spending and 20% of total national healthcare expenditures. NHE data estimates that gross Medicare spending will grow from about $800 billion in 2019 to about $1.66 trillion in 2028. Kaiser Family Foundation (KFF) says net Medicare spending will grow from $583 billion in 2018 to $1.26 trillion in 2028.[19-2, 19-3]

Where did the money go? The KFF says that in 2017, Medicare had a gross expenditure of about $688 billion ($705 billion, according to NHED) that was spent as follows:[19-3]

- ○ 30% for MA plan payments; this is about right given enrollment in the program
- ○ 21% went to inpatient costs for the traditional FFS program
- ○ 14% went to outpatient prescription drugs in the Part D program
- ○ 10% went to physician payments
- ○ 7% went to hospital outpatient services
- ○ 4% went to skilled nursing facility (SNF) visits
- ○ 3% went to home health visits
- ○ 11% to all other services

The profile of those on Medicare is one of ill health. That makes sense, as the program covers those who are aged or those with disabilities or serious disease states. Most have multiple chronic conditions and limitations in their activities of daily living. It is also the case that many have low incomes. A few statistics from KFF based on 2016 surveys:[19-3]

- ○ 32% had a functional impairment
- ○ 25% reported being in fair or poor health
- ○ 22% had five or more chronic conditions
- ○ 15% were under age sixty-five and living with a long-term disability
- ○ 12% were ages eighty-five and over
- ○ 3% lived in a long-term care facility
- ○ Half of all people on Medicare had incomes below $26,200 per person and savings below $74,450.

Like Medicaid, Medicare is an entitlement. If someone meets the eligibility criteria, continues to meet them, and pays his premiums, then he gets coverage and is entitled to the benefit generally for the rest of his life. This is a source of contention for some policymakers because the entitlement nature of the system will mean huge costs or unfunded liabilities in the future.

Also, because traditional Medicare is a FFS environment, there are little or no controls on utilization or authorization, with the exception of Medicare Administrative Contractors (MACs), formerly Fiscal Intermediaries (FIs). These entities handle claims payments and make policy determinations about what is covered in the program in each region. These are called local coverage determinations (LCDs). Over time, the Centers for Medicare and Medicaid Services (CMS) assesses these LCDs and may adopt them as national coverage determinations (NCDs). MA plans are obligated to follow NCD rules nationally and LCD rules where they serve members. But beyond deciding if something is a covered benefit, there is no prior authorization, *per se*. Also, with few exceptions, there is no care coordination or care management.

While Medicare has comprehensive coverage, it does have a significant cost-sharing burden. There are premiums, deductibles, co-insurance, co-pays, and out-of-pocket costs for uncovered services, such as dental, eyewear, and chronic long-term care. As a general rule, traditional Medicare FFS covers about 80% of your costs after premiums. There are also no absolute caps on your costs in Parts A and B, unless you are in an MA plan (more on this in the next chapter). There are some caps on costs, however, for everyone in the Part D retail drug program (with minimal co-pays/co-insurance), whether in FFS or MA.

The KFF reports that in 2016 Medicare FFS beneficiaries paid $2,640 in premiums for Medicare and other policies that help them cover costs of healthcare. They also paid $3,166 in out-of-pocket costs for cost-sharing and other services.[19-3]

Medicare beneficiaries in the traditional FFS program either pay these costs out of pocket or have the following to fill in the major cost-sharing holes in the FFS system.[19-3]

Employer-sponsored retiree insurance that wraps around Medicare—The actual benefit varies greatly from employer to employer. So, the amount that a Medicare beneficiary may pay in residual cost-sharing could be extremely high (for skimpy retiree coverage) to little or nothing (for benefit-rich retiree coverage). This applies to about 30% of Medicare beneficiaries.

Medicare Supplement—This applies to about 29% of Medicare beneficiaries and is further explained a few paragraphs from now.

Medicaid Dual Eligibility—This applies to about 22% of Medicare beneficiaries. As outlined in the previous chapter, the dual eligibles get partial or full help (depending on income and eligibility in other government programs) paying for premiums, deductibles, and cost-sharing. Some of these dual eligibles may also be fully eligible for Medicaid and therefore receive benefits in Medicaid that are not covered in Medicare. There is an Extra Help program for Part D prescription drug benefits, also known as the Low-Income Subsidy (LIS) program, that helps with premiums, deductibles, and cost-sharing for dual eligibles and others of low income.

Other coverage—applies to about one percent of Medicare beneficiaries.

No Coverage (and therefore paying out of pocket)—applies to 19% of Medicare beneficiaries.

The Medicare Supplement policies (also known as Medigap and Medicare

Wrap) are actually commercial products that pay for cost-sharing in Medicare. The types of Medigap policies are standardized in federal law and apply in most states. These are then regulated by state insurance departments. There are ten plan types in most states.[19-4]

The federal government uses a letter system to denote the types of Medicare Supplement insurance. These policies have to cover the same things across state lines. Each plan covers different amounts of the cost-sharing in Medicare.[19-4]

People can get confused between Medicare *parts* and Medicare supplement *plan types*. Indeed, we know that there are Medicare Parts A, B, C, and D, and there are also Medicare supplement plan types or Plans A, B, C, and D. *How is anyone supposed to keep all this straight?* I think the three states that don't use the federal lettering system (Massachusetts, Minnesota, and Wisconsin) are easier to understand.

A plan does not have to offer all Medicare supplement plan types in each state, but if they do participate in a state, they must offer Plan A and must also offer Plan C or Plan F if they offer any plan. Plans generally differ based on the benefits they wrap coverage around and the amount of residual cost-sharing covered. Plans in federal law are Plans A through N except for E, H, I, and J. Beginning January 1, 2020, Plans C and F are no longer available to most new Medicare enrollees because of the Affordable Care Act (ACA).[19-4]

Even basic Medicare Supplement plans (ones that pay for some but not all of the cost-sharing) can be pricey. Those that fill in *all* the cost-sharing holes in traditional Medicare can be unduly expensive each month.

If you are enrolled in MA, you cannot have Medicare supplement as MA plans essentially provide the "buy down" for much of the 20% FFS cost-sharing as part of the plan design.

Now let's get into the details of Medicare, which comes from my research over the years, unless specifically cited.

Qualifications for Medicare Part A[19-5]

Medicare Part A is what most people think of as inpatient services. The rules of the road for Part A begin with the requirement of being age sixty-five or older and a U.S. citizen or a permanent legal resident for at least five continuous years. In addition, a person must be eligible to receive Social Security or Railroad Retirement Board (RRB) benefits. Nowadays, many Medicare enrollees don't have to be actually receiving Social Security or RRB benefits because the regular retirement age for Social Security for some Americans has now risen to above sixty-five.

Every American pays a federal payroll tax to the tune of 1.45% (beyond the 6.2% for Social Security). This is placed in the Medicare Part A Hospital Insurance Trust Fund to help sustain that part of the Medicare program. In addition, your employer is also charged a matching 1.45% that is placed into the fund. Since the passage of the ACA, there is an additional 0.9% contribution to Medicare by high-wealth individuals. There are not additional government appropriations for hospital-related Medicare services.

In order to be eligible for Part A, most people must have the Medicare payroll tax withholding paid by them or a spouse for at least forty quarters (ten years). These quarters do not need to be consecutive. If there are forty quarters paid in, there is no premium for Part A. Less payroll history may be needed if you are disabled or have ESRD or ALS. If someone has less than forty quarters of qualifying work history, a person may still be able to join Medicare Part A by paying a premium each month (but they would also have to be in Part B). Part A penalties apply if a person required to pay premiums does not enroll on time. Some rare employer groups are exempt from Social Security and Medicare taxation and those employees would later have to pay a Part A premium each month as well.

You can also qualify for Medicare if you are sixty-five or older and your spouse meets the qualifications above even if you do not.

Once you satisfy the above, you are on your way to receiving Part A of Medicare, which automatically begins on the first day of the month you turn sixty-five.

Others may qualify for Part A without reaching age 65 or working the requisite timeframe. A person could qualify for Social Security Disability (SSD) or Railroad Retirement Disability (RRD) and be on the program for twenty-four months before getting Medicare. To qualify for SSD, you must have some work history, earned a certain number of credits under law, and have a qualifying disability.

In other situations, you may receive Medicare if you are disabled and wait up to twenty-nine months for Medicare. You can also have ESRD and receive or are eligible to receive Social Security or RRB benefits. (You could also qualify for SSD and receive Medicare.) You can have ALS and qualify for SSD. The waiting period may be waived under certain situations. A person of any age and certified as having ALS receives Medicare starting the month they receive SSD or RRD. Depending on the circumstances, someone with ESRD can obtain coverage after one to three months.

Qualifications for Medicare Part B[19-5]

Just having Part A and hospital-related coverage is not going to do much good later in life. There are doctors to see, outpatient surgeries, testing, and the like, so enrolling in Part B coverage—which most people think of as out-patient services—is critical as well.

The rules of the road for Part B are straightforward. Quite simply, if you receive Part A, then you are eligible to voluntarily enroll in Part B. Those who have to pay a premium for Part A must be sixty-five years or older and must be a U.S. citizen or a permanent legal resident for at least five continuous years.

Part B is voluntary. Beneficiaries have to sign up for and pay a monthly premium for getting Part B benefits. It also should be said that some people may only elect to have Part B coverage if they are not eligible for Part A.

In 2021, the standard Part B premium is $148.50 per month, although wealthier individuals have to pay more. This can be deducted from your Social Security, Railroad Retirement Board, or federal pension retirement check, or it can be paid directly to the Social Security Administration (SSA). If you are not yet getting a Social Security check, you must send the amount each month to SSA. These premiums go into the Part B/D Supplementary Medical Insurance Trust Fund along with government appropriations each year to sustain these programs.

The monthly premium is set each year so that the federal government subsidizes about 75% of Part B premiums while individuals pay the rest. In addition, there are deductibles and cost-sharing each year.

Penalties apply for those who enroll in Part B late or drop out and re-enroll. There are exceptions for those who are working beyond age sixty-five and delay enrollment.

When Someone Can Enroll[19-5]

As you approach age sixty-five, there is an initial enrollment period. This seven-month period begins three months before the month you turn age sixty-five and ends three months after you reach that age. During that time, you can enroll in Parts A and B, and you can also apply directly to a Part D plan for prescription drug coverage. Premiums are paid directly to the plan.

If you are enrolling because you are disabled or have ESRD/ALS, initial enrollment occurs in a similar seven-month period as the defined waiting period approaches its end. A person is auto-enrolled in Medicare Parts A and B after receiving Social Security disability for twenty-four months.

Other enrollment periods apply to those retiring after age sixty-five and certain other groups.

It is also important to remember that a Medicare beneficiary needs to enroll in the program on time, in order to avoid late enrollment penalties. This means you must enroll when you first qualify and have no other insurance coverage.[19-6, 19-7]

> For Part A, most people will never have a late enrollment penalty because they have worked their forty quarters and obtain it without a premium. However, as I noted, some people can pay a premium for Part A enrollment if they have insufficient work history. In this case, they must enroll when they are initially eligible for Medicare (usually age sixty-five) or pay an additional 10% per month on top of the premium owed. This penalty is paid for twice the period of time of the gap between when you were eligible and when you enrolled for Part A. If you enrolled two years late,

you will pay the 10% penalty per month for four years. Your penalty may increase each year as the regular premium does.

If you do not enroll in Part B when you are initially eligible for Medicare, then a Part B penalty may also apply. In this case, that penalty is not time-limited and might last as long as you are enrolled in Part B. The amount of your penalty may be up to 10% per year that you did not enroll. As an example, if you did not enroll for two years, your Part B premium would be 120% of the standard Part B premium each month. Your penalty may increase each year as the regular premium does.

If you do not enroll for prescription drug coverage when you are initially eligible, you may also have to pay a Part D premium penalty. The Part D penalty calculation is more complicated. A person must pay 1% of the national base beneficiary premium times the number of months between enrollment and when you were eligible to enroll. Your penalty goes up each year as the base premium changes.

In all of these cases, a person may have what is known as creditable coverage that would allow someone to enroll in Medicare later, such as employer coverage after reaching age sixty-five. In other cases, there may be special circumstances. You can apply to CMS and ask that penalties are waived.

The outrage—those nasty government bureaucrats and politicians levying penalties on me because I choose not to enroll when I am first eligible. Well, hold on for a second, these penalties are fair and reasonable. It is human nature for someone not to enroll in health coverage if they don't need it. If you are not regularly going to the doctor and if you do not have a health condition, why enroll and waste the money? But if only sicker people enroll, adverse selection sets in, costs in the insurance cohort go up, and premiums rise. Having people enroll on time, whether they need coverage at that point or not, smooths out overall costs and provides better stability in the system. Why should someone be able to step out of paying and only enroll when they need it? Thus, the penalties help compensate the system for the funding it did not receive over time and help pay for your costs now.

The Parts of Medicare

In this section we will dive deeper into the services covered in each part of Medicare. The truth is that once on Medicare, few average Americans even care about differentiating between Parts A, B, C, and D. The fact is they view it as their healthcare—period. However, the federal government does track the various parts methodically, and even has separate financing schemes for most of them. (Parts A and B are covered in this chapter; Parts C and D are covered in the next two chapters.)

Part A

This is the hospital and related services part of Medicare, supported by the Part A Hospital Insurance Trust Fund. As outlined previously, there is no monthly premium for most people to access Part A services. There are also no federal appropriations to the fund. It is entirely supported by annual payroll contributions. Alarmingly, the Medicare Trustees report that the Part A Trust Fund will only be able to pay full benefits until 2026, when the fund is depleted. The Congressional Budget Office confirms this prediction. Thus, to fund current benefits, there will need to be additional taxes, benefit reductions, and/or increased cost-sharing.[19-8, 19-9]

It is important to note that Part A uses what is known as a *benefit period* to determine if Part A inpatient hospital and skilled nursing facility (SNF) services are "qualifying" or not and what the cost-sharing will be. A benefit period begins the day you are admitted to an inpatient hospital, or to a SNF, and ends the day you have been out of the hospital or SNF for sixty days in a row. For the most part, you usually must enter an inpatient hospital before going to a SNF.[19-10]

Here are the services covered in Part A.[19-10, 19-11, 19-12, 19-13, 19-14, 19-15, 19-16, 19-17, 19-18] If needed, I updated premiums, deductibles, and cost-sharing with the latest figures for 2021 from official government sources. These figures go up each year based on inflation.

Inpatient Hospital Care

Beneficiaries receive inpatient hospital coverage, including a semi-private room, meals, nursing services, medications, and other services and supplies related to the inpatient occurrence.

Part A covers a variety of inpatient hospitals, including acute care hospitals, critical access hospitals, rehabilitation hospitals, long-term care hospitals, and mental health hospitals (190 days lifetime).

Rehabilitation hospitals and long-term care hospitals usually continue coverage after a stay in an acute care hospital.

An inpatient hospital stay under Medicare has capped coverage and major cost-sharing.

For the first sixty days, a beneficiary pays a deductible, which in 2021 was $1,484 per benefit period. For days sixty-one to ninety, there is a co-pay of $371 per day. If a hospital stay exceeds ninety days, beneficiaries can access sixty reserve days at $742 co-pay per day. But there are only sixty reserve days in a lifetime.

It is important to note that beneficiaries can have numerous benefit periods per calendar year, and they may pay multiple deductibles and co-pays for days sixty-one through ninety.

At the same time, a person could go into the hospital, be discharged and go back into the hospital. In these cases, the person may be within the same benefit period and may not pay the deductible again as they still have up to sixty days coverage.

Medicare will stop paying for your inpatient-related hospital costs (such as room and board) if you run out of days during your benefit period. To be eligible for a new benefit period, and additional days of inpatient coverage, you must remain out of the hospital or SNF for sixty days in a row. When you start a new benefit period, you will also have a new Part A deductible.

Overall, you can see that the hospital coverage can be very expensive, especially for those on limited incomes. You will see in the next chapter how MA plans insulate people from catastrophic hospital costs.

Skilled Nursing Facility (SNF)

To qualify for SNF care, you must have had an inpatient hospital stay for three consecutive days and must be admitted into a SNF within thirty days of discharge from the hospital. While most SNF stays occur upon discharge from the hospital, some occur post discharge to home and to avoid a readmission.

A SNF stay is for acute purposes only and does not include chronic nursing home needs. This is covered by Medicaid if you qualify.

A SNF stay includes a semi-private room, meals, skilled nursing services, rehabilitation services (if medically necessary), medical social services, medications, medical supplies and equipment, ambulance transportation for services not rendered by the SNF, and dietary counseling.

Medicare covers up to 100 days of SNF care per benefit period. The first twenty days have no cost-sharing. In 2021, days 21-100 were $185.50 per day. For anything over 100 days in each benefit period, the beneficiary covers all costs.

Home Health Services

Home health services are covered under both Parts A and Part B depending on circumstances. To qualify for Part A home health services, you must be homebound, need medically necessary skilled care in the home, have spent at least three consecutive days in the hospital or have a qualified SNF stay, and begin receiving care within fourteen days of discharge. For Part A home health, you can receive up to 100 days of daily care or an unlimited amount of intermittent care per benefit period.

Home health services include part-time or intermittent skilled nursing care (cannot be twenty-four hours per day), physical therapy, occupational therapy, speech-language pathology services, medical social services, and part-time or intermittent home health aide services (personal hands-on care as long as it is related to the treatment).

There is no cost-sharing for Part A home health services.

Hospice Services

Hospice care is a covered Part A service if a physician determines the beneficiary has a terminal illness with an estimated six months or less to live. Whether or not you are enrolled in traditional FFS or in MA, hospice is provided under Part A FFS through a certified hospice agency. As part of qualification, all curative treatments have stopped, and the hospice agency is rendering palliative care. You can give up hospice at any time. This can be received at home and for short durations in an inpatient facility.

Hospice services include doctor services, nursing care, pain relief medications, social services, durable medical equipment (DME), medical supplies, hospice aide services, homemaker services, physical and occupational therapy, dietary counseling, short-term inpatient care (if necessary for managing pain or symptoms), and short-term respite care.

Drug costs are five dollars per prescription. You pay 5% of any inpatient costs. Otherwise, hospice is 100% covered.

Part B

This is the outpatient and related part of Medicare and is supported by the Supplementary Medical Insurance (SMI) Trust Fund, which supports both Parts B and D. The fund is sustained by premiums paid by beneficiaries for both parts and appropriations from the federal budget. The premiums are supposed to be targeted to 25% of expected expenditures for the services, with the government picking up 75%. However, the reality is much the same for the SMI Trust Fund as it is for the Part A Trust Fund. As aging of beneficiaries and high costs in the inefficient system continue, more and more premium dollars and federal budget allocations will be needed to sustain the current benefit from year to year. At some point, benefits will have to be examined. Indeed, the Medicare Trustees project that the SMI-funded B and D expenditures/costs will go from 2.2% of GDP in 2019 to 3.9% within twenty-five years.[19-8]

As noted, beneficiaries must pay a Part B monthly premium (usually out of their Social Security checks for the Part B benefit). The standard premium applicable to most beneficiaries is $148.50 per month in 2021. There also is a deductible that applies each calendar year to all Part B services. The beneficiary must pay $203 in 2021 before any Part B services are covered by Medicare.[19-13]

After paying the annual deductible amount, there are few if any restrictions on obtaining services, except for whether it is a covered benefit or newly covered under the NCDs and LCDs noted previously. There are no benefit periods or qualifying events as in Part A.

Here are some of the major services provided in Part B.[19-11, 19-13, 19-18, 19-19] The services covered under Part B are so numerous that I cannot list them all here. For a complete list you can go to an Evidence of Coverage for an MA plan online or go to the "Medicare and You" pamphlet for the most current year (2021 is cited in this book). If needed, I updated premiums, deductibles, and cost-sharing with the latest figures for 2021 from official government sources. These figures go up each year based on inflation. Remember that in the FFS program, unless the service is a preventive screening with no cost-sharing, most services require a 20% co-insurance against the allowed amount for the Medicare service. Providers cannot balance bill over that as long as they are Medicare physicians accepting assignment. In the MA world, co-insurance may be changed to a lower co-pay for a number of services.

- Ambulance services, usually limited to emergency and medically necessary transport
- Ambulatory surgery centers and outpatient care at a hospital for the facility and physician costs
- Ancillary providers, such as chiropractic
- Outpatient behavioral health services

- ○ Chemotherapy, physician administered drugs, and related services
- ○ Durable medical equipment (DME)
- ○ Emergency and urgent care services
- ○ Home health services (covered under Part B when not qualified under Part A and a doctor believes they are medically necessary and someone is homebound; cannot be personal or custodial care unrelated to an acute illness; no co-insurance except on DME.)
- ○ Kidney dialysis
- ○ Laboratory services
- ○ Nutrition services
- ○ Physician services
- ○ Some prescription drugs (most are covered under Part D)
- ○ Prosthetics and orthotics
- ○ Preventive screenings
- ○ Radiology and imaging
- ○ Various rehabilitation services
- ○ Various therapies
- ○ Transplants
- ○ Vaccines

What is not covered?

- ○ Alternative medicine
- ○ Cosmetic surgery
- ○ Most dental care
- ○ Dentures
- ○ Eye exams tied to prescribing glasses
- ○ Routine foot care
- ○ Hearing aids

> ○　Acute long-term care, including personal and custodial care
>
> ○　Most non-emergency transportation
>
> ○　Most vision care

Let's talk a little about when Medicare is primary or secondary coverage.[19-11]

○　If you are sixty-five and older and have retiree health coverage from your employer, Medicare is primary and your retiree coverage secondary.

○　If you are sixty-five and older and you or your spouse is employed and you are covered on a group plan in a business with twenty or more employees, the group plan is primary, and Medicare is secondary. If the employer has fewer than twenty employees, Medicare is primary and the employer group coverage secondary.

○　If you are under age sixty-five and have a disability and are covered by a group health plan in a business with 100 or more employees, the group plan is primary and Medicare is secondary. If there are fewer than 100 employees in the business, then Medicare is primary and the group health plan secondary.

○　If you are a dual eligible, Medicare is primary and Medicaid secondary.

○　If you have ESRD and you are on Medicare, your group plan is primary for the first thirty months and then Medicare becomes primary.

○　There are other coordination rules that also apply to federal retirees, military retirees, and Veteran Administration benefits, among others.

As I have discussed often, the Medicare FFS system is very inefficient and wasteful. I go into greater detail about this in Chapter 30. About 57% of Medicare enrollees are still in the traditional program. The Medicare Trustees project that total Medicare costs will grow from 3.7% of GDP in 2019 to 6% of GDP by 2044, and then increase to 6.5% of GDP by 2094.[19-8] This is clearly unsustainable for the economy.

There is also little connection and improvement to quality in the system. This is by and large a result of the fact that the system is a transaction-based system where each service is paid a fee for the rendered service. As such, the providers pay little attention to treating the patient holistically. They are not getting paid to do so—only to move on to the next procedure or service.

Horror stories also abound as to the human toll due to the lack of care management in the system—an important piece of quality. The elderly and disabled have an exceedingly difficult time navigating the complex world of the health system. This is worsened by the complex rules surrounding benefits and eligibility. Confusion is the worst for the dual eligibles and others with low health literacy. Consequently, Medicare beneficiaries tend to access the system too late and at the most expensive point. Inpatient admissions are high due to exacerbation of disease states and conditions. We are a clear outlier compared with other countries. Other countries better monitor and maintain those with diabetes, asthma, chronic obstructive pulmonary disease (COPD), congestive heart failure (CHF), coronary artery disease (CAD), hypertension, and more.

Let's spend some time telling you how CMS is trying to reform the traditional FFS system. In fairness to CMS, the agency has gone down the path of trying to bring quality and cost controls to FFS through a series of pilot programs. For a more comprehensive list, you can go to CMS' Innovation Center website or to the footnoted KFF brief. But here are the major demonstrations that are in all fifty states in FFS.[19-11, 19-20]

- o Accountable care organizations (ACOs), where those in the traditional system are deemed members of an ACO based on attachment to given providers. If ACOs are successful in driving quality and lowering costs, then they share in some of the savings with CMS/Medicare.
- o Various bundled payments to hospitals, which seek to bundle hospital and post-inpatient care payments for various procedures. This is meant to ensure quality, better follow-up care, and reduced readmissions.
- o Primary care case management (PCCM), where primary care physicians (PCPs) get paid extra for conducting care management programs for their FFS members.

- ○ Various hospital quality incentives and penalties.
- ○ Various medical home models, which promote attachment to and care coordination by a PCP.

CMS says that about 61% of all payments in Medicare FFS are now tied to alternative payment schemes—other than traditional FFS payments.[19-21] But the verdict is out on how effective these reforms are or will be. And it is hard to argue that these pilot programs will ever reach the quality improvement seen in the rigorous Medicare Star quality program in the private, managed care program.

CHAPTER 20

Medicare Advantage Explained

art C of the Medicare program—Medicare Advantage (MA)—is the private alternative to enrolling in the Medicare traditional fee-for-service (FFS) program. MA must deliver the same Parts A and B services as the FFS program and may add additional benefits as well.

In addition, most MA plans also add the Part D prescription drug program benefits. A plan with no Part D benefit is called Medicare Advantage Only (MA-Only)—meaning only Part C (or Parts A and B). An MA plan with the Part D prescription drug benefits included is called Medicare Advantage-Part D (MA-PD).

Thus, think of MA-PD as receiving all of your healthcare services under one roof. In addition, MA-PD and MA-Only plans also provide other important services, such as case and disease management and care coordination, which are not available in traditional FFS.

A Medicare beneficiary who wants to enroll in an MA-Only or MA-PD plan still needs to enroll in Medicare as all other beneficiaries do. In addition, to join an MA plan, a Medicare beneficiary must be enrolled in both Parts

A and B, as MA plans are required to cover all services in both of these parts (there are some very small exceptions to this rule). Afterward, a Medicare beneficiary can enroll in an MA plan in lieu of being in the traditional FFS system. There are defined times that a person can enroll in an MA plan, which will be discussed later.

As noted in the previous chapter, MA is popular among seniors and the disabled. Over 43% of Medicare beneficiaries are in private MA plans as of early 2021 (based on an estimate of total Medicare beneficiaries at the time), while less than 57% are in traditional Medicare. Private estimates suggest that by 2025 about 50% of beneficiaries will be in MA plans. Between 2030 and 2040, that percentage could reach 70%.[20-1]

Here are the key facts to know about MA plans.[20-2, 20-3, 20-4, 20-5, 20-6, 20-7, 20-8] As applicable, I have updated certain figures to current values from official government sites.

> MA plans contract with the Centers for Medicare and Medicaid Services (CMS) to furnish all the benefits it covers for enrolled members instead of the members getting those services in the traditional FFS system. The only exception is when an enrollee needs hospice services, which is rendered in the FFS system. The member continues to receive some benefits from the plan. The MA plan receives a capitated (per member, per month, or PMPM) amount to furnish the benefits to each enrollee.

> In late 2021, MA reached almost 28 million of overall Medicare beneficiaries. This is over 43% based on estimates of Medicare beneficiaries at the time. Enrollment in MA in early 2021 increased by over 9% year-over-year and has more than doubled in a decade.

> Health plans are flocking to offer MA. About 2,100 more MA plans will be operating in 2021 than in 2017, a 77% increase. Overall, enrollees will be able to choose from more than 4,800 MA plans during 2021. The average number of MA plan choices per county will increase from about thirty-nine plans in 2020 to forty-seven plans in 2021, an increase of seventy-nine since 2017.

While it is difficult to attract private health plans in more rural states—due to the inability to create solid networks—MA plans thrive in more urban states. More than 40% of Medicare beneficiaries were in MA in nine states and Puerto Rico. In thirty states and Puerto Rico, more than 31% of Medicare beneficiaries were in MA. In 180 counties around the United States, about 10% of the U.S. population, over half of all Medicare beneficiaries are in MA plans. About 67% of enrollees in Miami-Dade County Florida (where I once developed a plan) are now in MA. In contrast, MA enrollment is low (20% or less) in twelve states and the District of Columbia. However, in some positive news for those in more rural areas, the number of plan options in rural counties will increase to 2,900 in 2021 from about 2,450 in 2020, an 18% increase.

In 2020, about 61% percent of MA enrollees are in HMOs, about 33% are in local PPOs, and 5% are in regional PPOs.

In 2020, more than 3.3 million enrollees were in the various special needs plans (SNPs).

In 2020, 60% of MA enrollees paid no additional premium beyond the Part B premium, with the average additional premium among all plans being $25 per month. Remember, this extra MA premium is because MA plans reduce cost-sharing (deductibles, co-insurance, and co-pays) and add benefits not covered by Medicare. For the most part, these premiums are far less than what a Medicare Supplement plan would charge to just fill the cost-sharing holes in traditional FFS.

An additional 5% of enrollees pay less than $20 per month. About 17% pay between $20 and $59 per month. About 18% pay over $50 per month. Average premiums for all MA plan types have dropped from $44 per month in 2010 to $25 per month on average in 2020. They are just $21 per month in 2021. With the exception of regional Preferred Provider Organization (PPO) plans, average premiums are dropping at the time of this writing.

Ninety percent of all MA plans are MA-PD plans and just short of 90% of MA enrollees are in such plans. Just 10% are MA-Only. A person who enrolls in an MA-Only plan either has separate drug coverage (e.g., a retiree plan), enrolls in a standalone Part D prescription drug plan (PDP) as if he were in traditional FFS, or pays out of pocket for drugs.

You must live in the plan's filed service area to enroll in a given plan. The service area is usually county based, but for some products it could be a region. While plans file in service areas and usually have networks, all plans are required to allow you to seek services for the following at any time and not limit you to in-network providers:

- ○ Emergency services
- ○ Urgently needed services
- ○ Hemodialysis
- ○ A thirty-day supply of prescription drugs

If someone had end-stage renal disease (ESRD), he or she could not enroll in an MA plan unless it was a SNP specifically geared toward ESRD (more on this later) or in another plan that was specifically allowed by CMS to enroll those with ESRD. However, as of January 1, 2021, those with ESRD can enroll in any MA plan.

MA plans must cover all Parts A and B services and cannot assess cost-sharing for these services that exceed the traditional FFS world. MA plans may use different methods of assessing cost-sharing but CMS watches to ensure that the overall burden is not greater than FFS.

As a way of controlling costs, most MA plans have networks and may use referrals and prior authorizations of both pharmacy and medical services. Seventy-nine percent of all MA plans had prior authorization requirements in 2019 but now, in 2020, 99% have such requirements.

Unlike traditional FFS, MA plans must have a maximum out-of-pocket (MOOP) cost threshold. The 2021 limits are $7,500 for in-network coverage and a combined in-network/out-of-network (OON) cap of $11,300 for products that have an out-of-network option. In 2020, the average MOOP limits for plans were the following, with MOOP averages trending downward since 2017:

- HMO Only (no OON): $4,486
- Local PPOs: in-network coverage is $5,622 and combined is $8,795
- Regional PPOs: in-network coverage is $6,493 and combined is $9,010

Note that the above MOOP only applies to Part C (Parts A and B services). Part D has a separate out-of-pocket limit that applies to both MA members and traditional FFS members. This will be discussed in a subsequent chapter.

MA plans add non-covered Medicare benefits. The most popular ones in 2020 and 2021 included:

- Eye exams and glasses—79%
- Telehealth—77%
- Dental—74%
- Fitness—74%
- Hearing aids—72%
- Over-the-counter (OTC) drugs—61%
- Meal benefit—39%
- Non-emergency transportation—34%

Major supplemental benefit additions were made by plans for 2021. A Better Medicare Alliance analysis by Milliman found that the number of plans offering supplemental benefits increased across thirty-six out of forty-one categories from 2020 to 2021. The most common benefits offered in 2021 include vision (96%), hearing (93%), fitness (92%), and dental care (87%). Fifty-seven percent of plans now offer a meal benefit, and 46% cover members' transportation to and from doctors' visits.

Another frequently added benefit is that MA plans help seniors and the disabled with their Part B premiums. This is known as the Part B rebate provision. MA plans use some of the premium they get from

Medicare for the member's health coverage and use it to buy down a member's Part B premium. There are three ways to get this benefit:

- If the member receives a Social Security check, the plan can ask Social Security to lower the Part B premium the member pays each month and divert some of the plan premium to cover it. (Thus the member's monthly check goes up.)
- If the member does not receive a Social Security check, Medicare will bill for the Part B premium. Medicare will divert some of the plan premium here as well and give a credit on the monthly Part B premium statement to the member, thus lowering the monthly bill.
- The plan can also reimburse the member each month for the amount of the Part B premium rebate. The member would get the full Premium deducted from his or her Social Security check or pay the full amount when billed by Medicare each month.

While CMS is not a huge fan of this last provision because it uses government money on a non-healthcare item, it allows it because it does help seniors and the disabled afford the Part B premium. As noted earlier, the standard Part B premium in 2021 is $148.50 per month. MA plans that offer the Part B rebate product generally cover $100 or more of the Part B premium in most markets.

These Part B rebate products are generally in markets where Medicare premiums paid by CMS to MA plans are high. This gives plans the flexibility to design benefits that include a Part B premium rebate.

Enrollees who take advantage of this usually are:

- Those on fixed incomes who struggle to pay the bills. The extra money in the Social Security check each month is a boon.
- Healthier people who anticipate lower overall health costs and don't need the rich added benefits in another MA product. They see value in the buydown of the Part B premium.

Before enrolling in one of these plans, seniors and the disabled need to think before they act. While receiving the Part B premium rebate appears extremely attractive up front, it could also be the case that opting instead for a richer benefit MA plan will save more money as cost-sharing will be lower and there may be greater medical benefits.

MA plans like to offer these Part B premium rebate plans because they do help attract healthier people. This provides critical balance between sicker enrollees and healthier ones and helps reduce adverse selection and overall medical expenses.

MA plans are subject to heavy CMS regulation. There is a rigorous compliance regime. Plans face heavy monetary penalties and other sanctions, including a freeze on marketing and enrollment, if rules are not followed. They are also subject to program audits and must ensure that prior authorization, appeals, and grievance cases are processed in a timely manner, that evidence-based criteria are used, and that they inform members and providers of decisions.

CMS also has a strong Star quality program, where plans with low quality can be terminated and those hitting four Stars or greater receive 5% bonus revenue that can be returned to members in the form of added benefits. At the beginning of 2020, 52% of MA-PD plans achieved 4-Star or greater ratings and 81% of enrollees were in such plans according to CMS. At the beginning of 2021, about 49% of plans are 4-Star or greater and about 77% of enrollees are in such plans. (CMS announced the number of quality-rated plans and enrollees in them skyrocketed between 2021 and 2022. However, this is in large measure due to the relaxing of measurement during the COVID-19 pandemic.) Overall, it proves that seniors are savvy consumers who gravitate to quality plans.

Plans are required to meticulously document benefits, coverage, networks, and formularies each year and monthly when updates occur. Again, plans face heavy fines and potential suspensions for not circulating documents to members and/or posting on websites. The key documents include:

○ The annual notice of change (ANOC), which outlines changes from one year to the next in benefits and plan design to ensure current members are aware and have the option of changing plans during enrollment periods.

○ The evidence of coverage (EOC), which is a several-hundred-page guide outlining benefits, plan design, and procedures the plan follows (prior authorizations, appeals, grievances, external appeals, etc.)

○ Provider directory, which outlines participating providers such as hospitals, labs, radiology, skilled nursing, home health, primary care physicians (PCPs), and specialists. These must be updated at least monthly on plan websites.

○ Formularies or drug lists—a plan's drug list changes each month based on new drugs coming to market and guidance from CMS. The published formularies must be updated monthly on websites and include covered drugs, the tiers or levels they are on, co-pay or cost-sharing amounts, and whether utilization management (UM) edits apply to that drug. These include prior authorization, step therapy requirements, and quality limits.

Recently, CMS has made some substantial changes to Medicare Advantage (MA) that provides for additional benefits to members and helps accelerate the MA growth seen lately. First, the agency now allows variability of benefits within MA plans based on chronic conditions or disease states. Plans now are allowed to waive cost-sharing and add services and benefits for certain conditions and disease states. In 2021, about 500 plans will offer up to 2.5 million MA enrollees with access to such benefits. CMS also has another demonstration for MA plans known as the value-based insurance design (VBID). This program has similar parameters and will have over 440 plans serving 1.6 million in 2021.

Second, MA plans can now also offer chronically ill patients a broader range of supplemental benefits that are not necessarily health-related but may help to improve or maintain health. These include ongoing meal delivery, transportation for non-medical needs like grocery shopping, and home environment services. In 2021, about 920 plans will provide up to 4.3 million enrollees access to these types of supplemental benefits.

Third, MA plans can now offer new supplemental benefits and extra benefits which are primarily health-related but tailored to specific needs to help maintain health. In 2021, about 730 plans provided up to 3 million MA enrollees with expanded primarily health related supplemental benefits, such long-term care services and supports. Previously, these were largely Medicaid-covered benefits.

Medicare Advantage (MA) Plan Types

Let's talk a little on the types of MA plans allowed by CMS. Generally, these plan types are similar to those in commercial plans, as outlined earlier, but with a few nuances for Preferred Provider Organization (PPO) and point of service (POS) plans in Medicare.[20-7, 20-9, 20-10, 20-11, 20-12]

Health Maintenance Organization (HMO) Plans: In MA, as with other HMOs, an enrollee is limited to obtaining coverage from a network provider except in emergent/urgent scenarios. MA plans have a few different HMO designs, including flexibility on primary care physician assignment and referral requirements. Generally, MA HMOs do have rather rigorous prior authorization requirements.

Preferred Provider Organization (PPO) Plans: As with other PPOs, MA enrollees have a generally wide selection for in-network care and are able to access out-of-network coverage from any enrolled Medicare provider. This of course is beyond the requirement for emergent/urgent care from any enrolled Medicare provider nationwide. They also tend to face fewer restrictions for in-network as with commercial PPOs. While seeking out-of-network care from commercial PPOs can be risky because there usually are no network or payment relationships with providers, in a Medicare PPO, out-of-network providers enrolled in Medicare

FFS cannot charge more than Medicare FFS payment rates for an MA member. That is a win for MA enrollees, who therefore have a safeguard against excessive costs when seeking out-of-network care. At the same time, cost-sharing for out-of-network coverage and MOOPs will be much greater than in-network care.

There are two different PPO products offered in MA. A **local PPO** is usually cheaper and your service area and network is usually based on the county you live in, although the network could be larger. A **regional PPO** is usually more expensive and your service area is regional (multiple counties, a state or the plan could even cross state boundaries). The network is usually much larger.

Point of Service (POS) Plans: An MA POS plan is unique and doesn't exactly parallel a POS in the commercial world. Designs can vary a bit in MA. The plan has a strict network HMO and rules for in-network care but has some out-of-network coverage beyond the emergent/urgent requirement. The plan can tailor its out-of-network benefits to certain benefits, as well as certain providers nationwide. These plans are not particularly popular as they are tough to understand and administer.

Medicare Cost Plans: These are only available in a few areas of the country and generally are being phased out. In this plan, you do not have to have Part A. You could only have Part B. These plans do set up networks and offer benefits in Parts A and B, but you can access out-of-network coverage by obtaining services through the FFS system. Thus, you may pay premiums and cost-sharing for services provided by the MA Cost Plan, but also pay cost-sharing and deductibles in the FFS system. A cost plan may provide Part D coverage or may be MA Only, in which case you can obtain coverage from a private standalone Part D plan (whether or not the cost plan provides it).

Medical Savings Account (MSA) Plans: These have small enrollment given the strength and cost-effectiveness of other MA products. The MA MSA plan combines a high-deductible insurance plan with a medical savings account that you can use to pay for your healthcare costs. The MSA plan uses a part of the premiums it is paid by the federal government to set up a medical savings account for you. You use these dollars to pay for your healthcare costs before you hit the deductible. When you hit the deductible, the MA MSA plan begins covering you for the covered benefits. MA MSA plans may also provide benefits beyond starts Parts A and B benefits. Generally speaking, you can access any Medicare provider. You will need to enroll in a standalone Part D plan for a drug benefit.

Private Fee-for-Service (PFFS) Plans: This is a bit of a dying breed of MA plans. In this case, an MA plan is set up in which you enroll and usually has both in-network and out-of-network coverage. PFFS plans can have networks but also leverage the Medicare FFS system and set up payment arrangements with these providers on behalf of its members. This gives you great latitude and flexibility, but the plan is more expensive than most types. You should always seek approval from your PFFS plan before you seek treatment from an out-of-network provider to ensure the service will be covered and the plan and the provider work together to ensure payment on your behalf. There is usually limited or no prior authorization for most medical benefits.

Special Needs Plans (SNPs): Quite simply, these are MA plans that focus in on dual eligibles (dual eligible SNPs or D-SNPs), those with certain chronic disease states and conditions (Chronic Condition SNPs or C-SNPs), and those in institutions or at-risk of institutionalization (Institutional SNPs or I-SNPs). Also note that there are Medicare-Medicaid Plan (MMP) demonstrations that focus on duals and sometimes those in institutions that combine Medicare and Medicaid funding and sometimes cover both acute medical care and chronic long-term care. SNPs will be discussed in detail in a Chapter 22.

Employer Group Waiver Plans (EGWPs): These plans combine the primary benefit of MA with a secondary benefit of an employer retiree coverage plan. Typically, when a retiree hits age sixty-five, the employer retiree plan requires them to enroll in Medicare. This is the case for public or private employers as well as union-sponsored plans. In some cases, the retiree plan will even pay for the Part B premium for the members. In essence, the Medicare benefit becomes the core retiree benefit and the employer retiree plan "wraps" its coverage around Medicare to fill in the holes—much as a Medicare Supplement would for traditional Medicare. This ensures that the retirees' Medicare and employer benefits are seamless—they deal with one entity for coverage.

EGWPs help employers reduce retiree costs as the MA benefit is usually richer than traditional Medicare. EGWPs can be either HMOs (about 25%) or PPOs (about 75%).

As opposed to the member enrolling in an MA plan on an individual basis, employers enter into agreements with MA plans and then members are enrolled into the employer-specific EGWP. Employers pay premiums to MA plans for the wrap program and members are only responsible for any residual premium and cost-sharing (and perhaps Part B premiums if the employer does not cover them). There are also some employers that contract with CMS to offer an EGWP directly without an MA plan (or may use a plan on an administrative basis only for some services). This means that some EGWPs are self-insured while others are fully insured.

Most of the rules that apply to mainstream MA plans apply to EGWPs, except that bidding is somewhat different. In addition, the network provided by the MA plan would usually be over a much larger geographic area than a traditional HMO or PPO.

Finally, EGWPs can be standalone Part D EGWPs and offer only Medicare drug benefits, MA-Only EGWPs and offer medical benefits only, or MA-PD EGWPs and offer both medical and drug benefits.

Program of All-Inclusive Care for the Elderly (PACE) Plans: These plans were developed many years ago and are rather independent of MA proper. But they look and feel like certain MA SNPs (think of a D-SNP and I-SNP combined), certain MMPs that offer acute and long-term care services, and even Medicaid managed long-term care (MLTC) plans that offer both acute and long-term care services.

PACE Plans are offered in some but not all states. These usually combine Medicare and Medicaid funding. A person may have Medicare or Medicaid or both in most states, but some states mandate Medicaid eligibility to be in a PACE plan. If you do not have Medicaid and your state allows you to enroll as a Medicare-only participant, a premium will be charged for long-term care and usually Part D.

The main goal of PACE is to maintain people needing nursing home levels of care in community settings (homes, community settings, and even PACE centers run by the PACE plan). You receive comprehensive Medicare and Medicaid services for medical and drugs as well as transportation and LTC services. PACE Plans are increasingly subject to many of the MA compliance rules set by CMS because most have Medicare funding and benefits included.

To be in a PACE plan, you usually must live in the service area, generally be fifty-five or older, on Medicare or Medicaid (or both), and certified by Medicaid as needing a nursing-home level of care.

Enrollment Periods

Those wishing to enroll in MA plans need to follow the same rules as all other Medicare beneficiaries when enrolling in Medicare proper. Then, they have additional rules to follow to join an MA plan. In general, there are certain, defined periods in which you can join an MA plan:[20-10, 20-13]

Initial Enrollment Period—When you are initially eligible to enroll in Medicare, you can also join an MA plan. But for most MA plans, you must have enrolled in both Part A and Part B.

General Enrollment Period—If you have Part A coverage and you get Part B for the first time during the General Enrollment Period, between January 1 and March 31 of each year, you can join an MA Plan as well. Your coverage may not start until July 1.

Open Enrollment Period—Every year, between October 15 and December 7, anyone with Medicare can join, switch, or drop an MA Plan. Your new coverage usually will begin on January 1 of the following year.

Medicare Advantage Open Enrollment Period—Between January 1 and March 31 of each year, you can switch to another MA plan or return to traditional Medicare FFS and join a private standalone Part D plan. You can only switch once during this period and your change usually becomes effective the first of the following month. If you are in traditional FFS as of January 1, you cannot switch to a MA plan or switch standalone drug plans.

Special Enrollment Periods—Certain Medicare beneficiaries have more flexibility to change throughout the year. In extraordinary circumstances, anyone may be able to ask CMS for an exception to switch an MA plan outside of normal enrollment periods.

Rate-Setting

So, how do MA plans get paid, why are they so successful, and how can they afford to create products for seniors and the disabled that offer far more than the traditional FFS benefits?

In large part, the answer is tied to a rather intricate process of rate-setting in the MA world, along with further incentives built in for high-performing plans from the Star program. In practice, the actual calculations of these items are significantly more complex.

First, CMS sets a county benchmark that is a percentage of the monthly cost of the average beneficiary in the traditional FFS program. Depending on where you are in the country, the county payment rate can be between 95-115% percent of the projected FFS cost. On average, MA rates are set at about 100% of FFS across the nation (some rural areas have higher rates against FFS to encourage MA participation there, while some urban areas are set below FFS rates). CMS evaluates plan bids against the benchmark.

Second, health plans in part determine the Medicare payments they receive. Each plan submits its bid to CMS specific to the Part C (and Part D, in the case of an MA-PD plan) coverage it intends to offer beneficiaries in each county it serves. The plan bids on what it believes its costs are for basic Medicare benefits. This will be the base rate. The Medicare Payment Advisory Commission (MedPAC, the congressional advisory group on Medicare) says that plans bid on average about 87% of the county rate benchmarks nationwide.[20-14]

Third, the plan also proposes enhanced benefits for its members that it believes it can fund. These added services include defrayed cost-sharing as well as additional services to the member such as dental, hearing, and vision. As long as the plan's base rate is below the county benchmark, it is allowed to keep a portion of the difference between the county benchmark and the cost of providing basic benefits to fund enhanced benefits. This is known as the rebate.

The higher a plan's Star rating, the greater the portion of the difference the plan gets to keep. For example, a 4.5- or 5-Star plan gets to keep 70% of the difference between its bid for basic Medicare and the county benchmark. That percentage must be returned to beneficiaries in the form of enhanced benefits. The federal government keeps the remaining 30% as cost savings to the Medicare program. Plans with a Star rating of 3.5 and 4, keep 65% of the difference between its bid for Medicare basic benefits and the county benchmark. A plan below 3.5 Stars gets to keep only 50% of the difference. If a plan bids above the county benchmark based on the base Medicare benefit and additional benefits it wants to offer, an additional MA plan premium would be charged.

Finally, plans rated 4 Stars or greater receive an additional 5% quality bonus to pass through to beneficiaries as well.

All told, the combination of the rebate and the quality bonus gives plans rated 4 Stars and higher a significant advantage in the marketplace. It can pass significant amounts back to its members in the form of enhanced benefits and lower cost-sharing. In 2017, per-enrollee spending in Medicare was just over $1,000 per month nationally. That means that high-performing plans can add well more than $100 per month (in some areas considerably more) to enrollee benefits each month to attract members. In 2021, MedPAC reported the national average was $139 to $140 in added enrollee benefits per month. Lower performing plans cannot add nearly as many added benefits. My calculation suggests at most they add about $65 per month on average.[20-14, 20-15, 20-16]

In short, CMS devised a rather brilliant system to align toward and reward quality. With their bonuses and rebates, higher-rated plans are able to offer increased benefit levels and lower cost-sharing that are appealing to beneficiaries. Higher rated plans grow faster and experience significantly less churn than health plans with fewer than 4 Stars. If the plan is run well, the increased membership adds to its profit margin each year. There is a direct correlation between Star rating and plan growth; doing the right things by beneficiaries leads to higher Stars and more business. In fact, about 80% of beneficiaries are in plans rated 4-Star and higher in 2021. (CMS announced the number of quality-rated plans and enrollees in them skyrocketed between 2021 and 2022. However, this is in large measure due to the relaxing of measurement during the COVID-19 pandemic.)

As an additional bonus, 5-Star plans can market to new members year-round and accept new members throughout the year. All other plans are more limited in their opportunity to enroll outside of the defined enrollment periods. What's more, top-rated health plans benefit from CMS's indirect marketing support when they promote 5-Star plans on their enrollment website. CMS also encourages enrollees to join highly-rated plans for the best service and healthcare outcomes.

Risk Adjustment

As if the previous section was not enough of a head-scratcher, there is one other component of the rate-setting system: risk adjustment. As has been mentioned in other chapters, rates increasingly take into account the relative health of the enrolled member. CMS has adopted a similar strategy for MA. Rates take into account the health or risk of the member, and CMS pays the plans accordingly.

The bid submission process noted previously—and in fact the plan's overall revenue—is heavily impacted by the plan's estimate of how its total population ranks in terms of health against the system overall. If its total population is healthier than the system, on average, then there is said to be "beneficial selection" with less overall revenue to the plan in the form of premiums from the federal government. If the plan's population is sicker than the system, on average, then there is said to be "adverse selection" and more money comes to the plan to help take care of the members.

As a quick explanation, let's say the population of Medicare has a 1.0 risk score as an average for the entire population. A health plan with healthy members may have an aggregate risk score of all members of 0.9. That means it would receive on average about 10% less revenue to adjust for its beneficial selection. A plan with an aggregate risk score of 1.1 would receive 10% more revenue on average to adjust for its adverse selection. In this way plans are compensated based on the health or risk of its members.

Risk Adjustment Simple Explanation

The risk adjustment system is known as the hierarchical condition category (HCC) system.

The rate-setting process just explained has a member-specific risk-adjustment factor or score tied to the base rate described in the last section. Within the risk adjustment factor are two components—demographic and clinical. Each member has a demographic component that takes into account age, sex, residence county, Medicaid status, and aged/disability status, among other things. Plans submit diagnoses to CMS through claims and encounter data. CMS assigns certain diagnoses (not all) on each member's claims/encounters to groupings of disease states and conditions. These are then given weights, which are added up to come up with the clinical component. The clinical component and demographic component are added together to derive the risk adjustment factor or score. The risk adjustment factor is then multiplied by the bid rate to come up with the member-specific rate.

Additional Detailed Risk Adjustment Information

CMS has designed a risk adjustment system for both Part C and D for most beneficiaries. It has very significant impact on revenue in Part C, and less so in Part D. There is a community and institutional portion of the main HCC model. There is also a separate risk model for those with ESRD.

Recently, CMS rolled out a new encounter data process to capture the diagnoses needed in the risk-adjustment system, migrating from a simple submission process to a sophisticated one, based on sending CMS HIPAA 837 X12 encounters. This has complicated things for plans and is leading to some plans losing revenue as the old system is phased out.

CMS is starting to audit plans' risk scores. Plans could face extrapolated penalties in the future if they do not have clinical evidence to support the encounter diagnoses reported to CMS. This is known as the risk adjustment data validation (RADV) audit.

FFS enrollees get a Part C and Part D risk adjustment factor or score calculation. Even though FFS enrollees are not in private plans, and are subject to payments, risk adjustment scores are maintained for these folks to ensure accurate payments in the MA world—and in case the FFS member enrollees enrolls in an MA plan.

CMS also places an arbitrary adjustment to the overall rates for MA plans based on its view that MA risk scores are "inflated" versus the FFS system. In the past, over many years, MA scores have come in higher on average than FFS enrollees. CMS argues this is due to encounter and risk score submission tactics by plans to arbitrarily increase scores. As such, a global adjustment to rates is made (this is known as the coding intensity adjustment, which is just below 6%). This is in addition to the below-FFS rates in some urban counties. Plans argue that MA risk scores are accurate as the plans work with providers to document all disease states. There is no incentive to do so in the FFS world. The truth is probably somewhere in between: (1) There is a disincentive to document all disease states in the FFS world and MA plans are much better at it, and (2) plans likely are somewhat too aggressive in its submission tactics. The encounter data migration (from the less sophisticated one) should rein this in. As well, if plans are too aggressive in their tactics, that will be seen in the RADV audit results.

Do MA Plans Save?

Many argue that MA plans do not save because their rates are based on those of the FFS model. This is not the case. Rates across the nation were meant to average about 100% of FFS after the reforms put in place in the Affordable Care Act (ACA). A piece of the difference between the county benchmark and the bid by each plan to provide the traditional Medicare benefit is given back to the federal government.

The Medicare Payment Advisory Commission (MedPAC, which advises Congress on Medicare policy) argues, though, in the aggregate MA payments are 1-4% higher (depending on the timeframe and whether quality bonuses and coding differences are factored in).[20-14, 20-15, 20-17] It says this is due to a few reasons, including higher risk scores in MA compared with FFS enrollees, the coding intensity adjustment for the above is set too low, and the quality bonus for MA is additive to the overall rate funding.

MedPAC has proposed to make numerous changes. The big policy ones are as follows:[20-14, 20-17, 20-18, 20-19, 20-20, 20-21, 20-22]

- ○ It wants to apply an additional 2% discount to MA rates to obtain savings due to the aggregate higher rates it believes exist. It argues MA should be more cost-effective than FFS.
- ○ MedPAC would like to blend MA rates using overall national costs and local county costs (e.g., 50% national and 50% local).
- ○ MedPAC would also gradually move to a total benchmark ceiling (including quality bonus) of 100%.
- ○ It would further reduce rates from the current 95% of FFS costs in heavily urban areas.
- ○ MedPAC would remove the ability of health plans to do chart reviews

and limit risk adjustment to encounter submissions.

○ It would refine the quartile (115% to 95% of FFS) benchmarks set in the ACA to avoid so-called cliffs (which drive much higher reimbursement for a few dollars difference in county FFS costs).

○ MedPAC also argues that the quality bonus program is flawed and needs a massive revamp, including removing the added funding for quality performance and taking it out of base fees, using peer groups to evaluate performance, and measuring performance at the local level today. It argues quality in MA cannot be meaningfully evaluated. My view is that CMS has done a good job at incremental reform and continues to boost quality in the program while balancing the impact on plans and members. MedPAC's recommendations could also be very administratively burdensome.

○ In part to offset some reductions above and to align with other quality bonus programs in Medicare, the rebate for added benefits would be increased to an average of 75% (from a current average of about 65% and a range of 50% to 70%) and delinked from Star quality program performance.

Many of MedPAC's recommendations deserve consideration. They have merit. But I do think MedPAC is taking a far too analytical approach to the issue. It fails to truly consider the impact that these far-reaching proposals would have. The MedPAC proposals taken as a whole would reduce plan offerings and materially impact benefits on which the poor and lower-income have come to rely. It also could reverse the course of MA growth, which is far better for the nation than the decrepit FFS system.

That said, delinking MA from county-by-county FFS payments in some form (either through blending or absolute bidding) may be important over time to bring greater efficiency to the healthcare system in Medicare and overall. MA plans could save more in high costs counties compared with FFS. (As an example, driven by utilization and waste due to the availability of hospital beds and other medical services, the Miami area's Medicare spending was $13,199 in 2017, compared with $10,317 nationally.)[20-23]

MA plans have had to adjust to rate reductions in the ACA and did so. They likely could continue to remain very profitable over time and attract members if rates are delinked from FFS.

But a reasonable rollout would be needed to continue the growth in MA, ensure high quality, and not disrupt the benefit enhancements on which members have come to rely.

CHAPTER 21

Why Medicare Advantage Is Good

Just in case you didn't glean it from the last chapter, let me state it more bluntly: I am no fan of the traditional Medicare fee-for-service (FFS) system. I believe that Medicare Advantage (MA) plans are the best way to deliver care in the Medicare system.

So, here is my admittedly biased take on why MA is good for seniors and the disabled, as well as for the health of the nation as a whole. It offers the best hope for controlling costs in the future and sustaining a relatively robust benefit for seniors and the disabled.

Before we jump into the meat of this, let's compare traditional FFS to MA and discuss some of the basic pros and cons of each system.

Medicare FFS Basics:

Services are delivered via direct contracts between the federal Centers for Medicare and Medicaid Services (CMS) and hundreds of thousands of providers nationwide. FFS enrollees have the freedom to see any enrolled Medicare provider in the nation. Demonstration projects or pilots in the FFS system are seeking to reform the process by reducing costs and improving quality. FFS enrollees receive Part D drug benefits via private insurers by enrolling in private standalone drug plans.

MA Basics:

CMS contracts with private health plans to deliver Medicare services. Plans go through an annual bid process. Plans then contract with providers. You usually have to see a provider in a network unless your plan has an out-of-network benefit or you have emergency/urgent situations. The CMS holds MA plans to quality and compliance standards. Plans usually cover medical and drug benefit, so you get all your coverage from one plan.

Here is my pros and cons list for FFS and MA:

Fee-for-Service: PROS	Fee-for-Service: CONS
Relatively open network—You can go to any doctor or hospital that accepts Medicare	Very expensive for those on fixed incomes (deductibles and cost-sharing), but can buy Medicare Supplement or Medigap policies (expensive, too)
You can join a Part D Plan—Prescription Drug Coverage with private insurance company	Little or no care coordination and beneficiary very much on their own to manage their care
No referral, prior authorization, or utilization management (UM) to go through	Little quality focus in program and very wasteful, which drives up costs for the nation and individuals

Medicare Advantage: PROS	Medicare Advantage: CONS
Usually covers well beyond traditional Medicare for little or no additional premium (reduced cost-sharing, added benefits, Part C maximum out-of-pocket [MOOP] cost, usually more expansive hospital benefit than FFS)	Usually confined to a network of providers. Any out-of-network access could be limited or expensive (although the cost may not be more than traditional FFS)
MA can provide very competitive Part D benefits by using Part C dollars to "buy down" D costs.	Must follow plan rules—authorizations, referrals, etc.
One-stop shopping for all your A, B, and D needs	
Focused on quality outcomes and member satisfaction	

So, now let's look at what MA does that FFS does not. This is the stuff that I think makes MA the right system for seniors and the aged as well as the right answer for America's healthcare crisis over time.

Proper claims payment and fraud, waste, and abuse (FWA) reduction. FFS has a largely retroactive process and it is notably fraud-ridden. MA plans invest a great deal in ensuring proper claims payment upfront and reducing fraud, waste, and abuse.

Prior authorization and appeals. While many champion the fact that access to benefits are unfettered in FFS, there is little doubt that over-utilization and inappropriate utilization are huge problems in the traditional system. In fairness to CMS, the agency has gone down the path of trying to bring quality and cost controls to FFS through a series of pilot programs, including accountable care organizations (ACOs), bundled payments, and more. But the verdict is out on how effective these reforms are or will be. Some data suggest little savings or even increased costs thus far in some of these reform programs.

In time, some of the demonstration programs may save a little, but not fundamentally change cost or quality trends. The use of prior authorization (PA) and utilization management (UM) is needed to take out inappropriate utilization and drive consumers to the most appropriate and least costly place of service.

While PA remains controversial, CMS and managed care plans are building the answer for the future, one that should satisfy both providers and members and reduce costs and inflationary trends.

CMS now mandates that private health plans use strict evidence-based criteria for denials of drugs and medical services and requires independent external reviews of denials if desired by the member. CMS audits this area thoroughly. This ensures significant accountability in plan decision-making.

Using technology, health plans are building electronic submission mechanisms and auto-authorization of PAs to reduce costs and turnaround times so that members and providers know whether a service at a given location or a given drug will be covered.

In the near future, it is also likely that health plans migrate to real-time claims processing, which will allow providers to immediately file claims at the time of rendering services, get real-time PA approvals if necessary, and see immediate evidence of claims payment.

Case and disease management. FFS has very little case and disease management. There are some care management pilots with physicians and readmissions penalties and some quality pilots with hospitals. But these are fragmented and not very robust. Plans increasingly center a great deal of spending and attention on monitoring chronic co-morbidities and interceding to stop exacerbation of disease states that lead to more expensive care. CMS is pushing plans to focus efforts on care management instead of exclusively on UM and plans are answering the call in a big way.

Quality improvement. I again note that CMS has gone down the path of trying to bring quality and cost controls to FFS through a series of pilot programs, but it is hard to argue that the pilots will ever reach the quality improvement seen in the rigorous Medicare Star quality program in the private managed care program. Case in point: about 80% of all MA enrollees were in high-performing plans in 2021. They have made a choice to seek out quality care.

Grievance and complaints processes. FFS does not have a thorough system and CMS has mandated a far-reaching oversight program in MA tied to prior authorizations and appeals.

Network management and provider credentialing. This is poorly performed by FFS and not governed by national accreditation bodies as private plans are.

Eligibility and member services. This is very rudimentary in FFS, but robust in private MA plans. This helps consumers navigate the healthcare system and understand all their rights.

A closing comment on those excessive and nasty administrative costs of health plans. Proponents of Medicare for All and those opposed to private plans tend to attack health plans for high administrative costs. They often cite a statistic that the traditional FFS system has administrative costs as low as 2%. This statistic is dubious at best as numerous other government agencies, including the Social Security Administration, help administer Medicare qualification and enrollment.

More important, administrative costs are now limited by the minimum medical loss ratio (MLR) dictates (which mandates that eighty-five of premium dollars in MA Part C get spent on medical expenses—explicitly limiting administrative costs and profit).

Further, administrative spending of about 10% (assuming a 5% profit) over time will reap the reward of lower base Medicare costs and additional benefits for seniors.

MA's Value Proposition

Now, let's tell you about the value proposition that MA plans have built for average Americans and with its CMS partner.

MA plans provide base Medicare benefits at huge savings by leveraging prior authorization, care coordination, and care management. Over time, this will bend the cost curve. FFS remains an inflationary monster because it has no real cost constraints.

MA plans roll most of the savings in providing major benefit add-ons, including reduced or eliminated premiums; reduced cost-sharing; adding inpatient days to prevent bankruptcy or altogether eliminating the day cap in the program; and providing myriad services not covered or poorly covered in traditional Medicare (dental, vision, hearing, and more). This saves average Americans hundreds if not thousands of dollars each year against what they would pay in traditional Medicare. For low-income folks, it is a godsend. Basically, it is an alternative social welfare program at no or minimal cost to the taxpayer.

Consider the following statistics: [21-1, 21-2, 21-3, 21-4]

Those sixty-five and older on traditional Medicare FFS were more likely to be a part of a family having trouble paying their medical bills than those who were on MA. For 2018, the Centers for Disease Control and Prevention (CDC) found the following with regard to adults aged sixty-five and over who were in families having problems paying medical bills in the past twelve months:

- 5.6% for those with private insurance
- 12.3% for those with Medicare and Medicaid
- 8.3% for those with Medicare Advantage
- 12.4% for those with traditional Medicare (no Medicare Supplement)

When it comes to those seventy-five and older, the statistics were as follows:

- 4.2% for those with private insurance
- 9.6% for those with Medicare and Medicaid
- 7.2% for those with Medicare Advantage
- 10.6% for those with traditional Medicare (no Medicare Supplement)

Similarly, a recent study by the Better Medicare Alliance, covering MA and Medicare FFS in 2016 found that MA members had total out-of-pocket spending of $3,198 compared to $4,474 for FFS members on average—a difference of $1,276 annually or about 29%. When looking at the percentage of enrollees who spend 20% or more of their income on out-of-pocket costs and premiums, MA members again did better than FFS enrollees—14.8% compared with 20.5% or 28% lower.

Further, a study by United Healthcare found that MA members spend as much as 40% less than those enrolled in FFS. The spending includes premiums and cost-sharing for those who have both medical and drug coverage. A FFS enrollee spent between $5,361 and $5,992 per year, depending on whether Medigap also was included. Spending for those with MA was just $3,558 per year.

MA plans improve quality through a wonderfully crafted CMS Star bonus program, a care management focus, additional targeted benefits, defined and accountable networks, and provider quality achievement incentives. People are flocking to high-quality plans, which helps improve outcomes.

A recent study by the Better Medicare Alliance shows that MA outperforms Medicare FFS on various preventive screenings and avoiding hospitalizations. When it came to vaccinations for pneumonia and the flu, MA members had 49% and 11% higher rates of vaccination, respectively, than their FFS enrollee counterparts. MA members had a 57% lower rate of avoidable hospitalizations for acute conditions than those in Medicare FFS. And 74% of MA members post-hospitalization had a follow-up clinical visit within fourteen days, while just 52% of Medicare FFS enrollees did so. The study also reported that MA members outscored FFS enrollees for diabetic eye exam rates and depression screenings.[21-5]

MA plans also reduce overall costs and the cost curve in the future by setting up accountable networks and processes. Indeed, they already show a record of savings against Medicare FFS in a number of areas. The Better Medicare Alliance study that showed better quality outcomes above also found that, among high-need, high-cost MA populations, inpatient hospital costs were

9-23% lower, compared with the FFS enrollees. It also found that Part D drug spending was 33-44% lower.[21-5]

Another study published in Health Affairs and led by the federal Agency for Healthcare Research and Quality (AHRQ) looked at 16 million MA members across 515 insurance contracts in 2014 and 2015. The study found that those enrolled in plans with higher Star ratings saw a 3.4% increase in the use of highly rated hospitals. Further, it found a 2.6% decrease in ninety-day readmissions and a 20.8% decrease in members who either returned to traditional Medicare or switched to another MA plan. The study surmised that the extra dollars given to high-performing plans likely drive the improvements. At the same time, the study left open the need to modify the Star program to further drive results.[21-6]

MA plans invest in care management activities that are beginning to emphasize prevention, disease management, and care coordination. This is often done through incentive payments and bonuses to providers. Shifting from UM to care management is critical to bend the cost curve and bring about quality. MA plans are working with CMS to change the paradigm. These services, too, help members navigate a labyrinthine healthcare system and obtain the right services at the right time.

MA plans also serve the dual eligible populations who are both elderly/disabled and low income. These populations consume a disproportionate share of the healthcare dollar in Medicare and Medicaid, but MA plans work on both the medical and social determinant aspects of these members to reduce costs and improve quality.

MA plans work with CMS to experiment on combining Medicare and Medicaid clinical pathways and finance. While Medicare for All bills have been amended to add certain chronic home and community-based services, it would not create linkages between acute medical care and Medicaid long-term care as many Medicare and Medicaid managed care plans are doing. The coordination is essential as America ages.

Another recent study from the Better Medicare Alliance finds that MA plans serve Medicare beneficiaries with more social risk factors compared with traditional Medicare. These risk factors, known as social determinants, may be greater predictors of health outcomes than underlying disease states themselves. Social determinants can be a number of different things, including socio-economic status, financial security, food security, housing status, health literacy, and more.[21-7]

The study also found that more than half of MA enrollees below the poverty line are in racial or ethnic minorities compared with 42% in traditional Medicare FFS. The study notes that this higher penetration of racial and ethnic minorities in MA continues even as income rises above the poverty level—31% in MA and 20% for FFS for the grouping from 100% to 199% of the poverty line.[21-7]

MA enrollees have lower levels of education and likely greater health literacy barriers—19% of MA enrollees and about 13% of FFS enrollees had less than a high school degree. Greater percentages of MA enrollees than FFS enrollees had food security issues and a primary language other than English.[21-7]

Perhaps the best testament to the program is how members feel. In a 1,200-member survey undertaken by the Better Medicare Alliance, respondents showed overwhelming support for MA, including record satisfaction in the following areas:[21-8]

- ○ Coverage (98%)
- ○ Networks (97%)
- ○ Plans performance during the COVID-19 crisis (98%)
- ○ Telehealth (91%)
- ○ Simplicity of the enrollment process (71%)

Ninety-five percent said it was important or very important to have a choice of plans other than traditional Medicare.[21-8]

MA is a Lucrative Health Plan Market

MA is growing and is a huge focus of insurers. While the health plan and insurance sector is robust and growing generally, there is no question that health plans are flocking to offer MA benefits given its unique value proposition. It is by far the most lucrative area for health insurers to enter. I noted several times that in early 2021 MA served over 43% of all Medicare beneficiaries. By 2025, that could hit 50%, and between 2030 and 2040 that could hit 70%.

The Kaiser Family Foundation (KFF) tells us why MA is the line of business to be in for health plans via a tremendous analysis regarding medical expenses and gross margins in various lines of business.[21-9]

> The three healthcare markets looked at were the 22 million strong MA market, the 14 million individual market (on-Exchange and off-Exchange) and the over 30 million group market (these are the truly insured products and does not include any self-insured ERISA plans).

> Kaiser looked at two financial bellwethers, the simple medical loss ratio (MLR) and annual gross margins. The data are averages from 2016 to 2018. To refresh, an MLR is the percentage of premiums spent on claims or medical expense. A gross margin is the amount by which premiums exceed claims costs per enrollee per year.

> Simple MLRs were the following for the period defined: MA (86%), individual market (84%), and group market (84%).

> The results make sense as the new minimum MLR requirements for individual and small group in the commercial world are mandated at 80% or 85%. In MA, the mandate is 85%. Note that the KFF did not calculate MLR per regulatory requirements. Thus, the word "simple."

> Annual gross margins were $1,608 for MA, $779 for the individual market, and $855 for the group market.

> While percentage MLRs are about the same for the three healthcare markets, gross margins in MA are about twice as much as in individual or group. This is because Medicare premiums are very high compared with

the commercial world. As such, the same MLR can derive very different gross margins. Here is a quick, simple example to demonstrate this:

- ○ Product A (proxy for MA): MLR 85%; Annual Premium Revenue $10,000; Annual Gross Margin = $1,500
- ○ Product B (proxy for commercial): MLR 85%; Annual Premium Revenue $5,000; Annual Gross Margin = $750

Since 2006, gross margins for MA have always exceeded the other two markets. KFF notes that gross margins vary across all three markets, including MA. KFF found significant variability in annual gross margins for MA plans, with 5-10% of plans even losing money in MA. While KFF did not elaborate much here, this is likely due to a number of reasons. There are significant revenue variances throughout the United States. Regions with lower FFS rates (upon which MA rates are partially based) could have lower gross margins unless the market is very efficient. New plans tend to have less experience and lower Star ratings than veteran ones. This not only impacts medical expense but overall revenue. CMS data consistently show how tenure means a lot to success in the MA world.

The KFF study makes it clear that MA is the place to be for health plans for a number of reasons. Premiums are high and they likely will remain so as long as the inefficient FFS world drives rates. Membership will grow as America ages and smart consumers realize the value proposition of MA compared with the traditional Medicare system. Plans seem to be getting the hang of the Star program, especially large and sophisticated ones, and this should drive revenue even more.

A cautionary note, though—the Star program is becoming much more complex with the introduction of very comprehensive clinical measures that monitor for episodes of care and transitions rather than just individual events or disease states. Plans cannot rest on their laurels and take for granted past and recent success. While plans can have low margins and even go into the red, the high-rate structure, coupled with Star premium revenue, should yield plans that do it right margins that are at least double of what they can be in most commercial products and the Medicaid line.

One last note on where MA growth is coming from. While there remains robust growth for the HMO product as plans continue to advertise their value proposition in more urban markets, a great deal of growth is also coming from the PPO product. For 2021, over 60% of MA enrollees are in traditional HMO products, with the remainder in PPOs. From January 2020 to January 2021, enrollment growth was basically evenly split between HMO and PPO products.

This product is attractive to wealthier individuals who face the healthcare cost crunch as they retire as well as for those who reside in more suburban and even rural markets.

I expect this trend to continue.

CHAPTER 22

Special Needs Plans

I n Chapter 18, I told you about dual eligibles. You can go back to that chapter for all the details. But here is a brief refresher on these individuals to help facilitate your understanding of special needs plans (SNPs) in Medicare Advantage (MA).

Dual eligibles are individuals who are eligible for both Medicare (because they are elderly or disabled) *and* Medicaid (because they have low income). There are full dual eligibles, who receive all Medicaid benefits, and partial dual eligibles, who only receive some benefits under Medicaid.

Dual eligibles tend to be much sicker than most other Medicaid and Medicare recipients. While the Medicare profile is much sicker, because of the age and disability of enrollees, dual eligibles usually are far more fragile medically than Medicare's overall cohort. For example, they tend to have multiple co-morbidities or complex conditions. They also tend to be impacted by social determinants of health or socio-economic factors that impact health outcomes.

Dual eligibles numbered about 12 million in 2017, or 20% of the Medicare population and 15% of the Medicaid population. However, they represented 34% and 33% of Medicare and Medicaid *spending*, respectively.[22-1]

Why Special Needs Plans Exist

So, with this brief refresher in mind, let's talk about why MA SNPs exist. They are very much driven by the fact that dual eligibles as well as a subset of other MA enrollees drive a disproportionate share of Medicaid's and Medicare's medical costs. While SNPs did not enjoy great support from the Centers for Medicare and Medicaid Services (CMS) and policymakers early on, they have since become endorsed thoroughly by the healthcare community.

Over time, SNPs should serve as the primary vehicle to begin merging Medicare and Medicaid funding streams for dual eligibles—and simplifying the process for them. As it is today, if a dual eligible is not in a SNP, they are fighting to access healthcare in two different systems with disparate rules. Given what often can be low health literacy for dual eligibles, the battle is that much greater for them.

SNPs will serve as a way to better coordinate care between the two programs. As I told you earlier, Medicare is usually primary for acute medical care, but Medicaid can be primary for long-term care *and* some other services. In today's environment, if you are not in a SNP, your care is not coordinated for acute episodes when you access both Medicare and Medicaid or between acute and long-term care—where Medicaid is the largest funder. As a result, the quality of care suffers.

SNPs serve as the best way to bend the cost curve. With better coordination of the funding and care coordination, the hope is that absolute dollar spending and inflationary trends for dual eligibles' and other high-cost MA enrollees' healthcare will come down over time.

So, what exactly is a SNP?

It is a type of plan within the overall MA program. CMS has added regulatory and clinical responsibilities to MA plans, given the fact that they serve far more complex members. All the standard regulatory and clinical requirements in an MA program also apply to SNPs.

Some SNPs can enroll members who are *not* dual eligibles. It is also true, though, that dual eligibles tend to dominate these products.

While most non-SNP plans offer additional benefits, CMS requires various enhanced coverage elements in order to qualify as a SNP. These include no or lower cost-sharing, closing the inpatient services gap in traditional Medicare, and longer coverage periods for specialty medical services such as acute skilled nursing and home healthcare.[22-2]

In addition, CMS requires that SNPs include enhanced mental health benefits and services; enhanced preventive health benefits such as dental, vision, and hearing; as well as social services—to address social determinant or social-economic barriers. They must also include transportation services and wellness and care management programs to prevent the progression of chronic conditions.[22-2]

There are three types of SNPs as noted below. In all three, the SNP is supposed to design benefits and services, including care coordination, to meet the unique needs of the individuals.

While SNPs are most commonly health maintenance organizations (HMOs) with network coverage only, they can also be preferred provider organizations (PPOs) with in-network and out-of-network benefits.

In addition to the standard enrollment rules for MA, plans must ensure members meet the specific requirements of the SNP, either meeting the Medicaid eligibility or specific clinical requirements. A SNP must also have Part D prescription drug coverage included.

The bidding and application process for a program to offer a SNP plan is basically the same as that of a regular MA plan, but it must also show how it meets the enhanced regulatory, benefit, and clinical requirements.

One enhanced requirement is the filing and approval of a SNP model of care (MOC). CMS has designated the National Committee for Quality Assurance (NCQA) as the policy body and approver of MOCs. Each MOC filing must meet a certain grade requirement and show how it meets and promotes the health and quality outcomes of the members' specific needs. The submission has both clinical and non-clinical requirements, depending on the type of SNP being offered.

SNPs are a fast-growing plan offering for a number of reasons. First the number of dual eligibles is growing in America and will continue to increase due to population growth and the aging demographic. Second, the costs of dual eligibles are much higher than the broader Medicare population. In Medicare, the financing scheme provides for positive adjustments to the demographic portion of the member rate for dual eligibles. In my work running Medicare plans, this seemed to equate to an add-on of 15% or more. And risk scores derived from clinical disease states drive even more revenue for dual eligibles and SNP enrollees.

MA plans make profit by driving down the cost of care for basic benefits. While duals and SNP members can mean greater risk, it also can mean enhanced margins for plans that implement a solid operating model.

CMS is pushing SNP growth—now that it is satisfied that the entities are accountable and driving quality. Various demonstrations, including the Medicare-Medicaid Plan (MMP) one referred to at the end of this chapter, are driving such growth.

In addition, plans are attracted to both the Medicaid and Medicare markets, given similar demographics of many enrollees and the ability to leverage networks and clinical operations. Dual eligibles are the critical link here.

Dual Eligible SNPs (D-SNPs)

In this type of SNP, eligibility is based solely on the member's status as both eligible for Medicare and Medicaid. You must be in one of the dual eligible categories—either partial or full—in order to enroll. Full duals are about 71% of all dual eligibles, with partials being about 29%.[22-1]

New laws and regulations require SNPs to work collaboratively with state Medicaid agencies in order to coordinate the provision of Medicare and Medicaid benefits.

In order to have a D-SNP in a given state, an MA plan must enter into a contract with the state Medicaid agency. The state Medicaid agency dictates the types of dual eligibles (see Chapter 18) that can enroll in the MA plan's SNPs in that state. There are a number of iterations and it gets very complex. States may allow a number of SNPs in their states covering various types of dual eligibles. In addition, MA D-SNPs must confirm the dual eligibility status on enrollment for each member and each month thereafter.

CMS had previously passed a rule mandating that MA SNP plans have financial and clinical integration with state Medicaid agencies, but it backed away to allow lesser forms of integration and stronger coordination models. In time, it likely will mandate full integration as the most efficient and effective model.

Below are various D-SNP models that exist today. Generally speaking, these fit into two broad categories—coordinated SNPs and integrated SNPs. A plan may coordinate cost-sharing and Medicaid benefits (usually with the state Medicaid agency's fee-for-service [FFS] program) as well as various clinical aspects, such as inpatient admissions and transitions of care. In some cases, the Medicaid benefit can be furnished by a different health plan's Medicaid managed care plan, which must be coordinated with a D-SNP.

In a more integrated approach, a plan may also receive capitation and cover—either directly or through a related plan—the Medicare cost-sharing covered by Medicaid for certain dual eligibles. Care management coordination also applies here. In addition, a plan may receive capitation and cover—either directly or through a related plan—this cost-sharing as well as other (but not all) Medicaid benefits. Care management coordination also applies in this situation.

The most integrated approaches are the following:

Fully integrated dual eligible SNP (FIDE SNP). This is slightly different than just being integrated with a state Medicaid agency as noted previously. In this case, the plan fully contracts and integrates with the state Medicaid agency to directly furnish all acute and chronic medical and long-term care services that the member qualifies for in each program. In some cases, a plan can be a FIDE SNP if it is in charge of some long-term care (LTC) services and coordinates any that are carved out. As of this writing, about 11% of D-SNP enrollment was in FIDE

SNPs. This allows the greatest care management coordination between the two programs possible.[22-2, 22-3]

Under the Bipartisan Budget Act of 2018, a cousin of the FIDE SNPs was created, known as a **highly integrated dual eligible SNP** (HIDE SNP). In this case, a health plan does not offer all Medicaid benefits, including long-term care and/or behavioral health services, within the MA plan. However, it does offer such services within a Medicaid plan of the same or a related entity. This allows for a high level of care management coordination.[22-3]

Chronic Condition SNPs (C-SNPs) [22-2]

C-SNPs are SNPs that seek to foster better care and quality for those with specific disease states or conditions. The idea is that by bringing people with common disease states or conditions together in one plan, benefits and services can be better targeted to meet unique needs of these individuals.

An individual does not have to be a dual eligible to enroll in a C-SNP, but many enrollees are. They prefer to be in a plan that focuses on their disease states or conditions rather than their dual eligible status.

CMS has outlined fifteen disease states or conditions for which MA plans can set up C-SNPs. As of this writing in early 2021, they include:

- Chronic alcohol and other drug dependence
- Certain autoimmune disorders
- Cancer
- Certain cardiovascular disorders
- Chronic heart failure
- Dementia
- Diabetes
- End-stage liver disease
- End-stage renal disease (ESRD)
- Certain severe hematologic disorders

- ○ HIV/AIDS
- ○ Certain chronic lung disorders
- ○ Certain chronic mental health disorders
- ○ Certain neurologic disorders
- ○ Stroke

C-SNPs should have enhanced benefits, networks, and cost-sharing specific to the disease states and conditions.

While it is quite common to have free-standing C-SNPs for a given disease grouping, CMS also allows plans to group certain disease states above into one CSNP plan. This is usually done for conditions that occur as co-morbid conditions in an individual. Some of these have been published for pre-approval, while others would take specific CMS approval.

MA C-SNPs must verify that individuals have requisite disease states on enrollment, either through member assessments or by contacting providers.

Institutional SNPs [22-2]

Institutional SNPs serve beneficiaries who have had or are expected to need the level of services provided in the following facilities for ninety days or longer. These include LTC facilities, including skilled nursing facilities (SNF), LTC nursing facilities (NF) and those with both levels of care (LTC SNF/NF). They also include intermediate care facilities (ICF) for the developmentally disabled and inpatient psychiatric facilities.

Upon enrollment, prospective enrollees do not have to be in such a facility for ninety days or longer. They can also be assessed to determine that individuals are at risk of such institutionalization.

A Medicare beneficiary does not have to be a dual eligible to enroll in an I-SNP, but many I-SNP enrollees do qualify for dual status.

Generally speaking, the goal of I-SNPs is to manage the overall acute care of these institutional or at-risk individuals in conjunction with their institutional or community long-term care provider. Many of the individuals are receiving long-term care coverage through Medicaid. The I-SNP must have an enrollee's facility or provider in its network. The model of care (MOC) filing provides for coordination of services with that facility or provider.

Medicare-Medicaid Plans (MMPs)

The Affordable Care Act (ACA) also created the Medicare-Medicaid Coordination Office within the CMS. One program created includes three-party contracts between CMS, a given state Medicaid agency, and a health plan in order to fully integrate the Medicare and Medicaid acute care funding. In some states, Medicaid long-term care is being included in the demonstration as well. These are called Medicare-Medicaid Plans (MMPs). These act much like FIDE or HIDE D-SNPs. They are subject to all of the general SNP requirements, all of the specific D-SNP requirements, and additional requirements laid out in the contract related to Medicaid in a given state.

All told, I see MA SNPs as a critical part of health reform moving forward. These SNPs enroll some of the most vulnerable and expensive populations—those who account for a disproportionate share of medical costs. Dual eligibles lay at the intersection of our two largest government programs. Cost reduction and quality outcomes must be a top priority if we are to fundamentally reform healthcare.

CHAPTER 23

The Medicare Part D Drug Benefit

W
e have arrived at the last chapter explaining the Medicare benefit. We have left the most complicated part—the recently added Medicare Part D drug benefit for last. So, let's get acquainted with the program.

Since its founding, Medicare has always been an important program for seniors. However, many seniors had a hard time affording their health coverage because retail drugs—those you get from the pharmacy—were not covered. This problem became especially acute as the use of prescription drugs increased over the years and prices for many pharmaceuticals leapt dramatically.

This has had numerous implications, including stories of seniors going without food and other basic needs because of the high cost of medications. Seniors also halved their drug supplies or skipped their drugs on certain days, reducing the efficacy or negating the benefits of the drug regimen. Seniors even ended up in high-cost emergency rooms or were admitted to a hospital because chronic disease states were not being managed or were exacerbated.

This led to the addition of the Part D benefit. The program was created in 2003 by the Medicare Modernization Act (MMA) under the George W. Bush

Administration. (Wow, a Republican expanded a social welfare program.) The program went live on January 1, 2006, a relatively speedy launch and in which I am proud to say I played a small part. Appointed by then-Department of Health and Human Services Secretary Tommy Thompson, I served on a federal commission that advised the administration on the integration of Part D with many existing state drug assistance programs that operated at the time. Some states continue to operate these programs and they wrap around the Part D benefit.

The program was not without its detractors—some arguing it was a massive expansion of a government entitlement, others stating it did not go far enough, and still others deeming it a giveaway to pharmaceutical companies and health plans. It also passed in close votes in each chamber of Congress, in great measure along party lines in the U.S. House and slightly less so in the U.S. Senate. In this case, Republicans controlled both chambers and championed the bill.

The policy argument in favor of establishing a Part D drug benefit is quite simple. While drugs can be expensive, not covering them can be even more so. Providing a reasonably comprehensive retail drug benefit will ultimately reduce overall health expenditures in Medicare by keeping chronic health conditions in check and reducing higher-cost services from occurring.

By any measure, the program has been successful. While drug costs continue to increase, overall inflation in the Part D program has been temperate. Enrollees have had low average monthly premiums. Premium increases were less than 4% on average from 2006 to 2018 and program costs were 45% below initial forecasts, or $350 billion less than the Congressional Budget Office's (CBO) estimate. In recent years, average nationwide premiums actually dropped, although they may increase in 2022. [23-1]

However, costs are beginning to outpace overall Medicare costs, leading to demands for drug price negotiation in the program. Over time, legislation has passed to reduce some of the costs that seniors pay. Finally, while Part D passage was not universally popular at the time, it enjoys widespread support today.[23-1, 23-2, 23-3]

While overall Medicare costs continue to rise, it is hard to argue that supplying a retail drug benefit hasn't reduced other costs, including inpatient and other high-cost services in Medicare. While the verdict is still out due to the short tenure of the program, some studies are already validating the savings. As noted, by providing drugs and driving medication adherence, other costs and services are being reduced. A 2014 National Bureau of Economic Research study found that Medicare Part D coverage led to an 8% reduction in hospital admission and about $1.5 billion in hospital-cost savings. Another study found that the Part D program led to a $2.6 billion reduction in overall medical expenditures annually for those with congestive heart failure who did not have prior drug coverage.[23-1]

Let's look at the Part D benefit and program more closely. The benefit is confined to what are known as retail drugs—the ones you get from a pharmacy. Remember that there are medical benefit drugs—those administered in a doctor's office or other facilities—and a few retail drugs that were always part of the original Medicare Part B program dating back to the 1960s. Unlike Part B, however, the Part D benefit is exclusively provided by private managed care plans.

One thing to know is that the Part D drug benefit spans both the Medicare Advantage (MA) program and traditional Medicare fee-for-service (FFS). There are four ways a person can obtain Medicare Part D coverage:

The senior or disabled individual is in the traditional Medicare FFS program and enrolls in a free-standing private managed care plan known as a Part D Prescription Drug Plan (Part D PDP or simply PDP). While the person obtains their medical benefits in FFS, the retail prescription drug benefit is obtained from the Part D plan. The PDP will reject coverage for medical or the small number of retail drugs covered under the Part B benefit and will send them back to the FFS program.

The senior or disabled individual is enrolled in an MA plan that does not provide Part D coverage. These are the so-called MA-Only plans. In this case, the individual is allowed to enroll in a free-standing PDP to get retail benefits. The MA-Only plans provide medical benefits, including the Part B medical and certain retail drugs, while the PDP covers the retail drug component.

The senior or disabled individual is enrolled in a Medicare Advantage-Part D (MA-PD plan), which has Parts A, B, and D under one roof. The individual receives all his or her medical and drug benefits from this one plan.

There are also employer group waiver plans (EGWPs) that also offer Part D benefits. There are MA-PD EGWPs, where an employer retiree plan has secondary coverage that "wraps around" the Medicare benefit for both medical and retail drugs. The retiree coverage provides enhanced coverage compared with the Part D benefit, offsetting some of the premiums, deductibles, and cost-sharing in the program. The EGWP plan receives funding from the federal government and retiree plan and crafts a benefit combining the Part D benefit and the extra benefits of the retiree plan. Retirees are only charged the remaining amounts for premiums, deductibles, and cost-sharing. There are PDP EGWPs, where an employer drug benefit wraps around the Part D free-standing retail drug benefit only.

In 2021, according to the Kaiser Family Foundation (KFF), about 48 million people took advantage of the Part D program. (As of September 2021, my calculation from available MA and PDP enrollment on the CMS website suggests that about 49 million had Part D coverage, with 24.9 million in MA-PDs and 24.1 million in PDPs.)[23-4]

The Part D program is voluntary. However, if you want it you must enroll on time for your Part D drug benefit (usually at age sixty-five). If you do not, you pay a monthly premium penalty for the rest of your life when you do sign up. You may defer coverage at age sixty-five if you are covered by another plan as an employee. You sign up for Part D with a private plan and pay a premium each month for coverage if in a PDP. If you are in an MA-PD plan, there is usually a consolidated premium, which could be as low as zero dollars per month. In addition, co-pays and cost-sharing are paid for each drug.

You generally enroll in Part D upon your initial enrollment in Medicare, and if you want to change plans, between October 15 and December 7 of each year thereafter.

MA-PD plans contract with the CMS to provide Part D coverage in health maintenance organizations (HMOs), preferred provider organizations (PPOs), and other products in counties and certain PPOs in regions. In contrast, PDPs apply to CMS to provide coverage in regions. In 2022, there are thirty-four regions, most of which were states or territories but in some cases groups of states. Individuals enrolling in Part D PDPs had between nineteen and twenty-seven plan choices.[23-4]

When the Part D program was adopted, the vast majority of prescription drug coverage was migrated from Medicaid to Medicare for dual eligibles. There are a small number of drugs not covered by Medicare that are covered by Medicaid in some states. In addition, Medicaid may cover over-the-counter drugs. Dual eligibles still have access to these drugs through Medicaid.

As mentioned in the chapter on dual eligibles, people with low or modest incomes can tap into the Low-Income Subsidy (LIS) program, also known as Extra Help. This helps individuals pay for premiums and cost-sharing. As noted, this is the parallel in Part D of the Medicare Savings Program (MSP) that helps people afford cost-sharing, deductibles, and premiums for Parts A and B.

I will outline the LIS program in detail later. Individuals receiving the subsidy are generally enrolled in what are known as LIS benchmark plans. In 2022, individuals have a choice of between four and nine plans, depending on their state. About 13 million enrollees receive the subsidy. The LIS program is more generous than the MSP program, covering people to 150% of the federal poverty limit (FPL) and with cost-sharing support for everyone (whereas MSP only covers premium support for some groups). Those who have certain MSP statuses are auto-enrolled in the LIS program.[23-4]

The Part D benefit is subsidized by the federal government as are much of the other parts of Medicare. In this case, the government pays for about 75% of overall costs (through funding to MA-PDs and PDPs) of the Part D standard benefit outlined in law, with individuals covering 25%.[23-4]

Each year, PDP plans bid to provide coverage in the regions as well as for benchmark status. Part of that bid process is setting a premium to be paid by all enrollees. I will get into more details about the benefit and financial structure of the program later. Suffice it to say that margins are limited in the Part D program; the federal government takes on a great deal of the risk. The base monthly premium in 2021 and 2022 for Part D is just over thirty-three dollars.[23-4]

The federal government also subsidizes employer prescription drug coverage as an incentive for those employers to continue to provide retirees drug coverage and not have them enroll in government plans. About 1.3 million individuals have employer-sponsored retiree plans with drug coverage that receive a subsidy from the federal government. For 2021, the employer gets about 28% of drug expenses between $480 and $9,850 per retiree.[23-4] The retiree plan has to be actuarially equivalent or better than the standard Part D benefit. The subsidy is up to the limit of the standard benefit.

When we discussed the pieces of the healthcare pie, I told you that retail prescription drugs are about 10% of total healthcare expenditures. In Medicare Part D that is somewhat higher—about 15% of net Medicare outlays (after individual costs). This is because seniors tend to have more disease states and therefore more drugs and ones with greater expense.[23-4] If you account for drug spending in Part B, the overall percentage of Medicare spending on drugs jumps to about 19%. Another interesting statistic is that, with the adoption of the Part D program, Medicare's share of the nation's overall prescription drug spending has increased from 18% in 2006 to 30% in 2017.[23-5]

There are also entities known as State Pharmaceutical Assistance Programs (SPAPs) that generally pre-date the 2006 launch of the Part D benefit. These state-funded programs formerly helped subsidize retail drug benefits for seniors and the disabled when the Part D benefit did not exist. Since that time, some SPAP programs have been phased out, since there is a national program now. However, some continue to exist, and they wrap around the national benefit by offering additional coverage to seniors and the disabled by covering some of the Part D premium and cost-sharing. In the states where these exist, the roughly 25% of costs that individuals generally cover is reduced. Usually, someone must apply for LIS first before being eligible for SPAP benefits. There are about sixteen states today that offer SPAP programs, some to a broad population and others for those with specific disease states, such as HIV/AIDS.[23-6]

Part D Benefit Structure

Let's now get into more details about the Part D benefit structure. As I alluded to earlier, it gets quite complex so I will not be covering every nuance. Some of the information below comes from my work over the years at MA plans, preparing bids and benefit designs. It also comes from my examination of a very comprehensive site on Part D maintained by the Centers for Medicare Advocacy, a group dedicated to advocating for and educating the public on Medicare issues, among other government and private sites.[23-4, 23-7, 23-8, 23-9]

Who offers Medicare Part D coverage: As noted above, Part D comes from either a standalone PDP plan or through an MA-PD plan. Some employers get subsidized by the federal government if they offer independent retiree coverage for prescription drugs.

Benefits: The Part D program covers retail prescription drugs only. The Part B medical benefit covers medical drugs and certain retail drugs. In some cases, drugs may be covered in both the Part B and Part D program and plans must determine what part of Medicare the drug should be covered under. This is called a Part B versus D determination. A good example: certain retail anti-nausea drugs are covered under Part B for those undergoing cancer treatment. At the same time, anti-nausea drugs may be covered under Part D for other disease states or conditions. In this case a B versus D determination would ascertain whether the anti-nausea drug is being prescribed due to ongoing cancer treatment. If so, it would be covered under the member's Part B benefit. If not, it would fall under the Part D benefit. The drug may still need to be prior authorized or reviewed for other utilization management (UM) requirements once the correct part of the Medicare program is determined.

There are some retail drugs that are excluded from the Part D benefit, but in some cases, plans can cover them as part of their administrative allocation. Good examples include over-the-counter, non-prescription medications as well as erectile dysfunction drugs (unless they are tied to an underlying disease state).

The standard benefit: There is a national standard benefit that Part D is based on, but most plans deviate from this and generally enhance the benefit. These are known as alternative and enhanced plans. The standard benefit has a fixed deductible that inflates each year. For 2021, the standard deductible was $445. After the deductible, the coverage is generally a 25%/75% split between the individual and government, respectively, for the initial coverage limit (ICL) phase, although plans can use co-pays as opposed to co-insurance.

The stages of Part D coverage: Part D was initially constructed to limit costs and therefore has an odd benefit structure. It has four phases. Note that those receiving a low-income subsidy (LIS) or Extra Help do not really have a true coverage gap phase. The stages are as follows:

- ○ **Phase 1—Deductible:** The member must meet any annual deductible in the plan design before any drugs are paid for by the plan. Some plans now design benefits to reduce or eliminate the deductible or not apply the deductible to generic tiers of the benefit. In 2021, the standard deductible was $445.
- ○ **Phase 2—Initial Coverage Limit (ICL):** In this phase, the plan and member share in costs until such time that a plan's outlays (not counting member cost-sharing) hit the ICL. For 2021, the standard ICL was $4,130 in plan costs. The cost-sharing here is dictated by the tier the drug is on and is usually a combination of flat dollar co-pays and percentage co-insurance. Some plans may increase the ICL in their benefit design under an enhanced benefit. Many plans offer zero dollars for the lowest, generic tier as well as sometimes all generic tiers.
- ○ **Phase 3—Coverage Gap or Donut Hole:** When someone enters this phase, they have much higher out-of-pocket outlays. In general, members are offered a discount on both generic and brand drugs from drugmakers and plans now have some required

outlays in the donut hole. For 2021, members received a 75% discount for brand drugs: 70% from the drugmakers and 5% from plans. For 2021, members received a 75% discount for generics, all from plans. Members exit the coverage gap when their true out of pocket costs hit $6,550 in 2021. (This amount jumped in 2020 due to expiration of a law that limited annual changes to the out-of-pocket threshold.) However, it is not exactly true that members pay that much out-of-pocket because the discounts on brands covered by drugmakers during the coverage gap are deemed spent by members along with actual member outlays. Subsidies from SPAPs, AIDS drug assistance programs and a few other categories count toward out-of-pocket spending as well. So, members hit the threshold more quickly. It is important to remember that members with LIS do not really have a coverage gap phase. They continue to pay the cost-sharing they did in the ICL phase.

Note that some plans are subsidizing drug costs in the coverage gap (for example, by eliminating co-pays on some generics). One last note: the coverage gap or donut hole phase was very large when Part D was initially launched. It was a huge financial burden for enrollees. A series of bills were passed to close the so-called donut hole to arrive at where we are today.

- **Phase 4—Catastrophic:** Once a person hits the catastrophic phase, most members pay only flat co-pays for all drugs. For non-LIS enrollees, in the catastrophic phase, members pay about 5% of total drug costs. The federal government and plans pay the rest. The government covers about 80% of the costs in this phase. LIS members already pay low co-pays in the ICL and coverage gap. When they enter the catastrophic phase, their costs are either eliminated or reduced.

For non-LIS members, in 2021, catastrophic co-pays for generic and preferred multi-source drugs were either 5% or $3.70—whichever is greater. For all other drugs, it is either 5% or $9.20—whichever is greater. Some plans even reduce costs to zero in the catastrophic phase for generics.

How does someone keep track of all of this and know where they are on this complex drug-spend journey? It is not easy, so the federal government has what is known as the true, out-of-pocket cost facilitator. This entity is connected with the pharmacy benefit manager (PBM) of each plan and is in charge of tracking and calculating with the PBM where a member is for each phase and what the cost-sharing should be for each drug purchase. This is quite important, since a member could have made a drug purchase that pushes them into the next stage and actual cost-sharing could be calculated in two different phases. This is known as a straddle claim.

In addition, members receive a Part D explanation of benefits (EOB), which shows monthly drug spending, cost-sharing, and where the member is on their phased Part D drug journey.

How do plans control costs? Plans use a variety of managed care practices to reduce costs and promote efficiency. I have discussed many of these in prior chapters, but some are specific to the Part D program.

The first involves the establishment of formularies and tiers. Formularies are drug lists that compose the covered drugs for a given plan. The Center for Medicare and Medicaid Services (CMS) mandates that PDPs and MA-PDs cover a broad range of drugs, including a minimum number in given categories. However, the actual drugs covered may be different from plan to plan, given pricing deals that plans may arrive at with drugmakers. So, consumers need to pick their plans wisely. Limiting access to certain drugs on a drug list or formulary should promote the use of the most cost-effective drugs for disease states and limit overall costs. Plans place drugs on various tiers and offer lower cost-sharing for the use of the most cost-effective drugs. Plans generally have three to five tiers, with the most expensive drugs usually on the higher tiers. Higher tiers often have percentage co-insurance, while those on lower tiers usually have fixed dollar co-pays. Cheaper generics are usually on lower tiers while most expensive brands are on higher tiers. This encourages the use of lower cost generics.

Another cost control practice involves prior authorization, step therapy, and quantity limits. Plans are allowed to put what we define as utilization management (UM) restrictions or edits on drugs to promote the use of the most cost-effective and efficacious drugs. Some drugs might require approval by the plan before their use (prior authorization). Others may require members try less costly drugs before another drug is allowed (step therapy). Still others may have quantity limits, and a member needs to seek approval to go over dosage amounts. UM changes usually occur at the beginning of each year but can change monthly with CMS approval based on new drug introductions. The CMS does not allow prior authorization of certain categories of drugs, known as protected classes (e.g., HIV/AIDS drugs).

There are exceptions. To protect consumers, Part D does require plans to allow members to petition the plan to cover a drug that may not be on the list. The plan must then determine whether the drug is needed for the individual's health despite not being on the set drug list or formulary.

CMS also requires plans to adjust cost-sharing if a given drug is necessary for a member's health and the cost is too high for the individual. In essence, plans need to determine if they will grant the member lower cost-sharing as if the drug were on a lower tier.

To protect individuals from the effects of changing established drug regimens without thorough medical review, CMS requires plans to offer what is known as a drug transition policy. If a formulary changes from year to year or a member changes plans, plans must cover at least a thirty-day or longer supply of the current drug so that the member can work with his or her doctor for a prior authorization, step therapy, or an exception to maintain the same drug.

As with MA and other lines of business, members have grievance rights and multiple levels of appeals if drugs are denied or not covered. Plans may also establish pharmacy networks and negotiate drug-by-drug discounts. Members can receive a thirty-day supply at a network pharmacy and a ninety-day supply at preferred network pharmacies or mail-order pharmacies at reduced prices. In addition, as a safeguard, CMS requires a thirty-day supply at an out-of-network pharmacy.

PDPs and MA-PDs also practice a great deal of clinical oversight of their members' drug utilization to improve quality and reduce overall costs in Medicare. Many of these are required of a Part D plan. This may include medication therapy management, where a member with high drug costs are identified and offered periodic medication reviews to ensure medication adherence and safety. It may also include monitoring for opioids and other addictive drugs and high-risk medications, as well as drug utilization reviews—to identify safety and interaction issues—and medication adherence monitoring.

Part D Low Income Subsidy (LIS) or Extra Help

As noted previously, those with low incomes receive an additional subsidy from the federal government to help pay for premiums and cost-sharing. The subsidy does not go directly to the member but is included in plan payments and plans must only charge LIS members according to the premium and cost-sharing rules of the LIS component of the program.

Generally speaking, individuals are eligible if they earn up to 150% of the federal poverty limit (FPL) for their family size. As also noted, there is a close association between the LIS and Medicare savings programs (MSP), which offers similar cost-sharing reductions and protections on the medical side. The MSP program is actually part of the Medicaid program for dual eligibles, where Medicaid covers premiums, deductibles, and cost-sharing for Parts A and B. The LIS program exists because retail drug coverage was moved from the Medicaid program to the Medicare program for all dual eligibles when Part D was created.

As with the MSP program, there are full and partial subsidies based on income. MSP dual eligibles and a few other categories that are not dual eligible are "deemed"—automatically granted an LIS status and they do not have to apply for such coverage. Others have to apply to obtain the LIS benefit.

There are four LIS subsidy status levels. These actually do not go in numerical order and are in order below from most generous to least. [23-4, 23-8, 23-10, 23-11] (Leave it to government to make it complicated.)

LIS Level 3—Individuals at this level are full dual eligibles. They are on Medicaid either in an institution or on a home- and community-based waiver program (such as home care) to avoid institutionalization. They have no premium, no deductible, and no cost-sharing in Part D.

LIS Level 2—This is the next most generous level if you are not institutionalized or at risk of institutionalization. These are full dual eligibles in the community with income under 100% of federal poverty limit (FPL). They have no premium, no deductible, and small, set co-pays per drug. In 2021, the co-pays were between $1.30 and $4.00, depending on the drug. There are no costs once the catastrophic phase is hit.

LIS Level 1—This includes those with higher incomes than Level 2. These are full dual eligibles with incomes between 100-135% of FPL and non-duals with incomes below 135% with low assets. They have no premium, no deductible, and small set co-pays per drug. In 2021, the co-pays were between $3.70 and $9.20, depending on the drug. There are no costs once the catastrophic phase is hit.

LIS Level 4—These are the highest income and asset individuals to receive LIS. Non-dual individuals have incomes less than 135% of FPL but with higher assets than Level 1, or are those with incomes below 150% with limited assets. Some individuals have no premium and others have a sliding-scale premium based on income. In 2021, these individuals had a ninety-two-dollar annual deductible. In 2021, their cost-sharing was co-insurance of 15% per drug. When the catastrophic phase hits, co-pays are either $3.70 or $9.20. These individuals must apply to receive LIS support.

Part D Financing/Rate Structure

I won't go into great detail about Part D's financing and rate structure, but here are a few key points. Margins in the Part D business are heavily regulated.

In addition, the government does take on a great deal of risk in terms of funding catastrophic costs and over-expenditures by plans.[23-4, 23-9, 23-12]

The Part D bid and financing is free-standing. As an example, even if an MA plan includes the Part D benefit in its offering, the Part D bid is technically a separate bid. However, MA plans are allowed to use part of the Part C premium rebate savings it gets (as described in an earlier chapter) to add to Part D benefits by reducing premiums, deductibles, and cost-sharing as well as enhancing the benefit. But technically, this happens on the Part C bid side.

The Centers for Medicare and Medicaid Services (CMS) pays plans for the standard benefit offering. An alternative benefit has to be actuarially equivalent to the standard benefit. Enhanced benefits are funded from savings the plan brings in offering the standard benefit.

CMS pays plans roughly 75% for the standard benefit. The remainder is financed by premiums paid by enrollees to the plan and cost-sharing paid by enrollees that reduce overall costs.

Actual rates are partially impacted by risk adjustment scores submitted by Part C plans or derived from FFS system claims. These risk scores were explained earlier. They are a major part of Part C funding but constitute much less of Part D funding.

Plans are also given additional premiums for the number and types of LIS enrollees they have. As noted above, this premium goes to offset premiums, deductibles, and cost-sharing for these low-income individuals.

Enrollees with high incomes must pay an additional premium. Plans are responsible to collect this (as opposed to in Part B where the government collects the premium) and it is deducted from their premiums paid by the government. In addition, any late enrollment penalties are also collected by the plan.

Plans also may receive prospective payments for two other areas. These may be reconciled after the conclusion of the applicable year. These are:

Reinsurance funding: These are the payments plans receive to fund 80% of the drug costs in the catastrophic phase. As I discussed, members pay about 5%, so plans are at risk only for about 15% of costs. Reinsurance costs to the government have steadily risen over time, from 14% in 2006 to 45% in 2020.

Risk corridor funding: Risk corridors are a standard insurance practice in many places and have been used since the 2006 launch in Part D. Risk corridors essentially limit overall profits and losses by having the federal government share in a piece of each. As profits or losses increase, the federal government takes a greater share. The current Part D corridors are set up as such:

- ○ If actual costs are between 95-105% of estimated costs from the bid, then plans shoulder all of the losses and keep all of the profits.
- ○ If actual costs are between 90-95%—or between 105-110%—of estimated costs from the bid, then the plan and the federal government share fifty-fifty in the loss or profit in that corridor. (This does not impact the first 5%, above.)
- ○ If actual costs are less than 90% or over 110% of estimated costs from the bid, then the federal government receives 80% of excess profits, or it pays for 80% of excess losses in that corridor. (This does not impact the first 10%, above.)

A number of proposals have already passed U.S. Congress to reduce the overall cost-sharing burden of Americans in Part D. At the same time, the sunsetting of a law that limited annual changes to the out-of-pocket threshold has caused the limit to jump from $5,100 in 2019 to $6,350 in 2020 (and to $6,550 in 2021). This will have an impact on non-LIS individuals with high drug costs, or about 2% of overall enrollment.[23-13]

Both sides of the political aisle have proposed changes to further reduce the spending and create incentives for plans to reduce drug costs in the program.

Thus far, nothing sweeping has occurred, although a series of proposals were moving through Congress at the time of this writing. Some proposals would eliminate cost-sharing in the catastrophic phase, cap the absolute amount enrollees would pay, and shift the amount the government pays in that phase to plans and drugmakers.[23-12, 23-13]

CHAPTER 24

The Medicaid Line of Business

O ver the years, Medicaid has become a polarizing subject in Washington. Many Democrats view Medicaid as their Holy Grail, but their no-holds-barred defense of anything government entitlement sometimes reminds me more of the comedic Monty Python version. Tinkering with it at all is sinful, no matter how much it needs reform. At the opposite end, many Republicans have a knee-jerk reaction to anything government-funded. If today's GOP were the rulers in the Orwellian novel *Animal Farm*, "Medicaid is Bad!" would be somewhere in the tenets of their "Seven Commandments of Animalism."

We'll address this polarizing subject in the next chapter. In the meantime, let me tell you all about the Medicaid program itself. I gave you some of the basics of the program in earlier chapters. Let's review some of that again and add additional details.

As we know, Medicaid was created in 1965 under President Johnson to serve poor and lower income citizens. It was created as Title XIX of the Social Security Act. As opposed to Medicare, the Medicaid program is a federal-state partnership. Nationally, the Centers for Medicare and Medicaid Services

(CMS) sets broad policies in terms of benefits and regulations for the program. Each state then has a Medicaid agency that creates and administers its specific state Medicaid program—with specific eligibility rules and covered benefits. Federal and state Medicaid expenditures in federal fiscal year 2018 were about $593 billion. The National Healthcare Expenditures website says Medicaid spending in 2019 was about $614 million. Medicaid enrollment statistics can be very confusing and disparate. I like to use CMS statistics. In this case, for federal fiscal year 2020 (ended September 30, 2020), full-year equivalent or average monthly enrollment in Medicaid was 76.5 million Americans. We do know that only a portion of enrollment increases due to COVID are included in this number and enrollment continues to climb due to the pandemic. This means that enrollment in Medicaid and its companion State Children's Health Insurance Program (SCHIP) together is now well over 80 million.[24-1, 24-2, 24-3]

The state Medicaid agency must file a Medicaid State Plan with CMS, which outlines the Medicaid program, eligibility, and certain financing in that state. It also may file waiver applications, which free states of some of the federal rules or expand eligibility. Some of the primary waiver categories are the following (they are named for sections of the SSA):

1915(b) Managed Care Waivers[24-4]—While a state can take other routes to establish Medicaid managed care in their state—including a state plan amendment and 1915(a) waivers—most file these 1915(b) waivers in order to waive additional rules and enroll additional population categories in managed care, such as dual eligibles. The waiver of certain rules of the road in traditional Medicaid include:

- Allowing states to set up restrictive networks and requiring beneficiaries to seek care from these networks
- Establishing an enrollment broker
- Adding certain benefits to the program
- Contracting requirements
- Expansion of population groups subject to mandatory managed care enrollment

1915(c) Waivers[24-5]—These allow states to create home- and community-based programs under Medicaid, including home care, adult day care, assisted living, and certain facilities for those with developmental disabilities. Many of the same rules above are waived and states must ensure that:

- The home and community services are cost effective against providing such services in an institution.
- There are protections for people's health and welfare and that provider standards are in place.
- These programs follow an individualized and person-centered plan of care.
- There are more flexible eligibility rules.

1115 Waivers[24-4]—Section 1115 of the Social Security Act gives the federal secretary of the Department of Health and Human Services (HHS) broad authority to approve experimental, pilot, or demonstration projects.

If a state gains approval for an 1115 waiver, then it generally is obtaining additional waivers beyond what is granted in the 1915(b) approvals. While 1915(b) and (c) waivers are relatively easy to get, 1115 waivers go through a strict evaluation process and take some time to obtain. These generally amount to substantial reform in a given state.

Presidents of both parties have used the 1115 process for their own political purposes. Democrats use them to expand eligibility and benefits, and Republicans usually do so to lower costs, restrict benefits, or have residents—even at higher income levels—pay some small part of their healthcare costs. As an example, some conservative states have sought the authority to expand to certain income groups with premiums and cost-sharing, which traditionally are not part of the program. Or they want work requirements to obtain Medicaid. President Biden opposes this move, which was heavily endorsed by former President Trump. Biden is busy unwinding work requirements and related GOP restrictions in Medicaid.

At its core, the 1115 process is meant to expand eligibility to individuals who are not otherwise eligible for Medicaid as well as provide services not typically covered by Medicaid. The process is also meant to use innovative service delivery systems that improve care, increase efficiency, and reduce costs.

Let's talk a little about who and what the federal government says states must cover and the discretion states have to cover others and additional benefits.

There are core populations that every state must support if they are to be a part of the Medicaid program. In these cases, you cannot have waiting lists or enrollment caps. A person who meets the qualification is entitled to receive all of their Medicaid benefits. Individuals can become Medicaid eligible based on their individual or family income and assets, which is modified for certain amounts, especially if someone is seeking coverage for long-term care and has a spouse. They may also do so by qualification in other government programs or by past and future expected medical bills.

There are over two dozen mandatory Medicaid groups. These generally include:[24-6]

- o Low-income children
- o Certain low-income families
- o Certain pregnant women and children
- o The disabled who receive federal Supplemental Security Income (SSI). Those receiving SSI first go on primary Medicaid and after a period of time (usually twenty-four months for most people) move to Medicare for primary coverage and Medicaid for secondary coverage.
- o Other aged, blind, and disabled individuals
- o Certain low-income Medicare eligibles

In addition, there are over forty optional coverage groups that states can elect to extend Medicaid coverage to, including:[24-6]

- ○ Other low-income children and/or families
- ○ Higher-income pregnant women
- ○ Individuals at higher incomes receiving certain home- and community-based care
- ○ Women with breast cancer
- ○ Individuals at higher incomes with high medical bills (the medically needy or "spend-down" category)
- ○ Up to 133% of the federal poverty limit (FPL) per the Medicaid expansion provision of the Affordable Care Act (ACA). (This actually computes to about 138% of FPL due to income and related set-asides.)

As with eligibility groups, there are mandatory and optional benefits. Mandatory benefits include:[24-7]

- ○ Inpatient hospital services
- ○ Outpatient hospital services
- ○ A strict regulation known as early and periodic screening, diagnosis, and treatment (EPSDT) for children. Many states complain that this is an unfettered mandate that allows coverage of almost anything.
- ○ Nursing facility services
- ○ Home health services
- ○ Physician services
- ○ Laboratory tests and X-rays

Optional services include:[24-7]

- ○ Prescription drugs (covered by all states)
- ○ Therapies
- ○ Optometry and optical services and benefits
- ○ Dental services
- ○ Dentures
- ○ Prosthetics
- ○ Certain alternative medicine

Given the low-income status of its enrollees, Medicaid largely has little or no cost-sharing, barring a few dollars, at most, for a physician visit or drug co-pay in some states. In addition, given the expansion of Medicaid over the years to higher income levels, some states are experimenting with charging premiums and higher cost-sharing.

Like Medicare, Medicaid is an entitlement. If you qualify for the program based on the eligibility rules in the state in which you live, you gain coverage. As long as you continue to meet those requirements, you cannot be removed or lose your coverage. You have the benefit regardless of the budget situation (surplus or deficit) in a given state.

There are two exceptions to this rule. Your coverage can end if you are in a discretionary eligibility group that the state later removes from its program. A state also can set up waiting lists for certain waiver programs. (This means that you don't get the benefit and keep it until you reach the top of the waiting list.) Many are concerned that the entitlement nature of the program will prove unaffordable for the nation and states over time. More on this later.

Unlike Medicare (which is paid wholly by the federal government), the federal and state governments share in the cost of Medicaid, based on each state's relative wealth, based on the state's per capita income, with a federal share minimum or floor of 50% (about a dozen states are in this category).[24-8]

The amount paid by the federal government, known as the Federal Medical Assistance Percentage (FMAP), will peak at just over 78% for Mississippi, technically the poorest state, in federal fiscal year 2022. For the most part, the District of Columbia is treated as if it were a state in these calculations but has a set 70% point FMAP in statute right now. Territories are treated differently and generally receive capped allotments. For FFY 2020 through FY 2022, the allotments are about 55%, although congressional bills may change this percentage periodically. This is the case despite the fact that citizens of these territories can be poorer than those in Mississippi. Note that the federal government may temporarily increase FMAP for extraordinary circumstances. As an example, states, the District of Columbia, and territories have been paid a temporary extra 6.2% reimbursement due to the COVID-19 pandemic since FFY 2020.[24-8]

Of course, for the Medicaid expansion under the Affordable Care Act (ACA), the funding formulary was changed for the expansion population only. From 2014 to 2016, the federal government paid 100% of the costs of expansion populations. The percentage was phased down beginning in 2017 and beginning in 2020 it will stay at 90%. So, for those enrolled as part of the ACA Medicaid expansion, a state receives 90%, while other enrollees are reimbursed at their FMAP percentage.[24-9]

Historically, the federal government has funded an average of 57% of Medicaid funding, with states picking up 43% of the tab. With the higher ACA reimbursement for expansion populations, the federal share has changed. The expansion population in FFY 2017 was about 14% of spending. By my calculations, the federal share of Medicaid spending peaked at about 63% and will be above 61% for 2020 and beyond. This does not include the temporary COVID-19 pandemic increases.[24-9, 24-10, 24-11]

The vast majority of people on Medicaid are children and healthy women. While there are high costs for things like high-risk pregnancies and emergency room visits, such costs are fairly low, per person. On the flip side, a distinct minority of the Medicaid-covered population are aged, disabled, and those in institutions who have high costs per person and are responsible for the vast majority of costs. About two-thirds of all Medicaid spending goes toward the elderly and disabled, which comprise fewer than one-fourth of beneficiaries.[24-11]

States may operate their Medicaid program as a fee-for-service (FFS) system, where the state contracts with providers and pays them for services rendered to beneficiaries. Alternatively, as is the case in most states now, state Medicaid agencies typically contract with private managed care plans to provide Medicaid benefits. The plans do so in their own networks and usually take on financial risk from the state. In other cases, plans may be hired to operate the Medicaid system in a managed way, but the plan is paid on an administrative services only (ASO) basis and acts like a third-party administrator (TPA). The state keeps the financial risk, in whole or part. Today, about 70% of beneficiaries are in comprehensive Medicaid managed care plans, with about 80% being in some form of private Medicaid managed care. About half of all spending in Medicaid goes to managed care organizations to furnish services on behalf of the states.[24-11, 24-12, 24-13]

Medicaid managed care is booming despite the fact that margins are often low. Medicaid state actuaries tend to set margins at a miserly 2% or so. As state budget director in Connecticut, I, too, asked my actuaries to set as low a number as could be justified, given the always-tight state budget climate. However, managed care plans continue to flock to the program, given the following facts:

- Medicaid provides crucial membership numbers over which to spread built-in administrative costs.
- Medicare is a lucrative market for them. Increasingly, more and more Medicare recipients end up being dually eligible for both Medicare *and* Medicaid.
- A well-run Medicaid managed care plan can still make money through the law of large numbers.
- States are also moving higher-cost populations, such as the aged and disabled and the institutional or at-risk of institution populations into managed care. These members have much larger costs and plans believe they can reduce costs markedly here.

How do private Medicaid managed care plans get paid by the state Medicaid agency? Usually, the latter runs a periodic request for proposal (RFP) or bid process and invites participation by numerous health plans. These submit information to the state—such as their experience, networks, operational and quality processes, and financial information—in order to qualify. Contracts are then awarded to a set number of plans for a three- to five-year period. The state may extend the initial term of the contract and not go out to bid for several one-year periods. Rates are usually inflation-adjusted in renewal years. As part of the bid process, plans usually submit pricing proposals based on an established reimbursement system that the state has in place. Rates are then either accepted or negotiated with the plans. The rates can consider the following characteristics of the enrollees or program parameters:

- ○ Regions or counties of the state that the plan will be in
- ○ Eligibility group of enrollees
- ○ Age of enrollees
- ○ Sex of enrollees
- ○ Risk of an enrollee

Plans are usually paid by the state per month on a per-member-per-month (PMPM) basis for each enrollee in the plan during a month. An upfront, monthly payment is usually made and may be supplemented later in the month for members enrolled after the first of the month. States have various rules related to if and how much a member is compensated if a member is enrolled after the first of the month.

Some states may also have supplemental payments for some or all health plans in addition to the core medical payments. These may include behavioral health, dental, vision, and non-emergency transportation.

Some states also carve certain costs from these rates because there can be extraordinary events and costs that can impact plans differently. They will pay a so-called kick payment for these events. Good examples of this are kick payments for pregnancies, delivery of newborns, and transplants. States may also carve out completely certain high-cost items and pay for them through the FFS system or process. A good example is Factor 8 for hemophiliacs.

More and more, states are also turning to risk adjustment to help set rates. Risk adjustment uses encounter data and diagnoses codes to determine the risk of an enrolled member. Each member receives a risk score. These risk scores are added up to determine an aggregate risk score per plan. The aggregate score for the entire population usually is set to 1.0. Base rates are set for the population, usually based on geography (county or region), demographics (age and sex), eligibility group, and other factors. Plans that have risk scores over 1.0 get a percentage added on to their base rates, while those with aggregate risk scores of less than 1.0 get reductions to their base rates. This is a way for states to reward those with sicker populations—even as budgets tighten and annual rate increases are limited. There are a few, popular Medicaid risk adjustment systems, including the encounter diagnosis-based Chronic Disability Payment

System (CDPS) and a companion based on pharmacy data known as MedRx. About half of state Medicaid agencies now use risk adjustment, with about 70% using CDPS, MedRx, or CDPS/MedRx.[24-14]

For many decades, the Medicaid program has suffered from poor quality and narrow Medicaid networks, which created access issues for enrollees. The advent of Medicaid managed care has helped begin to improve access and quality outcomes as plans were able to convince providers in their commercial and Medicare lines of business to join their Medicaid networks. Medicaid plans are increasingly focusing on quality initiatives as well. CMS is also holding states (and thereby plans) more accountable with several initiatives, including:

- Ensuring the actuarial soundness and adequacy of rates
- Encouraging the use of risk adjustment methodologies
- Ensuring the collection of encounter data for rate-setting and quality analysis
- Working with states to pursue and publish quality metrics. CMS has built out model scorecards for quality and other areas; they can be seen here: https://www.medicaid.gov/state-overviews/scorecard/index.html

Medicaid is also undergoing significant changes on compliance and quality, with the adoption of a major reform known as the Medicaid Mega Rule or Medicaid Uber Rule. Under this rule, managed care plans will now be held to much tougher standards related to their operations and approvals of coverage requests. The rule also mandates that each state has its own quality improvement or Star rating program, in which quality achieving plans will receive bonus revenue payments. The compliance and quality regime is expected to match that of the proven Medicare Advantage (MA) regime. Today, however, few states have these Star quality programs in place.

The Medicaid program also provides important hospital subsidies. This program is known as the disproportionate share hospital (DSH) program. It provides so-called safety net funding for hospitals that serve a large number of uninsured individuals as well as a high proportion of Medicaid recipients.

Currently, Medicaid reimburses at well below costs and substantially below Medicare and commercial. This funding is meant to compensate these hospitals and keep them financially sustainable. With the introduction of the ACA, major reductions were passed, given the fact that Medicaid coverage was expanded and Exchanges set up. This reduced the number of the uninsured. These DSH cuts were delayed along the way, but were set to go into effect in federal fiscal year 2020.[24-11]

You will see in the next chapter that I think, on the whole, Medicaid is a good investment and one that is integral to our healthcare future.

Americans constantly get Medicare and Medicaid confused. The terms are used interchangeably and shouldn't be. So, let's recap:

Medicare is:

- a government entitlement run only by the federal government
- enrollees are sixty-five and older or someone with certain disabilities
- a program for which you become eligible without regard to income or assets

Medicaid is:

- a government entitlement run jointly by the federal government and states
- a program for which the federal government sets policies and states can change them (with permission and within reason); states operate a Medicaid program in their state
- a program in which enrollees can be of any age and eligibility is usually based on income, assets, and at certain times eligibility for other government programs

Dual eligibles are:

- people eligible for both Medicare and Medicaid
- individuals for which Medicare is primary and Medicaid is secondary

- ○ able to be fully or partially dual eligible, depending on your income and qualifications for other government programs
- ○ a status in which Medicaid pays for the premiums and cost-sharing in Medicaid; how much is covered is dependent on your status as a full or partial dual eligible

There you have it!

CHAPTER 25

Why Medicaid Is Good

N ow that we have told you about the Medicaid program, I want to get back to that polarizing subject of my introduction in the last chapter.

I've told you that Democrats are ardent backers of Medicaid but seem to turn a blind eye to the need for any reform of the entitlement behemoth. On the other side, the pull-yourself-up-by-your-own-bootstraps Republicans (social barriers be damned) want to rip the program apart, arguing it is a financial boondoggle.

So, where do I stand? These Republican bones want to tell you that—drum roll please...

"Medicaid is good!"

This may not be artful or worthy of a literary award, but I hope my point gets across. It is heresy for most of my party, for sure!

I have come a long way over the years to endorse Medicaid. It is not so much about what we have today, but that I believe Medicaid represents, namely, the most cost-effective, stable way to deal with two crises:

○   An uninsured crisis that has meant terrible suffering for the up to 50 million people without coverage at various points in time

○   An aging demographic and looming long-term care crisis soon to hit this country

In short, I don't see any other system that can adequately deal with these issues in the future. At the same time, I do think it needs reform, given its huge, unfunded future liability (the cost of the program in the future), which will only mean eventual reduction of benefits for lack of affordability.

My "Medicaid is good" declaration is premised on a few assumptions:

If healthcare is not a right, it is downright close to it. As I write this, I can feel the collective grip of Republicans' hands around my neck. But frankly, I believe that a civilized society owes to all citizens the ability to access quality healthcare. And as I noted in the history of healthcare chapter, there were at least two Republican presidents that championed something akin to universal access to healthcare. Do you remember them? They were Teddy Roosevelt and Richard Nixon. I say, if it was good enough for Teddy and Dick, it is good enough for me.

The most affordable way to ensure access to quality healthcare is to ensure upfront health insurance access. Today, the American healthcare system has so many coverage gaps that tens of millions access care at its most expensive settings such as emergency rooms and inpatient facilities. In the end, this is more costly, is an extremely poor use of precious resources, and it does little to nothing to emphasize quality, care management, and prevention.

Unless we provide affordable insurance and reap all the benefits of upfront coverage, we will see the amount of our gross domestic product (GDP) going to healthcare reach or exceed 20%. Already, we are a huge outlier among developed nations, which range between 9-12% of GDP going to healthcare. In short, I believe policymakers are being penny wise and pound foolish when they think of reform in a static way versus a dynamic one. They seem to be focused on the short-term goal of cutting here and there to meet a bottom line. They need to think long term and ask the question: What system will it take to transform the paradigm—to emphasize quality, prevention, and care coordination—and ultimately bend the cost curve?

The next looming healthcare crisis of this nation, if it hasn't already arrived, is our aging demographic. Grandparents, and in time, this author himself, will collectively need billions of dollars in long-term care services but the nation is ill-prepared to meet the challenge. In a later chapter, I tell you about the crippling burden that the aging of America will mean for our healthcare system and the economy as a whole. The costs for both acute and long-term care will go up dramatically due to aging. The likelihood of use of long-term care services increases demonstrably as people get older. If some doubt the moral imperative of ensuring affordable coverage for all Americans, far fewer will argue that Grandma and Grandpa should be thrown out on the street because they saved an inconsequential amount to cover home care, assisted living, or nursing home costs.

The so-called Exchange or Marketplace construct will likely be a place of high costs, adversity, and instability in many states, no matter how well-engineered they may be. Medicaid offers a much better and more stable opportunity to cover the remaining uninsured Americans.

Even though Medicaid expansion costs initially came in well above original estimates (due to pent up demand for healthcare among the uninsured population), the average cost for expansion enrollees began to drop after the initial expansion in 2014. What is important to note is that the cost of providing care in Medicaid is substantially less than in the Exchanges—22% less in 2018 and projected to be 36% less in 2028.[25-1]

The overall lower Medicaid cost is the case despite Medicaid having a much higher overall actuarial value than the Exchanges. The higher Medicaid actuarial value is driven by almost no cost-sharing *and* a more comprehensive benefit. Admittedly, a good share of the lower cost can be attributed to very low provider rates in Medicaid, compared to the commercial world—which the Exchange rates generally follow. The low Medicaid rates are unsustainable if we continue to expand the program.

On the flip side, current Medicaid costs include massive Medicaid fraud, waste, and abuse (FWA), which some estimates suggest are as much as 25% of total spending. Such FWA is clearly preventable, but government has never been too invested in rooting it out except for turning over some populations to private health plans.

The bottom line is that there were 76.5 million Americans in Medicaid and 7.4 million in the related State Children's Health Insurance Program (SCHIP) in federal fiscal year 2020 (calculated on a full-year equivalent or average monthly enrollment basis).[25-2] This dwarfs Exchange enrollment. As of September 2021, enrollment in the state and federal Exchanges hit 12.2 million, in part due to the special enrollment period created by President Biden.[25-3, 25-4]

In summary, while Medicaid has many warts, it is at least a proven delivery mechanism that is relatively financially stable. With reform, it is capable of delivering the type of care Americans need in the future. It is also the place where all of our challenges, now and in the future, come together. Consider the following:

- Over 76 million people rely on Medicaid today.[25-2]
- Medicaid covers the deliveries of about half of all babies in the nation. It can do the most to lower infant mortality and morbidity and ensure a solid start for our children.[25-5]
- Medicaid already serves as a safety net for many who face financially catastrophic health events. Medicaid picks up the costs of these events for a temporary period of time.
- Medicaid provides critical programs and coverage for the most vulnerable in our society. No one can question the moral imperative to serve them.
- Already, Medicaid covers 40% of all long-term care costs in the nation. And this will rise considerably with aging.[25-6]
- Acute and long-term care services are fragmented and uncoordinated. Medicaid is the program that can best build a true continuum of care

and manage both types of services effectively.

○ Dual eligibles are individuals that qualify for both Medicare and Medicaid. They numbered about 12 million in 2017, or 20% of the Medicare population and 15% of the Medicaid population. However, they represented 34% of Medicare and 33% of Medicaid spending. This will only rise in the future. So, Medicaid will help coordinate Medicaid and Medicare funding streams, too.[25-7]

○ Over 21 million people have obtained Medicaid coverage since late 2013 (actual December 2013 monthly enrollment to average monthly enrollment for the federal fiscal year ending September 30, 2020.[25-2,] [25-8] They are relatively happy consumers. Contrast this with 12.2 million in the Exchanges, many of whom have been at risk of losing coverage in states with unstable systems in the recent past.

○ Given the overlapping populations, a properly funded Medicaid program also safeguards the Medicare program.

○ Last, people forget about the watershed Supreme Court Olmstead decision and numerous additional related decisions. These court cases essentially dictate that Americans have a right to safely live in the community and avoid institutionalization. For the most part, money is no object in these decisions. Without a strong Medicaid program, how would the nation meet these new and emerging mandates?[25-9]

My view is that there is a middle ground for compromise on Medicaid policy, one that leverages the proven stability of Medicaid and reforms it for the future, so we can meet the insurance access and aging crises. The major parties would be wise to simply sit down and hash out lasting reforms, tapping into that Medicaid stability I talk about.

Because there is so much mistrust between the parties on government entitlements in Washington, DC, here is what I would propose as a basis for reform and compromise:

Medicaid should not be a political bad word for anyone. Despite the rancor on Medicaid you hear from many Capitol Hill Republicans, Medicaid has significant bipartisan support. As of this writing, thirty-eight states and the

District of Columbia have expanded (implemented or adopted and have yet to implement) Medicaid to the levels prescribed in the ACA of 2010.[25-10]

Interestingly, many of these states had or now have Republican Governors. Many of these GOP Governors supported expansion or maintained the expansion after taking office. There were six major so-called politically purple, reddish, and red states (such as Missouri and Oklahoma) that recently expanded Medicaid via ballot initiative, and there could be more in the future. The COVD-19 relief package passed in early 2021 also has some temporary increases in regular federal matching funds if remaining states expand. The ideologues can call them big government Republicans all they want, but pragmatic and sensible GOP leaders, such as former Governor John Kasich of Ohio for one (who has served in both federal and state roles) do get it. It is time others open their minds.

Republicans will have to deal with preserving the Medicaid expansion. Overall costs are lower for Medicaid than the Exchange and disenfranchising people who now have healthcare should not be sanctioned. While it sets up an unlevel playing field, reward the thirty-eight states and District of Columbia that have expanded by preserving the 90% funding (it has been phased down from 100% and stays at 90% as of 2020). These states did the right thing when Obamacare was passed. Most states that expanded Medicaid would have to end their expansions should the federal government repeal the expansion. This has major impact on over 21 million enrollees who have gained coverage in Medicaid since 2013.

Democrats will have to deal with overhauling Medicaid; Republicans will have to deal with not gutting the program and truly preserving it so it can do what it needs to do in the future.

While we have huge challenges ahead in healthcare, the current Medicaid entitlement construct is not sustainable. Excess now will mean chaos and crisis later. More importantly, reforming Medicaid is needed to meet all the aging challenges we outlined previously.

Reform tenets should include the following. These come from my analysis of various proposals to reform Medicaid over time (especially the past several years), taking the best that is out there and creating what I think is a reasonable solution to the problem:

Preserve the expansion funding. Millions now rely on coverage through Medicaid and would return to the uninsured rolls if the expansion funding is repealed or somehow reduced.

Find a reasonable, policy-based option for the holdout states. Both Presidents Obama and President Trump played politics with Medicaid expansion. As noted above, thirty-eight states and the District of Columbia have expanded to 133% of the federal poverty level (FPL). Most holdout states are in the conservative South as well as in the Plains and Rocky Mountains. Since the ACA's enactment in 2010, this has led to the continuation of the haves versus have-nots phenomenon in Medicaid. Northeastern, Midwest, and West Coast states tend to have rich Medicaid eligibility and benefits, while other regions tend to have skimpy eligibility. Some of these southern states continue to have the barest of Medicaid eligibility.

Worried about the state budget impact, several states had considered or requested expanding to 100% of poverty in their states to provide a continuum for the uninsured—Medicaid up to 100% and Exchange coverage after that. This makes a great deal of sense, is consistent with federal law, and would help millions who remain uninsured. The Obama CMS leadership rejected this, demanding that states go all the way to 133% of poverty, which was a bullying tactic. Trump's CMS also turned down or discouraged most states from this middle ground as well—because they didn't want to see Obamacare succeed. Both acted selfishly political. Trump did clear an 1115 waiver for Georgia to go to 100% of FPL for Medicaid tied to work requirements. The Biden Administration is busy dismantling work requirement waivers, however. This compromise should be adopted, and Biden seems open to it.

Keep the entitlement for a time, as a transition, but then convert to a per-capita cap formula, which could send dollars to states in a far more flexible formula than could a strict block grant with inflation. This gives states time to plan and decide what their future Medicaid program should look like. In general, a block grant would be driven at the aggregate spending level, while a per-capita cap funding formula would be sensitive to enrollment and be set based on per-enrollee costs. In addition, a per-capita cap program could guarantee eligibility for certain groups, where a block grant likely would not.[25-11]

This is also time to meet head-on the rather ridiculous arguments made by the former Trump Administration, U.S. House, and U.S. Senate GOP, that their multiple proposals in 2017 and 2018 didn't actually represent cuts to Medicaid. Perhaps they did not, in the purest sense of the word, but of course they would have had huge impact. We know that to meet ongoing requirements almost every social service program needs to inflate over time. If you short fund the increase, it is tantamount to a cut. As Congressional Budget Office (CBO) scoring showed at the time, the potential loss of millions from the Medicaid rolls proves the point.

I admit that even a per-capita cap formula would mean savings from the current Medicaid program benchmarks. However, the per-capita formula offers the best approach to saving future costs so as to preserve the program for future generations, and at the same time provide sustainable funding to states to render important services. Certainly, a reasonable compromise can be found that is less expensive than the current Medicaid entitlement and that retools Medicaid to succeed and meets future demands, while still being fiscally responsible.

Any reform effort must recognize that states have much less financial room to maneuver than the federal government, especially in tough economic times. The formula should assume that the federal government picks up and consistently sustains a larger overall share of the program. Everyone should tighten their belt, but the rough allocation of risk and cost should be the same. The GOP wants to shift costs to states over time. Surely, we can come to a national consensus on a reasonable, future level of funding and the equitable breakout between the federal government and states.

The per-capita cap formula must be very nuanced and constructed to be sensitive to several factors. These include healthcare inflation and population growth trends (including within the various eligibility groups).

They must also include temporary recessionary trends (which badly hit states when Medicaid enrollment soars and rash decisions must be made), as well as aging demographics and extraordinary changes in healthcare, such as drug innovation, technology, and other similar trends. Given such complexity, a base year alone probably does not safeguard the states. Because of the factors above and the vagaries of picking a single base year for states, a periodic rebasing might need to be considered as well.

Some variability by state (and by eligibility groups) must be recognized in the Medicaid formula. While it can be argued that the formula should drive to or set national spending benchmarks, the reality is there is significant variation in costs—overall and within eligibility groups—between states today. Some of this is tied to variations in healthcare systems and infrastructure (for example, urban versus rural states), while others are related to state policies regarding the scope of Medicaid (for example, rich benefit states versus lean ones).

The annual inflation formula should be reasonably generous, yet provide for savings against the anticipated costs of continuing an unfettered entitlement. While any inflation factor will have its pros and cons, permanently using a "Consumer Price Index—Medical Plus X-percent Formula (CPI-M)" makes the most sense. This better recognizes the higher inflation in healthcare as well as the emerging challenges that Medicaid faces. This would best alleviate concerns at the state level.

Include in the formula reasonable categories of eligible expenses. Some expenses should not ever be factored in as they work against promoting quality and transformation. However, other categories of Medicaid spending should always be held harmless along the way, including payments made by Medicaid for dual eligibles' premiums, cost-sharing, and other actions.

We must also grapple with the fact that Medicaid is an under-reimburser. This actually adds to costs elsewhere in the system. Funding will be needed to fix this over time, using a phased approach.

Some states certainly will still argue that they want a richer safety net and that it should always be funded in part by the federal government—as it is now. I am not terribly sympathetic here, as long as reasonable effort is made to recognize legitimate differences in state costs and perhaps some consideration for additional investments already made by some states. (We can't pull the rug out from them now.) However, any future extraordinary decisions made by states in terms of benefits and scope outside a national norm or corridor should be borne completely by state taxpayers.

Funding Medicaid at a reasonable rate is important because private managed care plans need incentive to remain in the Medicaid market and carry the burden of reform. We know that traditional Medicaid fee-for-service (FFS) systems are decrepit and need to be phased out. Over the past few years, Medicaid managed care has proven a good model—with some regulatory urging from CMS and Medicaid agencies. It can ensure better access, improve quality over time, and be cost-effective. Indeed, the only vehicle out there that has a shot at managing the moving parts of coordinating Medicare and Medicaid acute and long-term care is Medicaid managed care. This is the key to future affordability. Without a reasonable funding formula and a chance at a reasonable margin, private health plans will not participate in long-term care or dual eligible plans. Over time, any private plans that stayed in to help states experiment in reform could very well abandon the programs if funding becomes insufficient—as more and more costs are shifted to state governments.

Let's truly reform the benefit to emphasize personal responsibility, have contributions by enrollees at reasonable levels, reward good behaviors, and penalize bad ones.

Free the states from the regulation stranglehold. Today, except in certain waiver situations, states deal with an obscene level of mandates and bureaucracy. Every member is given the same gold-plated benefit. This comes with excessive regulatory mandates (for example, early and periodic screening, diagnosis, and treatment, known as EPSDT). Regulations also include mandatory benefits, mandatory eligibility groups, and even the traditional non-discrimination mandate that dictates the same benefits to mandatory and voluntary eligibility groups. Freeing states from these burdens will allow them to truly innovate.

Think out of the box when it comes to such reforms. True innovation would recognize that perhaps every state is different in terms of its healthcare needs. Some states have older demographics than others. Some are more affluent or have naturally higher rates of insurance than others. State-tailored and flexible solutions have merit. States will fashion fair and sustainable benefits and program rules. Current law allows states to effectively bring Exchange/Marketplace dollars into Medicaid waivers to cover members. When the subsidy scheme is overhauled, this aspect should be preserved, as it could be very cost effective.

Here is another out-of-the-box idea. Make Medicaid funding, and perhaps Exchange funding, available to lower-income Americans to help them afford employer coverage.

In the great debate on what to do with Medicaid, both sides miss an important point. In the end, underfunding Medicaid does little to achieve our goal of a sustainable healthcare system and of serving aging Baby Boomers. Indeed, those costs will be there in the future anyway. With a dysfunctional and underfunded Medicaid system, such costs may be even more of a drag on society and the economy as a whole.

We must enact a reasonable federal policy infrastructure that emphasizes quality transformation and reduces costs.

A blanket devolution of authority to the states will likely mean that many states will lose sight of the need to enhance quality, prevention, and management in the healthcare system.

Set aside the politics and come to a common-sense consensus on a program that has served America well for over fifty years and undoubtedly will be one of the bulwarks of our healthcare system long into the future.

CHAPTER 26

The State Children's Health Insurance Program

I n late summer or early fall of 1997, I was just months into my appointment as deputy budget director of Connecticut. In addition to running vast parts of the state budget and bureaucracy, one of my missions was to get my boss, the governor, re-elected the following year. He had won the previous election with a minority of the vote in 1994 and was then trailing his probable Democratic opponent in early polls.

The task involved implementation of the State's Children's Health Insurance Program (SCHIP or CHIP). At the time, I asked myself, "What is this Title XXI children's health insurance thing?" I was just learning the intricacies of the federal budget and reviewing the recently passed Balanced Budget Act of August 1997. It had huge implications for state budgets and the financing of healthcare generally. Title XXI or the children's healthcare program was part of that mammoth bill.

This time was transformative for me in my approach to healthcare. While I still could be counted as a solid, fiscal conservative, it was one of my first forays into creating public policies that *expanded* social services. The program would be one of many subsequent catalysts in my political mission of softening my boss's political image and helping him sail to re-election, which he did in 1998. In addition, the insurance program also checked all the right boxes for a relatively conservative administration:

- ○ 65% of the funding for Connecticut was coming from the federal government.
- ○ It did not have to be an entitlement.
- ○ It allowed for premiums and cost-sharing as with commercial insurance.
- ○ It had families and government sharing in healthcare costs (as minimal as the cost-sharing may be for some). This reflected the personal responsibility that conservatives wanted to see in government social welfare programs.

As I researched the issues, I soon learned about the healthcare benefits that CHIP would have:

- ○ Providing children's coverage would be cheap and cost effective. It had tangible benefits in avoiding costs and improving quality outcomes.
- ○ Building on the existing Medicaid managed care infrastructure would be affordable.
- ○ We could close the healthcare insurance gap for tens of thousands of individuals for a relatively modest cost.

The creation of Connecticut's SCHIP plan was a success. Within weeks of our announcement, we negotiated with Democrats and Republicans in the legislature and called a special session to pass the bill in October 1997. It grew somewhat from our initial proposal but stuck to the core principles. Over time, it insured tens of thousands of children, some in Medicaid and some in SCHIP. We also created new branding and outreach, to help destigmatize enrollment in public programs. Medicaid was renamed HUSKY A and SCHIP was called HUSKY B. (HUSKY stood for **H**ealthcare for **U**nin**S**ured **K**ids and **Y**outh.)

SCHIP Explained

Following that introduction on how important the SCHIP program is to me personally, let's look at some of the details of the program.

As with Medicare (Title XVIII) and Medicaid (XIX), SCHIP is a title within the broader Social Security Act—Title XXI. It predominantly serves children but has been broadened in some states to serve pregnant mothers and families of children.

SCHIP is not an entitlement; it is a block grant to states to expand health insurance for children and others. The act has been reauthorized several times since its passage in 1997 as part of the Balanced Budget Act.

Many consider SCHIP as a complement to Medicaid. While it is a distinct program—not an entitlement—this characterization is reasonable. States have significant flexibility to design benefits and cost-sharing, but its coverage is comprehensive in nature. It covers preventive, diagnostic, and treatment services.

There are three models that states use for their SCHIP programs:

o   Use the funds exclusively to expand Medicaid for children and family members who are further up the income scale.
o   Use the funds exclusively for a separate, non-Medicaid program.
o   Use the funds in both Medicaid and in a separate program. It is not unusual for states to "round out" coverage for children in Medicaid first—up to certain income levels or ages—and then to cover others in a separate, free-standing program. In the case of putting those children or groups in Medicaid, little if any cost-sharing applies. In a free-standing program, premiums and cost-sharing usually apply. Generally, premiums and cost-sharing are modest compared with those of commercial insurance.

As of 2017, fifteen states (including the District of Columbia) used SCHIP funds only to expand Medicaid, while thirty-six states used a separate program or in combination with Medicaid. In 2015, more than half (56%) of children funded by SCHIP were in the Medicaid program.[26-1]

The program has reduced the level of uninsured children nationwide by millions. Calculated on a full-year equivalent or average monthly enrollment basis, about 7.4 million had coverage funded by SCHIP in federal fiscal year 2020, which ended September 30, 2020.[26-2] One reason for this is that states began outreach campaigns when the SCHIP program was launched and many children previously eligible for Medicaid enrolled in that program. In addition, with some states extending coverage to family members, this also led to increased enrollment among children. Just as importantly, SCHIP provides comprehensive coverage for children with chronic conditions that otherwise would likely be uninsured.

Generally, speaking states set their SCHIP income levels above those of Medicaid, which provides a bridge from Medicaid to SCHIP for children's insurance. Today, two states have Medicaid or SCHIP income levels less than 200% of the federal poverty limit (FPL) for children. Thirty states offer coverage up to 300% of FPL. Nineteen states, including the District of Columbia, offer coverage greater to or equal to 300% of FPL. It is also important to note that many states also allow children to enroll and pay full premium if their family income exceeds state limits.[26-3]

States receive an SCHIP block grant each year based on federal appropriations. States have two years to spend each annual allocation. The minimum states receive for Medicaid is 50% of program funding. When SCHIP was first passed, the base amount was 65% with a sliding scale that reimbursed states based on their relative wealth, up to 81% (8 percentage points greater than the poorest state's 73% Medicaid reimbursement). The Affordable Care Act (ACA) boosted the enhancement to 23 percentage points over Medicaid, making the range from 88-100%. This occurred for federal fiscal years 2016 through 2019. The regular rate dropped to an 11.5-percentage-point enhancement in federal fiscal year 2020 and went back to historic rates in federal fiscal year 2021. However, the COVID-19 pandemic led Congress to add extra funds temporarily through the end of the pandemic. States get an extra 4.34-percentage-point reimbursement.[26-4, 26-5, 26-6]

The governing entity for this program nationally is the Centers for Medicare and Medicaid Services (CMS). The governing agency within a state can be different. In many states, it is the Medicaid agency. In other states, separate government agencies or quasi-public agencies have been set up to run SCHIP. The rationale in these states is that they don't want it treated like the Medicaid entitlement. They want free-market healthcare principles applied.

As with Medicaid, the major delivery vehicle for SCHIP benefits in states is usually managed care plans. These can be bid as part of the Medicaid private plan procurement or bid separately by the Medicaid agency or independent entity in each state that runs SCHIP.

The SCHIP program rounds out the nation's health insurance system for children. I expounded on the value of Medicaid earlier. One other statistic to show SCHIP's and Medicaid's importance on children: 39% of all children in America get their insurance through either Medicaid or SCHIP. Today, about 95% of all children are insured due to the creation of SCHIP and the additional enrollment in Medicaid when SCHIP was adopted. Prior to the passage in 1997, 15% of all children and 25% of low-income children were uninsured.[26-7]

In my view, like the Exchange premium and cost-sharing subsidies, the SCHIP program serves as a model as to how the overall healthcare system could be reformed. In essence, it is a universal access program, where income is recognized as a determinant for the ability to pay. Premiums and cost-sharing, if any, are set based on that ability to pay. It also provides for a relatively cost-effective and efficient delivery system (Medicaid and free-standing programs) to deliver quality services. It also leverages private sector health plans.

Giving my wife the recognition she deserves

I wanted to tell a story and give my wife some long-delayed and overdue recognition. It has been a source of contention in my marriage for years—over twenty years now. Finally, I have the chance to give my wife proper credit for helping name the HUSKY Program in Connecticut.

It all started back in 1997 when three officials—state Department of Social Services Deputy Commissioner Michael Starkowski, state Medicaid Director David Parrella, and I—were meeting to design the program and outline the legislation for SCHIP in our state.

One late night, we realized the best thing we could do to excite families and push enrollment in the program was to come up with a clever acronym. At the time, both our men's and women's college basketball teams at the University of Connecticut were exceedingly popular, competing at the highest levels and winning national championships. We came up with the idea of naming the program HUSKY, after the teams' mascot. But we struggled with making it an acronym. Late one night we had come up with Healthcare for UninSured Kids. We were missing a Y—HUSK just didn't do it!

We were distressed, as we were unable to make "HUSKY" complete, so we retired for the night. I hadn't seen my wife for days, and I was talking to her through the shower door the next morning, telling her how we had failed. She shouted, "Youth." Dazed and still tired from the marathon policymaking session the night before, I asked, "What are you talking about?" "Youth," she repeated, "Healthcare for UninSured Kids and Youth—HUSKY." (My wife recalls that I also said, "That's brilliant!" Somehow, I don't remember that part of the story.)

There it was, the final piece of the puzzle. I promised to acknowledge the contribution for so long. I intended to at my retirement from state service, but I botched it. Now, with this book, I finally have my chance to right the long-standing wrong. Thanks, Donna. All the insured kids thank you, too.

After all these years, that lifts tremendous guilt off my chest.

CHAPTER 27

Obamacare Marketplaces/Exchanges

W̶e have arrived at the last chapter of our detailed review of the various health insurance lines of business in the United States. This covers the Marketplace or Exchanges set up under the Affordable Care Act (ACA or Obamacare) in 2010. (Throughout the chapter, I will use the words Marketplace and Exchange interchangeably.)

The goal of Obamacare was to reduce the level of uninsured through universal access to insurance plans. In 2013, before the law actually took effect, the uninsured numbered 44.1 million people. In 2019, that number was about 31.8 million. The number of uninsured actually went as low as 28.7 million in 2016.[27-1] This drop occurred due to two ACA insurance channels:

First, under the ACA, states can extend coverage in Medicaid to Americans if their family income is about 133% or less of the federal poverty level (FPL) for their family size. Thus far, just twelve states have not adopted expansion to this level.[27-2] Through December 2020, enrollment due to expanded Medicaid was almost 15 million. These numbers continue to increase into 2021. Another 1 million are in the Basic Health Plan option that some states set up under the ACA.[27-3, 27-4]

The second way, and the reason for this chapter, was the introduction of the Health Insurance Exchanges or Marketplaces. These are largely online insurance Marketplaces in each state targeted to individuals:

- without Medicaid
- usually without an employer nexus to insurance
- sometimes working for an employer whose coverage is too expensive or does not meet certain standards

There is also a small group component that I will cover later.

About 12.2 million were enrolled in the Exchanges (the federal Exchange as well as those run by states) in September 2021, after a special enrollment period initiated by President Biden. This is down from 12.6 million in 2016.[27-4, 27-5, 27-6]

In summary, about 28 million clearly have been insured due to the Medicaid expansion and creation of the Exchange program in the ACA. HHS also says another 4 million who were previously eligible for Medicaid coverage have enrolled in the program due to the outreach and enhanced funding efforts under the ACA.[27-4]

But if our uninsured number in 2013 prior to the ACA was over 44 million, then why is our uninsured number still about 32 million if between 31 and 35 million have been covered? The difference is a result of others losing coverage since 2013. Note, too, that in other chapters, I have relied on different sources because of the subject matter being covered; thus, numbers may be slightly different but tell the same story overall. (As an example, the national health expenditures data puts the uninsured at 32 million in 2019—in the end, the uninsured percentage nationally is still in the 10% range.)

So, despite the major effort to cover everyone, there are still holes and policy flaws. More on this in an upcoming chapter.

Since Medicaid was already covered in an earlier chapter, let's go into details about the ACA's introduction of Marketplaces. Much of the following information is based on my actual experience, being among the first to design Exchange plans when they were first introduced in 2013 for the 2014 coverage year.

Marketplace/Exchange Details

This section will cover eligibility for insurance coverage on the Marketplace and the major federal role and structure set up for the delivery of individual contract insurance—something that was once the exclusive purview of states. It will also discuss the mandated benefits and designs in the Exchanges, as well as the various subsidies given to individuals and small businesses to help Americans afford coverage. Finally, we will cover small business SHOP coverage on the Exchange, plan qualification, and annual benefit and rate filing.

Eligibility

I won't go into too many details here; but, generally speaking, Americans are eligible for coverage in the Exchange if: [27-7]

- they are U.S. citizens, nationals, or otherwise lawfully in the country
- they are not incarcerated
- they do not have access elsewhere to qualifying or affordable coverage

Residents of U.S. territories have the option of setting up their own programs, but generally are not part of the national marketplace. The District of Columbia is treated as a state.

Individuals earning below certain income levels, as described later, are also eligible for premium subsidy support. A subset of this group is also eligible for additional subsidies to offset cost-sharing in their plans.

All individuals must be accepted into the program, regardless of health status, and enrollees cannot be charged more due to their health status. Plans can no longer reject coverage or have waiting periods for pre-existing conditions.

Generally, people can enroll in the Marketplace only once per year. This is usually done online or via telephone, although brokers can play a role as well. The open enrollment is currently held between November 1 and January 15. However, someone may be able to enroll in other parts of the year (e.g., if they lose coverage or under other special circumstances).

An important note: As we discussed, not all states have expanded Medicaid to individuals earning up to 133% of the federal poverty level (FPL). While the law is meant to enroll the uninsured with incomes at 133% of the FPL or more, you can still obtain coverage and subsidies if you are over 100% of FPL. This is an important safeguard for residents of states that have not expanded. However, there are actually those in states that are in a coverage gap—they do not earn enough (100% of FPL) to get Obamacare coverage through the Exchanges and earn too much to be on Medicaid because the state did not expand coverage.

One last point: A small subset of legal immigrants who do not yet qualify for Medicaid can obtain coverage on the Exchange if they have incomes under 100% of FPL.

Marketplace Structure

Prior to the adoption of the ACA, the provision of individual coverage (where individuals enter into contracts with health insurers for benefits for them or their families) was the exclusive domain of state insurance regulators and other state agencies. The states regulated these plans' solvency, the types of insurance they could offer, including its benefits and rules. Each of the fifty states had different rules. Some states required rich benefits, while others allowed bare-bones policies. Many states allowed benefit limitations and exclusions as well as annual and lifetime caps on services.

The ACA changed all that and brought individual coverage into a fifty-state uniform program and structure. The federal government essentially holds great control over the establishment of any Insurance Marketplace or Exchange in a given state. If a state elects to set up its own Exchange, it must enact the federal rules governing the ACA but retains some discretion in policymaking regarding administration and state benefit requirements. If a state does not elect to set up its own Exchange, the federal government will enroll those eligible in that state via the Federally Facilitated Exchange (FFE) or Marketplace (FFM). There is also a hybrid option where states largely run their own Exchanges but utilize the federal website and infrastructure. As of this writing, thirty states use the FFE/FFM model, three states use the hybrid approach, and eighteen states and the District of Columbia operate their own State Exchanges (three states moved from hybrid to fully state in late 2021).[27-8]

All the same federal benefits and rules as well as other ACA dictates apply whether it's a State Exchange, a hybrid, or Federally Facilitated. It is also important to note that someone does not have to enroll via the state's Marketplace or Exchange. Americans can enroll off the Exchange through a broker or directly with an insurance plan. But whether you enroll On-Exchange (via the federal or a state website) or Off-Exchange (direct with a broker or a plan), the same benefits and rules apply. The small exception is if you have a grandfathered plan, as noted in Chapter 17 (where those who had plans effective prior to the ACA can keep their plan design with only some ACA mandates applying). In addition, On-Exchange and Off-Exchange product offerings are both considered non-grandfathered, meaning all the ACA rules must be followed.

Benefits and Design [27-9, 27-10]

Health plans must be deemed qualified health plans to meet the rules to furnish insurance in the Marketplace. The CMS issues specific benefit and network rules, among others, that these plans must follow. Plans must meet specific benefit offerings to offer Marketplace plans. These offerings were constructed to ensure that Americans can correctly compare plans. The construct ensures that whether you enroll in plan A or plan B, the offering will be relatively the same (i.e., while cost-sharing may differ between the two, the overall consumer financial outlay is roughly the same and the benefits roughly similar). These are as follows and are known as "metal" plans:

Platinum: At this uppermost tier, benefits are constructed so that 90% of the benefit cost is covered by the plan and 10% by the individual. Obviously, premiums for these plans will be the highest. The percentage of the benefit cost is known as the plan's actuarial value (AV).

Gold: Benefits at this level are constructed so that 80% of the benefit cost is covered by the plan and 20% by the individual. Premiums will still be high.

Silver: Here, benefits are constructed so that 70% of the benefit cost is covered by the plan and 30% by the individual. This is also known as the benchmark plan (the plan type that the federal government targets subsidies for and assumes most Americans will enroll in). Premiums will be more modest.

Bronze: Benefits are constructed so that 60% of the benefit cost is covered by the plan and 40% by the individual. These premiums will be among the lowest and are usually meant for younger, healthier people.

Under Thirty Catastrophic: To encourage enrollment of young people and reduce adverse selection (where sicker enrollees drive up overall costs and premiums), those under thirty (and those that qualify for a hardship exemption) are allowed to purchase catastrophic plans on the Exchanges. These are similar to high-deductible health plans (HDHPs). The AV of these plans are generally even less than a Bronze plan. You are unable to get a premium subsidy if you enroll in this type of plan; however, these plans offer a comparatively low premium and still offer the protection needed in the case of a catastrophic event and the plan's discounted pricing when you need to access services.

To be in the Marketplace, a plan must offer at least a Silver and a Gold plan in each given area that it wants to offer coverage.

Under the law, these metal plans all must still cover what are known as essential benefits. Each metal plan may have higher or lower cost-sharing, but these benefits must be covered fully in each metal tier. The benefits that must be fully covered, largely without limitations, are as follows:

- Ambulatory patient services
- Emergency services
- Hospitalization
- Maternity and newborn care
- Mental health and substance use disorder services, including behavioral health treatment
- Prescription drugs
- Rehabilitative and habilitative services and devices
- Laboratory services
- Preventive, wellness, and chronic disease management services, which must be offered free of charge and without a deductible applying
- Pediatric services, including oral and vision care
- Mandatory dental coverage for children

Individual and family maximum out-of-pocket (MOOP) costs are capped from year-to-year for all enrollees. Lower MOOPs apply to cost-sharing for subsidized individuals. Deductibles are dependent on the metal tier you are buying. Deductibles can be combined (medical and prescription drug) or separate. Deductibles are also lower as you move up the metal tier rankings.

Plans may offer additional services beyond these. In addition, states may prescribe additional services or scope of services be covered beyond what is noted previously. This gets quite specific, but generally this is done by setting benchmarks for coverage in each state.

Everyone must receive a Summary of Benefits and Coverage (SBC) in a prescribed format.

Those are the basics, but there are numerous other requirements, including network requirements, that would make anyone's head spin. Every year, plans must prove that they meet network adequacy, cover all required essential benefits, and that their metal offerings meet the percentage AV standards.

ACA Subsidies Defined

The ACA provides vital tax credits for those with more limited incomes so they can afford individual and family coverage if their employers do not offer it, or if the coverage is not affordable. Although these are tax credits, as outlined in the next section, they have immediate effect. In fact, they are *advanced* tax credits, meaning that the health plan receives payment from the federal government up front, on your behalf, so that you are not paying first and getting the tax credit later.

There are two kinds of subsidies available under the Affordable Care Act (ACA):

Premium Subsidies [27-9, 27-10, 27-11]

Americans at or under 400% of FPL for their family size are eligible for premium subsidies. The subsidy goes directly to the plan in which you enroll. The plan must offset your premium based on the subsidy for which you qualify. The amount of assistance is on a sliding scale and applies to enrollment in the Silver benchmark plan. Individuals or families that enroll in richer metal plans must pay 100% of the difference between the Silver benchmark subsidy rate and the higher metal plan premium. In addition, the subsidy is targeted to the second lowest premium benchmark plan in the region or county of enrollment. Therefore, someone enrolling in a plan that bid higher, would also pay the difference between the target premium for the second lowest Silver benchmark plan and the higher premium Silver plan they enroll in. On the flip side, if someone enrolls in a Bronze plan, they could apply the full amount of the subsidy to that health plan and pay less. It is important to note, though, that those with limited incomes may not be eligible for cost-sharing subsidies if they are not enrolled in a Silver plan.

An example of the scaled premium assistance for a family of four is in the following table. (For clarification, the family of four poverty limit—100%—for 2021 is $26,500, meaning 400% of FPL is $106,000.[27-12]) Note that some of the sources used here published their articles before the most recent poverty guidelines were finalized. I have adjusted the figures below to the most updated values.

Family Income		Percentage of Income Paid Toward Premium
Percentage of FPL	**Top Amount**	
Up to 133%	$35,245	2.07%
133% to 150%	$39,750	Between 3.10% to 4.14%
150% to 200%	$53,000	Between 4.14% to 6.52%
200% to 250%	$66,250	Between 6.52% to 8.33%
250% to 300%	$79,500	Between 8.33% to 9.83%
300% to 400%	$106,000	9.83%
Over 400%	—	(no subsidy)

About 87% of all enrollees in early 2019 were eligible for a premium subsidy.

If someone receives a subsidy and it is later determined they were not eligible for it—or for that range of subsidy—then there are repayment penalties in tax law (this was suspended for 2020). There are also penalties for not offering affordable and qualifying coverage, depending on employer size. Further, there is an individual penalty in the law if you do not obtain qualifying coverage. But that penalty has been zeroed out for the time being.

I have argued in the past that those at the lowest end of the scale may receive too much, whereas those earning between 300-400 % of FPL clearly get too little. At the low end, families are paying $546 to $726 per year for premiums. How is it that a family of four earning $79,500 to $106,000 can afford $7,775 to $10,367 per year before any subsidy kicks in and then pay cost-sharing beyond that. Consequently, the premiums for the uninsured for those earning 300-400% and above is extremely high. Indeed, the number of uninsured middle-income families has increased markedly, due to the instability of Exchanges in many states and the rise of premiums through 2018. From 2016 to 2019, unsubsidized enrollment in the Exchanges declined by 2.8 million people, a 45% decline.[27-13]

Cost-Sharing Subsidies (CSRs) [27-9, 27-10, 27-11, 27-14, 27-15]

Cost-sharing reductions are available to those making between 100-250% of FPL. To obtain the advantage of these subsidies, a person in this income range must enroll in a Silver plan because only these plans have special designs to account for the need to lower cost-sharing for lower-income groups.

In essence, the actuarial value (AV) of the special design plan is increased from the standard 70% to various levels up to 94% of AV to provide better affordability to lower-income enrollees. Enrollees are also mandated to receive lower deductibles and MOOPs, in addition to lower cost-sharing. Again, the subsidy goes directly to the health plan to offset your cost-sharing immediately through the special plan design. The CSR eligibility and special Silver plan types are as follows:

- ○ 100-150% of FPL—special Silver benefit with an AV of 94%
- ○ 150-200% of FPL—special Silver benefit with an AV of 87%
- ○ 200-250% of FPL—special Silver benefit with an AV of 73%

About 52% of all enrollees in early 2019 were receiving a CSR subsidy.

Small Business SHOP [27-16, 27-17, 27-18]

As I noted earlier, the Marketplace also has small business offerings. Plans can also apply to offer Small Business Health Options (SHOP) products. Plans post offerings on the Exchange, but most of the interaction between plans and even employees are done in a traditional manner, directly with health plans.

Businesses must be between one and fifty full-time equivalent workers (FTEs) to purchase coverage on the Exchange (in some states you may be able to have up to 100 FTEs). Small businesses with twenty-five FTEs or fewer are able to obtain tax credits—up to 50% of the employer share of premiums—for offering benefits to their employees through the Exchange. The average salary must be about $50,000 or less. The credit is scaled against average salary and number of employees. The plan must pay 50% of total premiums. They must also offer benefits at least to all full-time employees that work thirty hours a week or more, but not necessarily to dependents.

Most small businesses purchase through other channels. All of the ACA requirements apply to SHOP plans as well. SHOP is open to small businesses year-round. As with most employer coverage, employees are only able to enroll as new hires, for life-changing events, or at that employer's open enrollment.

SHOP is not available in every state. If an employer offers SHOP, then it may be possible to decline it for you and even for dependents. You may then be able to enroll in the individual Marketplace.

Temporary Increases in Premium Subsidies and Prospect for Permanent Enhancement [27-19, 27-20]

When President Biden took office in January 2021, he undertook several initiatives to expand Marketplace enrollment expansion. He held a special enrollment period in 2021 due to the COVID-19 pandemic that had already enrolled over 2.5 million through mid-2021. He also added tens of millions to outreach, marketing, and so-called community facilitator dollars to encourage enrollment. Last, the COVID 19 relief bill passed early in his tenure increased the generosity of Exchange premium subsidies temporarily. For 2021 and 2022, the bill lifts the cap on Exchange premium subsidies, which is now 400% of the federal poverty limit (FPL). This allows more middle-income earners to qualify for a subsidy. Next, for 2021 and 2022, the bill makes more generous premium subsidies for those between 100% and 400% of FPL and caps the family income contribution at 8.5% for everyone. It eliminates family premium contributions for those up to 135% of FPL. The bill also deems those on unemployment as eligible for the highest Exchange premiums subsidies, meaning these displaced families pay no premium. Here are the temporary increases in premium subsidies:

Income Levels	Permanent Law	2021 COVID-19 Relief Bill Temporary Enhancement
Less than 133% FPL	2.07%	0%
133-150% FPL	3.1-4.14%	0%
150-200% FPL	4.14-6.52%	0-2%
200-250% FPL	6.52-8.33%	2-4%
250-300% FPL	8.33-9.83%	4-6%
300-400% FPL	9.83%	6-8.5%
Over 400% FPL	N/A	8.5%

Democrats want to make these enhancements permanent (or at least extend them) and were trying to find funding under budget rules at the time of this writing in mid-2021.

A U.S. Senate Democratic bill would make the premium subsidies in the COVID-19 relief bill permanent, tie CSR subsidies to Gold plans as opposed to Silver, and enhance and extend CSR subsidies to 400% of FPL. The premium subsidy changes would match what has been adopted temporarily for 2021 and 2022. The CSR changes would be as follows, which would enhance the AV of plans for many of modest to middle income.

Current ACA CSR Subsidies:	Senate Democratic Proposal:
100-150% of FPL—94% Actuarial Value (Individual/Family pays 6%)	100-200% of FPL—95% Actuarial Value (Individual/Family pays 5%)
150-200% of FPL—87% Actuarial Value (Individual/Family pays 13%)	200-300% of FPL—90% Actuarial Value (Individual/Family pays 10%)
200-250% of FPL—73% Actuarial Value (Individual/Family pays 27%)	300-400% of FPL—85% Actuarial Value (Individual/Family pays 15%)

The Urban Institute says that an additional 4.5 million could be covered if the Senate bill were passed. It would save enrollees an average of $1,400 a year. It would cost about $350 billion over ten years. The bill would also permanently fund the CSR subsidies to plans that were eliminated by the Trump Administration. Since the move by Trump, plans have had to hike all Silver premiums as they are still required to fund the lower cost-sharing in mandated CSR plans.

I am a proponent of not only affordable universal access but affordability of benefits. I am not sold on the major expansion of premium and cost-sharing subsidies. Some of this may be needed but perhaps not all. However, studies show cost-sharing that is too high is a barrier to seeking care, something that might cost the system in general more over the long term than enhancing lower-income Americans' premium and cost-sharing subsidies.

Plan Qualification and Annual Bidding

Plans bid annually in a joint process overseen by the federal government—via the Department of Health and Human Services' Centers for Medicare and

Medicaid Services (HHS-CMS) and state insurance departments. HHS-CMS plays the lead role, with state's largely approving rates after the federal government does so. States oversee licensure and solvency.

Depending on the state, plans apply to offer coverage by county, region, or statewide. Benefit and actuarial submission usually occur in the first half of each year for the succeeding year. As noted, open enrollment is in November and December of each year.

At a minimum, plans must submit a Silver and Gold plan to be in a given county, region, or state. Many plans battle it out to be the two lowest premium plans in the Silver category in order to win as much membership as they can. Plans submit both standard plans as well as cost-sharing reduction (CSR) Silver plans for individuals with incomes at or below 250% of the federal poverty limit (FPL).

As with Medicare Advantage (MA), risk adjustment is used in paying plans. Member rates are adjusted based on the health status of the individual, in part because people can no longer be barred from obtaining coverage because of pre-existing conditions. In this case an Exchange version of the hierarchical condition category (HCC) system is used. The ACA only allows plans to set rates based on geography, gender, and age (within certain ratios).

Assessment of Exchanges

The Exchanges got off to a very rocky start. First, rates skyrocketed as the country was essentially converting from an underwriting system (where people were accepted, rejected, or receive increased premiums based on health status) to a community rating one (where everyone is accepted and the healthy in essence subsidize the ill). Second, the Obama Administration was criticized heavily for not fully funding two important risk and revenue stabilization programs, namely risk corridors and reinsurance, that were supposed to aid plans from 2014 to 2016. Finally, the Trump Administration took a number of steps to clamp down on enrollment, challenged CSR subsidies, and otherwise impacted financial stability due to its overall opposition to the program.

Notwithstanding all this, the Marketplace has stabilized nationally. Initially, premiums skyrocketed with the new community-rating approach. They continued to climb given uncertainty over the risk programs' funding. In 2018, premiums also rose due to the uncertainty related to CSR subsidies. In 2019 and 2020, however, premiums stabilized and in some cases actually fell. In fact, in 2020 premiums went down between 2.5-3.5% nationally for a forty-year-old in all metal tiers. This was in large measure to make up for the over-correction in 2018. In 2021, premiums for a forty-year-old dropped again between 1-4%. Quarterly gross margins have steadily improved in the last few years. Unfortunately, enrollment decreased due to the massive premium hikes in 2018. This largely was for those who could no longer afford unsubsidized coverage. [27-21, 27-22, 27-23, 27-24]

Plans and providers bolted from the Exchanges early on but are coming back. For three straight years (2019 to 2021), insurers have been returning to the program or expanding their footprint. In September 2020, Cigna announced it would expand its offerings by 50% in 2021—adding 79 new counties to reach 220 in total. The biggest player in Obamacare, Centene, announced it would add 400 additional counties in 2021, an over 50% increase in its geographic footprint. Several Blue Cross and Blue Shield plans and Oscar Health also announced plans to expand in 2021. [27-25, 27-26, 27-27]

For 2021, across a sample of twenty states, a study found thirty insurers entered the program, and sixty-one insurers expanded their service areas. There are an average of five insurers per state in the program as of 2021, up from 3.5 in 2018. (The peak was six in 2015.) The range in 2021 is between one and thirteen plans. In 2021, 78% of enrollees (living in 46% of all counties) will have a choice of three or more insurers. In the national Exchange states, there are 181 plans for 2021, an increase of twenty-two insurers. [27-28, 27-29]

While it is early, there are preliminary reports that many of the plans noted will further expand their footprint in 2022. CVS Health's Aetna subsidiary has also announced plans to re-enter to the Exchanges in 2022. [27-30]

Despite this better outlook, the Exchanges remain challenging in some states. In 2021, fourteen states still will have two or fewer plans (down from seventeen in 2020) and some insurers do not participate statewide in many states. The good news is that the number of national Exchange enrollees who have just one plan option has decreased from 29% in 2018 to 4% in 2021.[27-28, 27-29]

As I have alluded to in previous chapters, despite being from the Republican party, I support universal access to affordable insurance. There are economic and moral imperatives here. So, the ACA was a worthy endeavor. At the same time, I do think the ACA and the Marketplaces in particular have flaws and need reform. In some ways, we have too much of a good thing for some citizens, and not enough of it for others.

PART FOUR

The Future of U.S. Healthcare

We have come to the last quarter of the book. With the exception of explaining why health insurance is important, why Medicaid is good, and why Medicare Advantage (MA) is good, the book thus far has been largely informational and analytical. The coming pages take a different track. In most of them, I plan on expressing my views on what is wrong with healthcare in America and where we might go. Here is how it will be laid out:

- In Chapter 28, we will discuss what is wrong—what is dysfunctional about American healthcare.

- ◦ In Chapter 29, I will turn to some positive signs that point to possible reform.
- ◦ In Chapter 30, I will outline the various forms of healthcare in the developed world and what elements America may have of each.
- ◦ In Chapter 31, I will tell you why I think a single-payer system in America (aka, Medicare for All) is destined for failure.
- ◦ In Chapter 32, I will give you some ideas for what the solution to our crisis may be.
- ◦ Then, we will close with the consolidation craze, the drug debate, and aging in America.

CHAPTER 28

Our Dysfunctional Healthcare System

In the previous twenty-seven chapters, you have learned a few things about the American healthcare system. America has so far rejected the institution of a nationalized healthcare system in favor of a predominantly employer-based system. Relying on employer-sponsored coverage creates gaps for those who do not have a connection to private-sector businesses or public employment, leading to vast numbers of uninsured. Over the years, efforts were made to create several social welfare programs for healthcare, including Medicare, Medicaid, and the Affordable Care Act (ACA). This has reduced the number of uninsured. As such, government spending now represents a majority of our healthcare expenditures. However, we continue to have a great number of uninsured.

So, is America's healthcare system dysfunctional? For the most part, yes. On one hand, we can claim to have the most advanced, on-demand healthcare system in the world. In America, the ability to be cured of disease and medical conditions is perhaps unparalleled. The ability to tap into the healthcare system quickly is also greater than any developed country. There is one big caveat to all this. You must be able to afford to do so and have access to the healthcare system. You have to have robust health insurance (a double expense—first to buy the pricey coverage and then to have dollars left over for what are often still major out-of-pocket costs) or the means to simply pay for your healthcare out-of-pocket.

If you don't have such access or resources, then you don't do as well from a health perspective in the United States as you would in other developed countries. As such, America's overall healthcare outcomes and results are among the worst in the developed world. Our healthcare system costs the most and our aggregate outcomes are among the lowest.

It is a curious dichotomy. The wealthy in America have good outcomes, if they want them. There are many non-U.S. residents from developed nations who travel vast distances and spend much wealth to seek healthcare in America. But, when you look at it from the perspective of many Americans—or, perhaps more precisely, average Americans—our performance is pitiful. The average American receives limited or inferior care. Too harsh? You be the judge.

The American health insurance system is fractured and inefficient. While I do not favor giving up on an employer-based model, the reality is that too many of us don't have a strong enough nexus to employment to rely on this system exclusively. It's true that various public programs like Medicare and Medicaid were set up to fill the voids. However, the uninsured measured in the tens of millions before the most recent public health insurance experiment—the ACA—was passed. Even with substantial progress after that, we still have tens of millions who are uninsured.

To compound the problem, we have dozens of insurance vehicles, each with what I call its own GPS—and the navigational system for each is pretty much broken. As the late, great Uwe Reinhardt, a brilliant economist who has helped form many of my thoughts, said in his book *Priced Out*, the American healthcare system "is almost beyond human comprehension."[28-1] It has layer upon layer of overlapping rules and missed handoffs. It is arcane and exceedingly complex. Our insurance system includes multiple types of products, plans, coverage, benefits, and cost-sharing rules. It is extremely expensive. It is obscure, lacks transparency, and, consequently, people have a hard time navigating the system. This leads to expense, waste, and poor outcomes.

We have put a series of dirty Band-Aids on our healthcare system. The problem is that the system is not just cut and bruised. We cannot treat our system as if there is just a small infection. In fact, the patient is hemorrhaging and the system cannot survive as we know it.

The American healthcare system is the most expensive in the developed world. We are a clear outlier in terms of spending when compared with other developed countries. According to national healthcare expenditure data for 2019, America spent 17.7% of its gross domestic product (GDP) on healthcare, or about $3.8 trillion.[28-2] If our healthcare system were a country, it would be the fifth-largest economy in the world.

Other developed countries' healthcare expenditures are generally from a low-end of 9% to a high end of just over 12% of GDP.[28-3, 28-4] America's system is expensive in comparison to other developed countries. In 2013, on a per-capita basis, America spent more than double of other OECD nations ($8,713 in the U.S. compared with $3,453 for the OECD average).[28-5] That trend has continued. In a study using 2019 data adjusted for purchasing power parity, per capita healthcare consumption in the United States was $10,996 versus $5,697 in select other developed countries, which is over 92% more.[28-6] Even if you argue that more is better, our healthcare system is at least 50% more expensive and perhaps twice as expensive as the rest of the developed world.

What does this mean for the average American? It means that premiums and out-of-pocket costs continue to rise each year, which prices families out of quality coverage. To understand the impact, let's turn to the largest area of coverage in America, large group employer coverage, and the Peterson-Kaiser Family Foundation Health System Tracker.[28-7] Here are some recent statistics:

- Total health spending by and on behalf of a family of four with large employer coverage in 2018 was almost $23,000.
- In 2018, the average family spent $4,706 on premiums and $3,020 on cost-sharing (deductibles, co-insurance, and copayments), for a combined cost of $7,726.

- ○ Over the past decade, health spending by families has increased twice as fast as wages. Family combined premium and out-of-pocket spending was up 135% from 2003 to 2018. Employee costs increased an average of 9% per year from 2003 to 2018.

- ○ The increase in family costs has been driven in part by rising deductibles, an increasingly prominent feature of the employer benefit design. Deductibles have surged from 2003 to 2017, up from 20% of cost-sharing to 51%. Co-insurance has remained roughly steady, with co-payments as a percentage of out-of-pocket costs dropping. This contributes to concerns about lack of access to early and preventive coverage.

- ○ Thankfully, the family costs in the last five years of the study were more tempered, increasing 18% from 2013. Still, that is against an 8% general inflation increase and a 12% increase in workers' wages over the timeframe.

- ○ The large group employer funding percentage is only slightly down from 2008. Employers paid about two-thirds of the cost of health coverage in 2018 and shared a reasonable part of the cost of the increase. Employer premium increases were 115% from 2003 to 2018. As such, the cost increases are huge for these employers to handle and threaten economic growth.

Another study looked more broadly at employer coverage, finding that health insurance premiums in the United States also are increasing. From 2005 to 2015, premiums for family coverage increased 61%, while worker contributions to those plans increased 83%. A surge in deductibles was also found.[28-5]

What is interesting about these statistics is that we are in a relatively low period for overall health inflation in the large group employer world. I told you about the 1990s backlash against managed care that led to more flexible or liberal managed care plans in the 2000s. This led to a surge in costs. In 2007, the inflation trend was 11.9%. Healthcare inflation had moderate increases from 2008 to 2019, from 9.9% in 2008, slowing down to 5.5% in 2017. It ticked up to 5.7% in both 2018 and 2019 and was expected to go up to 6% in 2020 (a pre-pandemic prediction).[28-8]

A Commonwealth Fund study of 2019 employer plan premiums shows something similar and concludes that health plan premiums are taking up much more of an employee's take-home pay:[28-9]

- Employee premium contributions and deductibles increased from 9.1% of incomes a decade ago to 11.5% in 2019.
- Premiums and deductibles were over 10% of employees' incomes in thirty-seven states in 2019, compared to ten states in 2010.
- In nine states, premiums and deductibles were 14% or more of household incomes.
- Average deductibles accounted for 5% or more of median income for people living in twenty states.
- The single coverage average premium contributions nationally were $1,489 in 2019.
- Family coverage average premium contributions nationally were $5,719 in 2019, within a range of $3,685 to $8,202.
- The average deductible for single coverage was $1,931, within a range of $1,264 to $2,521 in 2019.

While we pay the most, the United States has among the lowest health outcomes and lacks quality. Earlier we talked of the dichotomy of our healthcare system. We have the most technologically advanced, on-demand system in the world that attracts patients from all over the globe. Yet, on various health outcome measures and quality indicators, we perform terribly against our developed nation peers. We get little value for our money. Here is how we stack up in recent years. We are among the lowest in the developed world on a number of common measures, including the following:[28-3, 28-4, 28-10, 28-11, 28-12]

Life expectancy—At just above seventy-nine years, we rank forty-sixth in the world, out of about 190 nations. This is lower than the vast majority of developed nations and even lower than many less-developed nations.

Most developed nations have two to five more years of life expectancy. For 2017, the Commonwealth Fund reported U.S. life expectancy at 78.6, with the developed world average at 80.7.

Share of older adults—Similarly, the percentage of people sixty-five to seventy-nine and eighty-plus is less than other developed nations. About 12% of our population is in the first grouping, with 4% in the latter. In other developed countries sampled, those percentages range from 12-15% and 4-6, respectively.

Infant mortality—The U.S. rate is 5.9 deaths per 1,000 live births. The average rate for developed nations is 3.9 deaths per 1,000 live births. The U.S. ranks thirty-three out of thirty-six developed countries. (Note that there is significant deviation between states, with top performing states at about the developed world average, and the worst-performing state at about 9 deaths per 1,000 live births.)

Obesity—Various studies put obesity rates for American adults at between 31-40%. We know that obesity is a major contributing factor to various disease states, such as diabetes, hypertension, other heart conditions, and stroke. The developed world average obesity rate is 20-21%.

Healthcare-related avoidable deaths—The United States also performs poorly against a sampling of developed nations. The U.S. had 112 avoidable deaths per 100,000, while the other countries in the developed world surveyed between fifty-five and eighty-five.

Other performance measures—As you will learn later on in this chapter, we perform very poorly on wellness, prevention, primary care access, and disease management. Consequently, we have high hospital admission rates for exacerbation of chronic conditions.

One of the few areas that the U.S. shines is the smoking rate, which is about 12% for those age fifteen and above, compared with about 20% for other developed countries.

Despite spending the most on healthcare, we have a high level of uninsured and underinsured. The dollars we spend should be more than enough to cover all Americans. Most developed nations have crafted systems that cover about 99% of their citizens. Unfortunately, because our system is so fractured, the level of uninsured in America is high. Even with the advent of the ACA in 2010 (when over 44 million were uninsured and about 28 million gained coverage), the United States sits at about 90% of all Americans with health coverage, or about 32 million uninsured. (Statistics vary, but I am using the 2019 CMS national health expenditure number.) The number of uninsured individuals is projected to rise to 37 million by 2028. These are pre-COVID-19 pandemic numbers. In addition, the aging of America likely will drive further increases in the uninsured unless we develop policies around the looming crisis.[28-2, 28-13, 28-14, 28-15 28-16]

What do the uninsured look like? [28-14, 28-17]

Most are lower income and have at least one worker in the family. But the uninsured crisis does hit the middle class. Here is the breakout of the uninsured in 2018:

o   Under 100% of the federal poverty limit (FPL)—23%
o   100-199% of FPL—28%
o   200-99% of FPL—32%
o   400% and over of FPL—16%

Given State Children's Health Insurance Program (SCHIP) coverage as well as more generous coverage for children under Medicaid, adults are more likely to be uninsured than children.

Blacks and Hispanics are at higher risk of being uninsured. Over 50% of the uninsured are people of color. (It is worth noting that the ACA had a profound impact on helping minority groups gain coverage.)

People cite the high cost of insurance as a reason for being uninsured. 45% of those uninsured said this is so.

Many do not have access to employer coverage. Others do not have access to Medicaid in states that have not expanded. Some are not aware of the Medicaid entitlement and the Marketplace subsidies and still others are not eligible for Marketplace subsidies.

Of the 12 states that have not expanded Medicaid under the ACA, people earning under 100% of FPL but above the state's Medicaid income eligibility (on average 40% of FPL across states) are in a coverage gap—unable to be on either Medicaid or the Exchanges. This has led to a curious predicament where those with lower incomes are not entitled to coverage while those with higher incomes are. As of this writing in early 2021, there are about 2.2 million people in this category, while others put this number at over 3 million. Seventy-six percent of them are in Texas, Florida, Georgia, and North Carolina. Interestingly, in the 12 states, there are 400,000 people who are eligible for Medicaid and 1.8 million for the Exchanges who are also not enrolled in health insurance.

Undocumented immigrants are ineligible for Medicaid or Marketplace coverage.

An important issue is the fact that we also have an underinsurance problem. (I never thought I would agree with Bernie Sanders on something—but there it is.) Since the ACA passed, the overall number of uninsured has dropped and the long-term uninsured rate has declined, as have gaps in coverage (The COVID-19 pandemic has temporarily impacted this somewhat). However, the percentage of people between nineteen and sixty-four who are underinsured in America remains at about 45%, including those who are uninsured. This is the same as it was before the ACA went into effect. In fact, the number of underinsured in America has risen, mostly related to erosion of employer coverage and the higher cost-sharing noted above. This amounts to about 87 million underinsured in 2018. And, as you will see below, being either uninsured or underinsured has profound effects on accessing care at the right time, along with overall costs and outcomes.[28-18]

The costs of the American healthcare system threaten our overall economic competitiveness. Overall, American companies are at a great disadvantage, compared with their foreign counterparts. Here are a few reasons:

While the tax deductibility of health insurance for employers is a huge subsidy, it only covers part of the costs of providing employer-based coverage. This is because it is taken as an ordinary business expense and a deduction. It is not a dollar-for-dollar tax credit. The corporate tax rate is now 21% as of this writing, meaning businesses get just 21% off the cost of providing healthcare to their employees.[28-19]

Beyond the absolute costs of health coverage, American companies also fund, in employer premiums, the massive cost shift from Medicare and Medicaid. Because rates in government programs are low—sometimes lower than actual costs—providers demand higher commercial rates. This rolls out in the cost the employer pays and what you pay in premiums.

It is also not the case that other developed nations' businesses pay higher corporate taxes. The 21% tax rate was lowered recently from 35% (it could go back up to 28% under Biden's pending tax proposals). Thus, America re-aligned its corporate tax rate to be more competitive with other countries, although states charge corporate tax rates as well. These may not be in place in other countries. Although Europe has some outliers in terms of corporate taxes, the average corporate tax rate there is 22.5%. The global average is 21.4%.[28-20]

The greatest cost of other developed nations' health systems is paid by a mixture of income and value-added taxes (VAT) and not by business, *per se*. While VATs do impact the costs of goods, these taxes are passed ultimately to the consumer and are not really a corporate tax. While one could argue these so-called high VATs create a drag on consumer spending and corporate growth, it is also true that America does have sales taxes at various levels on some of the same goods. I would note that some nations, such as Germany, do have businesses contribute directly to healthcare costs for employees, but the amounts per employee are much more modest and tend to be capped at a percentage of payroll (similar to the FICA and Medicare tax in the United States).

In sum, the direct taxes on American businesses and other developed nations' businesses are not vastly different. But American businesses are paying healthcare premiums not shouldered in other developed nations by businesses.

So what is the impact? Let's examine the macroeconomic level. The size of the healthcare pie is already large. Annual healthcare inflation tends to ebb and flow, but one thing is clear: there almost always is inflation (not deflation—COVID-19 is the exception) and growth in costs almost always outpaces growth in the GDP as well as in people's incomes. Thus, healthcare spending will grow as a percentage of the economy over time. While growth in costs have slowed somewhat, national healthcare expenditures and inflation will accelerate again in the near term. Spurred by aging and other factors, projections suggest we will spend about $6.2 trillion on healthcare by 2028, about 19.7% of projected GDP. [28-2]

You can argue that certain healthcare spending can be "positive" or "dynamic" spending. However, it is also the case that the already huge GDP health burden (about 18%), the singular costs shouldered by American business in the form of employer healthcare premiums, and the unfettered increases in healthcare costs do "crowd out" other forms of investment that would otherwise grow the economy and spur innovation. As with a household budget, there is only so much money to go around and only so much growth in income from year to year. If healthcare spending outpaces the growth in your budget (in this case growth in GDP), fewer dollars are there to grow in other areas (such as jobs and investment).

Here is a good example. If a company is on the verge of investing in a new piece of machinery that can grow its business and add jobs, but the healthcare bill for next year has come in with a 10-20% increase (not unheard of in some years for health bill increases), then the business owner may have to forego that machinery purchase and all those new jobs. Multiply this by thousands of businesses and it can be a recipe for disaster at the macroeconomic level.

Our nation's economic growth could stagnate under the weight of the overall burden, the increasing healthcare cost, and other public- and private-sector burdens. We can look to Europe for visible examples of where this has happened. European countries tend to have a heavy public sector burden that creates a drag on the economy. The investment "crowd-out" is one reason among many (others are demographic aging and lack of major population growth), that economies in Europe grow at a much slower rate—when they do grow—compared with the United States.

It is easy to see how the United States might end up like Europe. Over time, profligate spending, unfunded government liabilities (such as Social Security, Medicare, Medicaid, and public pension and healthcare liabilities), and the drag of ever-increasing healthcare costs could all come together to create this problem here. Indeed, our gross public debt as a percentage of gross domestic product (GDP) is roughly at the European Union average. With the COVID-19 crisis, it will soon shoot up even more.[28-21]

The costs of the American healthcare system threaten our individual health, well-being, and prosperity. At the micro level or on the personal front, why does it matter? As I noted, healthcare costs tend to outstrip personal income growth. Each year, seeking to deal with high inflation in healthcare, businesses may force you as a consumer to pay more premiums. But if healthcare costs outstrip your income, you must make up the increased premiums from somewhere else. This includes the loss of disposable income.

Businesses may also reduce benefits or increase cost-sharing—making you come up with even more money from somewhere else and putting you in the class of underinsured. The business may drop coverage altogether as costs increase. Or you may drop coverage due to costs. In these cases, you end up among the uninsured. If you are on a public healthcare program such as Medicare or Medicaid, something similar could occur—your premiums could go up, your cost-sharing might increase with your private plan, or government could reduce benefits.

Higher costs or loss of insurance has known impacts on health outcomes and well-being. We don't seek preventive services. Disease states exacerbate. You end up accessing healthcare during a crisis when costs are the highest, namely at emergency rooms and inpatient care facilities. You can't afford the cost of care, often even if you are insured. You can't pay your bills. You are among those who declare bankruptcy due to medical debt. Your good name is ruined. It takes years to build back your credit.

Here are a few more facts about the impact of being uninsured or underinsured.[28-18, 28-22]

Due to the ACA, the number of people aged nineteen to sixty who reported skipping a test, treatment, or follow-up, not filling a prescription, having a medical problem but not seeking care, or not getting specialist care declined from 43% before to 34-35% following the bill's implementation. But that still is more than one-third of people who fail to access the system appropriately due to barriers.

Due to the ACA, the number of people aged nineteen to sixty-four who reported having problems paying a medical bill, were contacted by a collection agency for unpaid medical bills, entered into payment plans, or similar scenarios declined from 41% to 35%-37%. But again, more than a third of people struggle with the overall cost of healthcare.

Continuous coverage means a greater likelihood that you will seek appropriate preventive care; if you are underinsured or uninsured, you may forego it. Consider the following:

Insurance coverage status	Have regular source of care	Blood pressure checked	Cholesterol checked	Seasonal flu shot	Females receiving a pap test	Females receiving a mammogram	Received colon cancer screening
Insured all year; not underinsured	93%	94%	79%	48%	73%	71%	63%
Insured all year; underinsured	94%	94%	76%	44%	70%	71%	60%
Insured but had coverage gap	84%	89%	63%	30%	72%	48%	38%
Uninsured	68%	72%	44%	20%	53%	32%	35%

A more recent study by Peterson-Kaiser Family Foundation Health System Tracker found similar results related to the uninsured for the 2019 calendar year:

- High costs meant about 1 in 10 adults delayed or did not get care, with minority groups having even worse rates.
- Those in worse health are twice as likely to delay or forego care.
- For those who are insured, care delay or avoidance is below 10%, while those who are uninsured delay or forego care at a rate of 30% or greater.
- Those below 200% of the federal poverty limit have an almost 18% rate of delaying or foregoing care.
- Over one-third of those who are uninsured do not have a usual place of care, such as a primary care physician.

Why are we the most expensive yet perform so poorly overall? There are numerous factors that make us the most expensive and result in failing grades on healthcare:

Because we are the richest (in aggregate), biggest, and most developed nation, **the U.S. healthcare system tends to shoulder greater burdens**. New healthcare advances are often introduced or experimented with here first. In addition, because America has an open healthcare marketplace, including few if any price controls, healthcare entrepreneurs recoup much of their investments from Americans. Clearly, this has its pros and cons. We get many advancements sooner, but we seem to pay a much higher price than elsewhere. In essence, we take on the burden of funding some of the rest of the world's healthcare systems, because we are big and because other nations, by using price fixing, effectively refuse to pay for it.[28-5]

Related to the above, **the United States has an on-demand, expansive, and high-technology-focused healthcare system.** Americans demand the best now in so many ways. The healthcare system's on-demand nature adds considerably to our costs, since much of the treatment may or may not be needed, resulting in saturation of services. An example of such on-demand services includes expensive same-day or same-week medical resonance imaging (MRI) and other high-tech radiology.

The mere presence of advanced technology fuels demand. For example, with limited exceptions, the United States has the most MRI machines per capita at around 38 per million citizens, while the average in select developed nations was between 9 and 31. (Japan did exceed the United States, however, at fifty-two). MRI exams per million were also much greater in the United States than in most developed nations. Most had a range of 35-76 exams per 1,000 population. France had 96 per 1,000. The United States had 110 per 1,000. Only Germany had more, at 114. Another study puts the developed world average at just below 60 per 1,000, with the United States at 121 per 1,000. Germany was higher at 136.[28-3, 28-4, 28-5]

I have already said that on a GDP and per-capita basis, America is a huge outlier for costs of its healthcare system. **America has profoundly high prices, and this is perhaps the greatest reason for the disparity in overall costs between the United States and other developed nations.** Apart from the set fees we see in the Medicaid and Medicare fee-for-service (FFS) programs as well as a few other smaller government programs, America has few price controls. A lack of price transparency—the fact that the average person has no idea of what prices are like in the system—also adds to costs. Let's dive deeper.[28-2, 28-3, 28-4, 28-8, 28-23, 28-24, 28-25, 28-26]

One study of employer benefit costs found that utilization has hovered around 0% growth since 2006. Another study found that utilization by individuals with employer-based insurance dropped by 0.2% from 2013 to 2017, but prices increased 17% over the same period.

Various studies have shown that hospital spending per discharge is well out of line due to high hospital prices. As we learned earlier, hospital costs are about one-third of overall healthcare spending. One study shows a range of $5,000 to $14,600 per discharge for select developed nations. However, America has an average discharge cost of over $21,000. Another study puts the average discharge at just below $10,000 for developed nations versus almost $30,000 for the United

States. Between 2007 and 2014, hospital inpatient prices increased 42%, and physician inpatient prices grew 18%.

There are similar results for specific procedures involving physician and hospital costs. Physician and clinic costs are about 20% of healthcare expenditures in the United States.

○ Hip replacements: The U.S. average is over $29,000 versus select developed countries' range of $15,500 to $19,500 per discharge.
○ Angioplasty: The U.S. average is over $31,600 versus select developed countries' range of $7,300 to $13,700 per discharge.
○ Cataract surgery: The U.S. average is over $3,530 versus select developed countries' range of $2,114 to $3,145 per discharge.

While some hospital mergers bring efficiency and quality, multiple studies have shown that hospital mergers lead to higher prices. In the twenty-five metropolitan areas with the highest rates of consolidation as measured by the Federal Trade Commission (FTC), prices increased by 11% to 54% following mergers. It is also true that hospitals and health systems are acquiring physician practices to have greater leverage in the market, which drives higher prices as well as physicians now practice at high-cost hospital-owned locations. By early 2018, almost half of all physicians in the United States were employed by hospitals or large healthcare systems.

The Medicaid and Medicare FFS programs set fees for providers. This helps private Medicare and Medicaid plans control costs. However, private plans in the employer world have a hard time benchmarking prices against those government fee schedules. As such, hospitals and other providers often force private plans to pay exceedingly high reimbursement based on inflated provider market fees. A recent RAND study looked at claims from 2016 to 2018 in 49 states and over 3,000 hospitals, adding up to $33.8 billion in hospital spending. It found that private insurers, on average, paid 247% more for hospital care than Medicare. The range was 200-325%.

Drug prices in the United States compared with the rest of the developed world are indeed obscene. Retail drugs account for only about 9% of healthcare expenditures. However, medical drugs (administered in hospitals, on an outpatient basis, or in physician's offices) are buried within other categories. All told, it is a growing part of healthcare spending and one that is garnering the most public attention. Several factors lead to these obscenely high drug prices:

Much of the rest of the developed world effectively fix prices that will be paid for brand medications. If drug companies are unwilling to negotiate or accept those prices, then the drug is simply not included in the system. Even in private universal access systems, such as Germany, effective ways are found to provide cost controls on drug prices through negotiation or a price list.

There is some price fixing for certain U.S. programs, such as the federal supply schedule (FSS) for certain healthcare programs and the Medicaid drug rebate program. There are also negotiations between health plans and drug manufacturers. However, for the most part, drugs are not price controlled in the United States. This leads to exorbitant prices and exceedingly high annual inflation. Drug companies can largely ask what they want and increase prices from year to year with impunity.

The drug business lacks transparency, with its array of middlemen and distribution channels—each of these shadowy entities taking its piece of the pie and inflating prices. These include the manufacturers, wholesale distributors, pharmacy benefits managers, drug rebate aggregators, and more.

Despite some reforms, **drugmakers advertise with abandon.** Consequently, they sell physicians and patients on expensive brand drugs when legacy drugs—those on the market for decades— could control disease states just as well, and sometimes better.

While reforms have been made, **drugmakers still stop cheaper generics from coming to market quickly**.

Estimates of drug costs in the United States versus other developed-world countries can differ markedly, but it still amounts to a huge difference. In one study, individuals globally saved 56% compared with Americans on select drugs. That means Americans pay more than double for those same drugs. Just north of us, Canadians paid $772 annually compared to Americans' $1,112—a 31% difference. A report from the U.S. House of Representatives Ways and Means Committee says that costs are actually orders of magnitude higher. It finds that prices are almost four times higher than the average in eleven similar countries. The committee analyzed 2018 pricing data of seventy-nine drugs sold in the United States, the United Kingdom, Japan, Canada (Ontario), Australia, Portugal, France, the Netherlands, Germany, Denmark, Sweden, and Switzerland. Average per-capita spending in the eleven countries was $626 compared with $1,220 in the United States.

America has a lack of focus on primary care, prevention, and health education, combined with a relative paucity of physicians. The number of practicing physicians is comparatively low in America. A study shows that in 2018, the developed world had 3.5 practicing physicians per 1,000 population, while the United States had only 2.6. Doctor consultation rates here are low compared to the average in the developed world. In one study, it was found that America has 4 physician consults per capita, while the average for developed nations is above 6, with some having 7-10. In another study, the developed world physician visits per capita was 6.8, with the United States at 4. Statistics also show that in addition to having too few primary care physicians (PCPs), we are over-specialized. Given the huge costs of medical education, more medical students want to become brain surgeons, plastic surgeons, or heart surgeons, rather than primary care doctors. We tend to under-reimburse for primary care and over-reimburse for specialty visits in our system. This leads to major costs as well. According to the Organization for Economic

Cooperation and Development (OECD), this lack of investment in primary care means that America spends just 5% on primary care versus an average of 14% in other developed nations.[28-4, 28-5, 28-11, 28-27]

A study by the Association of American Medical Colleges (AAMC) concludes that the United States could see a physician shortage of between 54,100 and 139,000 by 2033. This includes a shortfall of primary care physicians (PCPs) of between 21,400 and 55,200 and specialists of between 33,700 and 86,700.[28-28]

The COVID-19 pandemic may create even more complications on the primary care physician front. A new survey from the Larry A. Green Center and Primary Care Collaborative says that the status of primary care has been terribly impacted by the COVID-19 pandemic. The survey had 636 responses across 47 states.

The study reports that, in August 2020 alone, 2% of primary care practices closed and another 2% are considering bankruptcy. Ten percent of primary care practices are uncertain of their solvency for the coming month. Worse, consider the following:[28-29]

○   21% had furloughs or layoffs
○   20% of primary care clinicians are considering leaving primary care
○   28% lost 30–50% in FFS revenue
○   46% have seen a 30–50% drop in patient volume
○   24% stopped quality initiatives
○   13% said they were uncertain of their future in the profession

Our rates of chronic diseases are high, and they are not well-managed. Obesity, diabetes, and other disease states significantly add to the costs of the healthcare system. According to the Centers for Disease Control and Prevention (CDC), between 75-90% of all healthcare spending can be tied to treatment of chronic diseases or conditions. The percentages for Medicare and Medicaid are 96% and 83%, respectively. People with chronic conditions are over three times more costly. Those with complex conditions are over eight times more costly. Sixty percent of adults have a chronic disease and 40% have two or more. A study of eleven countries (including the United States) shows an average chronic disease burden of 17.5% of the population, while the United States is at 28%. A United Healthcare review of employer claims shows an extrapolated cost of $2.5 billion to treat employees' asthma, diabetes, hypertension, mental health and substance abuse, and back disorders over the course of two years. It says that 60% of employees struggle with at least one of these conditions.[28-8, 28-11, 28-30, 28-31, 28-32]

America has little care coordination and management, which exacerbates disease states and consumption of healthcare at high-cost places of service. Because of the lack of primary prevention and wellness and little focus on population health, Americans access care in greater rates at the most costly levels when there is a crisis. In one review of selected developed countries, 35% of American patients reported issues with coordination of their care. While some nations performed equally or nearly as bad, others scored much better, with just 19-30% reporting care coordination issues. Consequently, our use of hospitalization due to disease state exacerbation or crises is remarkably high. Of select developed countries, most had discharges per 100,000 population for diabetes episodes of between 60 and 153. For hypertension, it was 18 to 61. America had 204 per 100,000 for diabetes and 159 for hypertension. Only Germany fared worse in the group (well above even the United States in both categories).[28-3, 28-4, 28-33]

Part of the problem is that we have high rates of readmission for these disease states and because, more significantly, we lack care coordination for care transitions and discharge. Good care transitions and discharge would pick the optimal, post-hospital place of service to receive care. Increasingly, it may be home as opposed to a skilled nursing facility. They would also ensure that care is set up, delivered, and monitored for outcomes and risks of readmission. We don't have that. Nearly 20% of all Medicare discharges had a readmission within thirty days. Avoidable readmissions are costing billions each year.[28-3, 28-4, 28-33]

America has a patchwork system, which in part drives high administrative costs and duplication. As I have said, I am not an advocate of eliminating our employer-sponsored coverage system, but some reforms need to occur to eliminate the overlapping and duplication in our system overall. With each separate program or insurance scheme comes administrative costs of operation, enrollment, paying claims, and more. The plethora of competing plans within each scheme also drives up administrative costs.

As Uwe Reinhardt notes in his book *Priced Out,* **there is no political consensus on the fact that affordable, universal access is a social good**—as it is in every other developed country. The lack of affordable universal access adds costs to the systems because the uninsured and underinsured forego treatment and later access care at expensive places of service. They are then unable to pay their bill and these costs are borne or spill over into the overall system.

To be sure, people self-ration because they cannot afford healthcare. **But broadly, the U.S. system itself does not ration care.** It is anathema to American values. One can debate the appropriateness of some or all of this rationing, but the lack of rationing adds to costs. In other developed systems, there is implicit and explicit rationing. Explicit rationing examples include the fact that certain developed healthcare systems do not cover certain drugs and certain services will just not be given to individuals based on certain policies. Implicit rationing includes waiting lists or times to receive certain treatment, such as hip or knee replacement.

Fraud, waste, and abuse (FWA) are rampant in the U.S. healthcare system, in part tied to the tremendous duplication and overlap described previously. Traditional estimates of FWA used to say it was about 10% of total annual healthcare spending—hitting Medicare, Medicaid, and the commercial lines of business. But recent studies have re-evaluated old assumptions and calculated a much higher number for

FWA. An abstract by the *Journal of the American Medical Association* notes several prior studies that estimated it to be as much as 25% of healthcare spending.[28-34] The conclusion is that despite recent government crackdowns and health plan efforts, the percentage attributable to FWA likely remains unchanged. According to the studies, the FWA breakdown is as follows:

- Failure of care delivery—$102.4–$165.7 billion annually
- Failure of care coordination—$27.2–$78.2 billion annually
- Over-treatment or low-value care—$75.7–$101.2 billion annually
- Pricing failure—$230.7–$240.5 billion annually
- Fraud and abuse—$58.5–$83.9 billion annually
- Administrative complexity—$265.6 billion annually

America also has significant healthcare costs associated with social barriers to good health. These are things like food security, income and socio-economic status, housing security, and health literacy.

That FFS reimbursement system I have talked about ad nauseam adds costs as well. The more a provider supplies in terms of services, whether it is needed or not, the more he gets paid.

Aging is and will continue to influence high costs. Aging will mean an explosion in both acute care and long-term care health costs and spending.

Both our tort system and government regulation add to healthcare costs. A tort system is the ability to sue for a civil wrong. In this case, people can sue healthcare providers for malpractice. While there has been an effort at the state and federal levels to rein in the expansiveness of this right, and the awards that can be made, it remains a cost contributor. Government regulation, where the state and federal governments require the addition of benefits or mandates processes, also adds to the cost of healthcare.

The phenomenon of social good versus individual rights also plays a role. In the United States, the relatively free ability to sue someone in the healthcare system for damages, compared with that of other nations, adds to the cost of tort lawsuits and medical malpractice insurance.

Let's sum up with two last points to put this in context. Uwe Reinhardt's book *Priced Out* discusses a study brief, the most recent of which was published in early 2021, by the Agency for Healthcare Research and Quality, which sums up why we are so dysfunctional. Perhaps along with price, our lack of primary prevention, wellness, and care coordination seems to be the biggest problem we have that drive high costs and low quality. We are driving people to expensive forms of care late in their medical episodes. The most recent survey looked at the U.S. civilian, non-institutional population's share of spending in 2018. The so-called concentration curve of healthcare spending is phenomenal.[28-35]

- The majority of spending in the United States is concentrated in a small percentage of the population.
- In 2016, 1% of the survey population consumed about 21% of total healthcare expenditures, while the bottom 50% accounted for only about 3%.
- 5% of the population accounted for about 48% of total healthcare expenditures.
- Inpatient hospital care was about 36% of spending for persons in the top 5% of the spending distribution.
- Individual, per-capita healthcare consumption for 2016 was as follows:
  - The top 1% of consumed $72,212 or more, annually, with a mean of $127,284
  - The top 5% consumed $26,355 or more annually, with a mean of $58,609
  - The top 10% consumed $14,651 or more annually, with a mean of $38,980

- o The top 30% consumed $3,776 or more annually, with a mean of $18,027
- o The bottom 50% consumed less than $1,317 annually, with a mean of $384
- o Aggregate healthcare consumption for 2018 was as follows, with total expenditures for the surveyed group being about $1.979 billion:
  - o The top 1% consumed $415 million
  - o The top 5% consumed $956 million
  - o The top 10% consumed $1.272 billion
  - o The top 30% consumed $1.765 billion
  - o The bottom 50% consumed about $63 billion

Second, a preeminent study from The Commonwealth Fund in 2021 spoke to the overall ranking of the U.S. healthcare system and the problems it has. As it had in the past, Commonwealth compared the U.S. system to ten similarly developed nations' systems. Its findings should sound familiar. The U.S. system ranked eleventh overall. It ranked last in access, equity, administrative efficiency, and healthcare outcomes. The best it did was in care process—second. In other words, we have a huge value problem—the highest cost with few quality outcomes. [28-36]

I will discuss more about the differences in healthcare systems in Chapter 30, but the study shows that outcomes are also not tied to *types* of systems. There are socialized, government-run systems (public run and largely public care provision), as well as single-payer systems (public run with largely private care provision), and universal access systems (public mandated but private health insurance and care provision). Each of these models performed at the top of the Commonwealth list. The top four performers were Norway, the Netherlands, Australia, and the United Kingdom—representing all three types of systems.

To summarize the big issues that make our system so expensive and dysfunctional, I would offer three things:

We have no price controls. At heart, I am a price control skeptic and Republicans will wail against them, but the reality is that the healthcare system is not a functioning free market for so many reasons. As well, every other developed country has them, whether they have socialized medicine, single payer, or private universal access systems. They use a combination of master price negotiations and international reference pricing. We need to get our arms around and grapple with price because it impacts access and quality outcomes. What we have now simply does not work.

Our high level of uninsured and underinsured creates costs and poor quality. We need to get everyone covered to emphasize upfront care.

We need to shift to care management and population health. We need to emphasize wellness and prevention to identify and treat underlying disease states and conditions earlier. This will help us overcome our status as a developed nation with among the worst health outcomes.

CHAPTER 29

Progress Toward a New Paradigm

The last chapter was full of statistics about why our healthcare system is dysfunctional and, admittedly, fairly depressing. Now, I want to go a little lighter and show you why there is some hope for our system as a whole. There are some positive trends in the healthcare system that can serve as a foundation for reform and move us toward a new healthcare paradigm.

The Emerging Public-Private Partnership

Let's talk first about what I view as a growing, public-private partnership model emerging in the United States.

While some parts of the left wing of the Democratic Party continue to advocate for a Medicare for All system and the elimination of private health plans, the more moderate members of that party (including President Biden), along with the Republican Party, support the continued provision of care through private health plans. There is a chance that a Medicare for All system could come into play; but, as I suggest in a future chapter, I predict it would be disastrous for America's healthcare system. Cooler heads will likely prevail as the proposal works its way through Congress. And, as I have alluded to, while some polls show Medicare for All as popular, digging into the poll statistics suggests America really does not want to get rid of private health plans or their personal insurance.

In fact, the more moderate minds on Capitol Hill on each side of the aisle have actually been working on a public-private healthcare model for years. This goes back decades. In my many years of working in government and the private sector, I saw this firsthand as I visited key senators and congresspeople about various government healthcare programs. These lawmakers and key policymakers within various Democratic and Republican administrations are slowly but surely creating a system where the federal government—in partnership with states—drive accountability and quality in the healthcare system, while private health plans largely deliver care. There is a clear, behind-the-scenes consensus on this.

As I have noted throughout the book, private health plans continue to grow in influence in both government and employer-based care. The majority of healthcare in America is furnished through employer-based coverage using private health plans. In Medicare, private Medicare Advantage (MA) plans now account for over 43% of enrollment of beneficiaries and could reach 70% in the next fifteen to twenty years. Medicaid now has about 75-80% of all care through private plans and this percentage is rising as well.

Lawmakers and policymakers have designed a system where the federal government, principally through the Department of Health and Human Services (HHS) and the Centers for Medicare and Medicaid Services (CMS), essentially oversees all policy for the healthcare system and issues various dictates to health plans to reduce costs and improve quality.

There is no question that the accountability and quality measures have done many things, starting with changing how America thinks about healthcare. CMS has also enacted important policy changes to reduce costs and improve quality. CMS is establishing an over-arching policy framework across Medicare, Medicaid, and certain commercial products, especially the Affordable Care Act (ACA) Marketplace Exchanges.

Essentially, what this does is allow the government to exercise reasonable stewardship over the healthcare system and expenditures (as it occurs in some form in every other developed country) but rely on innovation in the private sector (health plans) to drive change.

Given its wide breadth of responsibility, it is clear that CMS is the pivotal player in healthcare oversight and future healthcare reform. We will see that CMS is driving all lines of business to a common compliance, accountability, and quality standard. I am a huge fan of the strides the agency has made in Medicare and it should have similar success in Medicaid and the Exchanges. The Obama Administration published a far-reaching Medicaid reform rule, (called the Medicaid Uber Rule) that looks and feels like what has occurred on the compliance and quality front in Medicare. In time, CMS will roll the same out in the Exchanges. I would also predict that CMS, HHS, and the Department of Labor will continue to press greater accountability and quality in self-insured employer plans.

This will be supported by forward-thinking corporations who put a premium on associate health and well-being. While at times plans complain about the rigor that has been put in place, there is little doubt that it is the only way to bring accountability to the system, root out waste and inefficiency, and improve quality. Building a national program based on quality is the only way to truly bend the cost curve and begin seeing national healthcare expenditures as a percentage of gross domestic product (GDP) that is more in line with other developed countries.

I go into greater detail below about these accountability and quality measures, but the setting of a new national policymaking infrastructure is the most important, over-arching development thus far. It needs to be understood and championed.

Medicare Compliance Accountability

With private MA plans beginning to lose support in Congress and in government in the 2000s, CMS began formulating an aggressive compliance and regulatory agenda. The focus was to ensure that plans meet reasonable timeframes to answer members' and providers' requests for coverage of drugs and services, consistently use evidence-based criteria, and have a member-centric outlook and low tolerance for beneficiary harm.

What has emerged over the past decade is a finely tuned and constantly honed compliance regime. While plans take issue with the extensive nature of the dictates from time to time, there is no question that it has restored faith in private, managed care in Medicare and bolstered overall support from the public. It is one of the main reasons that MA plans have been so successful and have grown markedly.

The compliance regime prioritizes the following factors:

Ensuring that each plan has a comprehensive compliance program to carry out the various regulatory dictates. Plans also must focus on various healthcare waste, fraud, and abuse laws.

Requiring plans to offer fairly aggressive turnaround times from the receipt of a request for a drug or service and the plan decision on whether to approve or deny such requests. In the drug world, these timeframes are between twenty-four and seventy-two hours for the initial request, while they range from seventy-two hours to fourteen days for medical services.

Ensuring that each service or drug request is evaluated by appropriate clinical personnel using evidence-based criteria, consistently applied across the entire population.

Ensuring that members and providers are notified of the decision on each case with a clear and concise communication using defined regulatory templates. This includes outlining next steps for a drug or service denial and ensuring members and providers understand all appeal rights.

Ensuring members have internal and external appeals processes. These include aggressive timeframes to decide internal health plan appeals.

These appeals must be conducted by a qualified clinician who did not review the original request. In addition, a member has the right to appeal a second denial to an external review entity, which will decide whether to sustain or overturn the plan decision based on evidence-based criteria.

Having a comprehensive complaint and grievance program to address members' concerns about quality and service provision.

Fully investigating all complaints and grievances to ensure operational improvements.

Ensuring ongoing transparency with members, including accuracy of enrollment, benefit, network, and drug list information as well as frequent publication of drug, benefit, and provider network changes.

Following strict rules related to drug formularies, utilization management (UM) practices, drug safety, and appropriate transitions of drug therapy.

Ensuring that plans follow a strict model of care (MOC) for its special needs plans (SNPs) for various vulnerable populations within Medicare.

Having ongoing submission of complex universes and regulatory reports to ensure compliance and oversight by CMS.

Being subject to periodic program audits and annual monitoring, which can result in significant civil monetary penalties and suspension of enrollment and marketing for sever violations.

As noted previously, the Medicaid Uber Rule promises to bring a similar compliance regime to Medicaid over the next several years. The Obama Administration sponsored the overhaul and, surprisingly, the Trump Administration did little to disturb its implementation. Also, as the owner of nationwide Marketplace Exchange policy, CMS will apply similar rules governing the ACA. In the end, we will have an extremely compliance-focused policy paradigm—one that will drive accountability throughout the healthcare system.

Medicare Quality Focus

In the 2000s, in addition to turning a blind eye to government compliance mandates, Medicare private plans were also accused of caring little about quality outcomes. As such, CMS also pursued an aggressive quality attainment program. Over time, the Star quality program emerged, and it has become transformational for the MA and Part D programs. Over time, this Star program is scheduled to be rolled out to Medicaid, via the Uber Rule, as well as the Exchanges.

Much more has to be done at the transaction or provider level to focus on quality. But for the time being, CMS has built a strong MA Star measures program in MA and Part D centered on the following factors:

Reporting by health plans on various clinical, administrative, and customer survey measures.

A quality bonus program in MA for plans that score 4, 4.5, or 5 on the 1-5 Star scale. The bonus is equal to 5% of premium. In addition, plans that score 3.5-5 get enhanced premiums in the rate process. These additional dollars are retained by the higher quality plans compared to lower scoring plans (which must rebate more in savings back to Medicare). In both the 5% bonus case and the retained premium incentive, plans must pass the amount on in the form of enhanced benefits to enrollees. But the plan benefits from much greater enrollment. I have personally followed the Star scores over the past decade and have recorded the following:

○ In 2010, on the passage of the ACA and the overhaul of the Star program, only 14% of plans had attained 4-Star or greater status. Even with a much more robust set of quality measures being introduced over the past decade, in 2020 52% of plans were 4-Star or greater. In 2021, 49% of plans are 4-Star or greater. (CMS announced the number of quality-rated plans and enrollees in them skyrocketed between 2021 and 2022. However, this is in large measure due to the relaxing of measurement during the COVID-19 pandemic.)

- ○ Seniors and the disabled have become very savvy and have followed the quality progress. In 2010, just 24% of MA enrollees were in plans with 4 Stars or greater. At the beginning of 2020, 81% of enrollees were in such plans. At the beginning of 2021, 77% of enrollees are in such plans.

CMS brilliantly set up the MA Star program by tying quality achievement to added revenue and requiring that it be allocated to additional member benefits. This fills in numerous benefit holes in the traditional fee-for-service (FFS) program, which is a godsend for many lower-income seniors and the disabled. In essence, MA has become one of the greatest social safety net programs in America.

The Star program drives plans to achieve high quality so as to grow membership. High-scoring plans have a huge premium advantage and can out-compete lower performing plans by offering much better benefits. Although percentage margins are largely fixed in regulation now (see the section just below), high-performing plans will still see larger financial margins as enrollment grows.

As noted, CMS is also constantly refining the quality program. Tougher and tougher measures are emerging. This is especially true on the clinical front. Plans struggled in the past to excel on basic clinical measures, such as whether a diabetic received routine blood testing and whether blood sugar was under control. Over time, plans got better and better. But CMS is now rolling out clinical measures that are both complex and comprehensive. Plans are now assessed—or will be—on measures that include reducing readmissions, preventing hospital admissions for chronic disease states, discharge and care transitions, care coordination, and medication reconciliation after hospitalization.

Financial Accountability

Congress, HHS, and CMS have also driven a substantial amount of financial accountability with the passage of laws and rules requiring minimum medical loss ratios (MLRs) across all lines of business. These laws and rules addressed a long-standing concern that health plans charged high premiums but did not spend the necessary amount on medical services, instead pocketing it as margin. Years ago, insurers did make fairly substantial margins, sometimes double-digit percentages from year to year. However, the new rules essentially set the minimum amount of premium spent on medical services at 80-85% of premium, depending on the line of business and product. These rules now apply in MA, Medicaid managed care, ACA Marketplace Exchanges, and in small and large group risk markets. (ERISA plans are self-funded, so the concept does not apply.)

If a plan does not spend the requisite amount of money on medical services, it must rebate the difference between what was spent and the percentage of premium required to be spent back to employers for employer coverage, individuals for various individual coverage, the federal government for Medicare, and state Medicaid agencies for Medicaid.

These rules have had a number of positive impacts:

○ They help control premium increases over the long term.
○ They help reduce overall costs by tightening what is available to pay providers.
○ They keep plans accountable by requiring a set amount to be spent on medical services.
○ Combined with the compliance and quality measures, minimum MLRs help bolster faith in employers and in the public at large. While health plans are still demonized, they are less so with this and other reforms.

Broken down, with a minimum established for medical services and sales and administrative costs, plans might now see a margin of no more than 4-6%, depending on the line of business. This is substantially down from the past, but enough to have a vibrant and innovative marketplace. Health insurers now have among the lowest margins for healthcare players.

Could the idea be used in other areas of healthcare?

Medicaid Overhaul

As mentioned previously, CMS is also busy overhauling Medicaid. Most states now are predominantly using Medicaid managed care as the vehicle to deliver most services. Historically, whether it was the traditional Medicaid FFS system or private health plan models, Medicaid quality was abominable. Over the past decade or so, CMS and states have paid much more regulatory attention to compliance and quality issues. Incremental progress has been made and some states have strong oversight regimes. (This is especially the case in big states like New York, California, and, increasingly, Florida.) These are being used as models for CMS and states seeking to bring accountability. The reforms revolve around compliance, reporting, penalties, and some quality rating experiments. And as outlined, the Medicaid Mega or Uber Rule will further drive changes in all these areas by bringing a Medicare-like account-ability regime to Medicaid in all fifty states. A mandatory quality rating system similar to Medicare Star will be required.

These reforms are especially important in Medicaid for two reasons: (1) the notable barriers to good health the population has, including significant socio-economic or social determinant barriers and (2) the aging of America and the need to ensure cost-effective and quality long-term care services.

Driving Efficiency

CMS and health plans are also pushing for greater efficiency in the utilization management (UM) world. Plans are mired in old technology, including—believe it or not—an over-reliance on fax machines. CMS is pushing hard for electronic medical record system adoption to facilitate electronic prior authorization (ePA) submission in both the pharmacy and medical world. Pharmacy ePA is doing well, given a national standard that providers and plans can follow, but there is not yet a uniform medical service submission standard. This is coming (see the interoperability discussion below for a new medical prior authorization requirement).

Many plans have yet to truly assess efficiency in their organizations and make the kind of technology investments that can be game changers in the area of administrative costs. However, given the tight margins in most lines of business, health plans are beginning to leverage technology to reduce administrative intake costs and drive electronic submissions of service requests and to obtain critical information regarding hospital admissions, hospital discharges, and transitions of care. Increasingly, HIPAA and the Health Level 7 Fast Healthcare Interoperability Resources (HL7 FHIR) electronic communication standards are helping drive such communication. This helps reduce administrative costs, drive efficiency, and improve compliance.

Legacy systems are being sunsetted, and plans are increasingly turning to universally available and reliably hosted platforms that feature the following:

- Efficient intake of cases, including electronic intake whenever possible, optical character recognition, artificial intelligence, and machine learning
- Automatic authorization of requests using algorithms and evidence-based criteria
- Robust member history to reduce errors and provide unprecedented insight
- Auto-population of case-received dates and the countdown to due dates through dashboards, alerts, and other functionality
- Automated workflow and monitoring throughout the case's life
- Automated correspondence generation, correspondence triggering (in most cases), and correspondence monitoring to ensure compliant and timely fulfillment
- Barcoding and auto-generation of medical necessity outreach, representative appointment, and waiver of liability requests
- Real-time effectuation of approvals and tight integration with other

fulfillment vendors (via fax, letter, and interactive voice response to ensure timely fulfillment)

o System auto-population of fields whenever possible

o Audit-ready out-of-the-box regulatory reports

o Superior availability through a secure hosting infrastructure

It should be noted that technology is linked increasingly to greater satisfaction among members and providers.

Care Management and Population Health Focus

Since the introduction of modern insurance back in the days of the Blue Cross and Blue Shield Associations, managing utilization and its costs have been the focal point of health plans. This was the case whether in extracting concessions from providers for volume commitments or in scrutinizing requests for authorization of services. But while utilization management (UM) will always be here (hopefully in a very efficient manner), shifting to care coordination, care management, wellness, and prevention is critical to reducing costs and improving quality in our system. Thus, CMS is also attempting to get plans to shift their long-time focus from UM to care management initiatives.

CMS is planning a national strategy to bring a model of care to all members in some form, regardless of their line of business. The elements of this overall transition effort can already be seen in a number of initiatives from CMS and in state Medicaid programs:

The rework of the MA special needs plans (SNPs) was the first of these efforts. Only a decade ago, SNPs seemed to be on their death bed, viewed by Capitol Hill and CMS as plan marketing vehicles that had little quality or cost-reduction benefit. They survived via a series of last-minute legislative extensions. During this period of limbo, CMS began a fundamental redesign of the program, including:

o Reining in the disease states allowed for Disease-Specific Chronic

Condition SNPs.

○ Requiring closer coordination with state Medicaid funding streams and policy for dual eligible SNPs.

○ Instituting a rigorous model of care (MOC) for all SNPs. The National Committee for Quality Assurance (NCQA) must approve the MOC and review it over time as well.

○ Expanding its audit scrutiny of SNPs and formulating numerous best practices for timeliness of assessments, ongoing individualized care plans, activities of the interdisciplinary care teams, and ongoing stratification and interventions for members.

Similarly, in the Medicaid Uber Rule, many Medicaid beneficiaries will require an initial assessment to determine risk and morbidity. Those found to be of increased risk will get additional assessments and will also have ongoing treatment plans similar to care plans. Care coordination rules for those in need of various long-term care services will be even stricter and more complex.

The establishment of the dual demonstration plan pilots, also known as Medicare-Medicaid Plans (MMPs) for dual eligibles, was the next step. Paralleling the SNP reforms above, MMPs seek to form an even greater integration of Medicare and Medicaid funding streams and, in some states, both acute and long-term care spending. The duals pilots are rooted in CMS' belief that accountable, care management-focused managed care across the two government programs can finally tackle the dual eligible quandary. Dual eligibles numbered about 12 million in 2018, or 20% of the Medicare population and 15% of the Medicaid population. However, they represented 34% of Medicare and 33% of Medicaid spending.[29-1]

But CMS is worried about an additional problem that can be seen in both Medicare and Medicaid: other beneficiaries with chronic conditions. Members of this group drive overall costs and these individuals are not solely dual eligibles. Those with chronic disease states account for 96% and 83% of costs in Medicare and Medicaid, respectively.[29-2] So how does CMS go beyond the focused reform of dual eligible programs to tackling the need to focus better care management and prevention on the overall population, especially those that drive costs and have poor outcomes?

One step is the introduction of the value-based insurance design (VBID) initiative in MA to have greater focus on members who have multiple disease states. Traditionally, mainstream MA plans have been one-size-fits-all for enrollees. Everyone has the same benefits and cost-sharing. With the VBID, plans may fashion benefits and services for a subset of their population in need of additional interventions. In this case, plans offer additional benefits and incentives as well as reduce cost-sharing to encourage the use of value-added services (PCP, specialist, and other preventive services). In addition, plans wrap disease and care management around these revised benefit offerings. The VBID can be viewed as the first step in CMS' desire to target appropriate benefits and care management services that match a Medicare enrollee's actual risk and needs. As VBID matures, CMS and plans are tacking more and more complex issues in the initiative.

CMS is also expanding MA plans' ability to offer supplemental benefits to drive healthcare changes. Like with VBID, uniformity has been waived for benefits and cost-sharing to help those with chronic disease states and conditions better afford healthcare and drive outcomes. Traditional supplemental benefits that are not necessarily health-related have been expanded to help maintain health. Other health-related benefits previously not allowed to be offered are now permitted to help reduce hospitalizations, ensure independence, and maintain health.

So, the stage is set. While major work must be focused on high-cost individuals that consume the vast majority of resources, CMS understands that a model of care for everyone is needed to fundamentally realign the system, reduce costs, and improve quality. In time, CMS will expect plans to perform the following on all insured individuals. These include:

- ○ **Assessing all members** for health risks and conditions
- ○ **Identifying and stratifying these populations**, based on socio-economic factors, health literacy, disease states, and financial and service risk
- ○ **Fashion interventions** appropriate to care needs for each member. This might be limited reminders and health education for some people and complex case management for others
- ○ **Identifying care gaps** to improve health outcomes

Leading employers are also promoting health and wellness and focusing on employee/associate well-being. These innovations include wellness programs, healthy living incentives, premium rebates, and onsite clinics. Employers are increasingly demanding accountability on health outcomes from health plans and providers. Some of them are leading the way on value-based purchasing or reimbursement with providers.

In addition, while I'm not a big fan of the decrepit Medicare and Medicaid FFS environments, CMS is trying to retool them through various initiatives to reduce costs and improve quality. One of the leading initiatives is the Medicare accountable care organizations (ACO) program, which features primarily provider entities coming together to form managed-care-like entities to reduce spending and improve quality on beneficiaries in their geographic catchment area. Similar pilots are under way in the Medicaid FFS arena.

Value-Based Purchasing and Arrangements with Providers

Consistent with the shift from UM to care management and quality, health plans have been quietly working with innovative providers and provider groups to develop what I call the next generation of managed care.

Naysayers will argue that this next generation looks like a return to the days of the late 1980s and early 1990s, when narrow-network Health Maintenance

Organization (HMO) plans were all the rage. But the latest trend is somewhat different as it truly focuses on implementing the wellness, prevention, and quality focus of managed care, which was not the case before.

Health plans are teaming up with these providers in new, value-based reimbursement arrangements where high-quality providers will obtain additional reimbursement both by reducing costs and by improving quality. These arrangements also will have global or partial risk arrangements with providers and groups. Networks may be narrower, as plans focus on top quality providers, but overall members should have great member experience and outcomes over time. So, yes, there will be tighter networks but also a focus on quality providers, wellness and prevention, quality outcomes, and aligned incentives.

Two good examples of value-based reimbursement that have been recently announced:

> Humana, a large MA insurer, reports that its leap to value-based payments from FFS produced significantly lower costs in 2019. This means savings, both to Humana and to seniors and the disabled paying cost-sharing, especially when compared to the decrepit traditional Medicare system. Humana documents lower hospitalization rates and bed days, lower emergency room visits, holistic care by providers, and a focus on social determinant barriers.[29-3]
>
> In the commercial world, Aetna announced that it now has a co-branded plan with Cleveland Clinic for its commercial line of business. The plan began being offered to employers in Northeast Ohio in ten counties in late 2020. The network is composed of Cleveland Clinic Quality Alliance's network of employed and independent community physicians. In addition, Cleveland Clinic's renowned cardiac center will be available in Aetna's nationwide network, including second opinions on a virtual basis. Aetna has built an accountable care model with the Cleveland Clinic network that will reward the providers if they meet quality and cost targets. The narrower network plan could mean employers save as much as 10% in healthcare costs.[29-4]

Slowly but surely, these value-based purchasing initiatives should begin replacing strict, transactional reimbursement.

In the Medicare and Medicaid FFS worlds, value-based changes are occurring as well. These include some hospital reimbursement reform (bundled payments, readmission penalties, and new episodic payments) as well as quality reporting and reimbursement.

Also note that there is more and more focus on drug costs—as pressure emerges to grapple with high drug prices. Chapter 34 will cover this issue in detail, so I will not elaborate now. Suffice it to say:

- Democrats have their views on price controls and negotiations.
- The Trump Administration promulgated some novel views on price control or caps, including international reference pricing, and began acting on them in the twilight of the administration.
- President Biden endorses the German model, which has national price negotiations as well as international reference pricing.
- Republicans are softening on drug price reform, but still seem overly protective of the drug lobby.
- Value-based reimbursement is emerging in the drug world.

Compromise could emerge over time.

I would also note that efforts are being made to deal with our primary care provider challenges. In the final days of the Trump Administration, it put in place a Medicare payment rule that shifted monies from specialty physicians to primary care and evaluation and management services. This helps begin to focus efforts on primary care and management of conditions and address over-specialization in our healthcare system.[29-5]

Price Transparency

There is also some movement on transparency. While legal disputes are by no means over, federal courts have given a preliminary thumbs up to the Trump Administration's price transparency executive order and subsequent rules focused on health plans and hospitals. My review of the executive order and rule finds hospitals now have to:

- Make all standard hospital charges public, including gross charges, payer-specific negotiated charges, minimum and maximum negotiated charges, and, most importantly, the amount the hospital is willing to accept in cash from a patient. This applies to all items and services and must include billing and accounting codes as well as descriptions. They must be in computer-readable formats.
- Post minimum and maximum negotiated charges for 300 common shoppable services in a consumer-friendly manner. This list must be updated at least annually. Shoppable services are largely advance-booked, outpatient services as well as some inpatient ones.

My review of the executive order and rule finds health plans will have to:

- Disclose, in a standardized online tool and paper format, price and cost-sharing information up front, to help members determine out-of-pocket costs for deductibles, co-pays, and co-insurance
- Disclose negotiated rates for in-network providers and allowed amounts paid for out-of-network providers

Hospitals and health plans argue that price transparency will absolutely cripple them and unsettle the healthcare world. They contend that the rules violate the confidentiality of negotiated rates with insurers and chill negotiations. They also say the rule's assumed costs are wildly too low, saying that actual costs could be twenty-six times the estimate. Finally, they claim that the rules could increase consumer confusion and increase costs. That is, people may see higher-priced providers and assume they are better.

I do not discount some of the concerns raised, but I am a proponent of price transparency and these rules. As discussed previously, one of the leading reasons the United States spends so much more than other developed nations on healthcare is due to the cost of services. A lot goes into that, but a lack of price transparency is clearly a major reason. Some providers simply are too highly priced. Certain providers have monopolies or near-monopolies, where they decide to charge anything they like. Too much care is delivered in expensive settings when costs and outcomes are better elsewhere. Finally, there is the real concern about surprise billing, whether you seek care in-network or out-of-network.

The price transparency rules will not change consumer or provider behavior overnight, but it begins the process. Indeed, there are real costs of implementation, but resetting the table in this area is key to seeing change down the road. We need to come to a day when consumers can view their choices in real-time—by provider, by site of care, and by place of service—to make more informed decisions. The Biden administration has stood behind both the provider and health plan price transparency measures. This has allowed some delay in certain health plan provisions given the complexity.

Congress and the Trump Administration also took a major step to stop surprise billing. The law, enacted in late 2020 and taking effect on January 1, 2022, applies to all insurance types, including self-insured employer plans. The law will eliminate all balance or surprise billing for emergency care, air ambulances, and in most cases where an out-of-network provider furnishes services in an in-network facility. However, some balance billing still is allowed, and a costly arbitration process was chosen over a simpler median in-network rate methodology. This means exorbitant prices may still be paid by health plans on behalf of members or by members. See Chapter 7 for additional details.[29-6] The Biden administration supports the measure, but it is allowing some additional time for the implementation of certain complex provisions.

Site-neutral Payments

A big blow to hospitals occurred in 2020 when a federal appeals court ruled that the Trump Administration's site-neutral payment policy regarding services in off-site, outpatient departments can be adopted in the Medicare program. Hospitals had challenged the HHS rule on various procedural grounds, arguing that the imposition of the rule violated the agency's rule-making ability. The verdict, however, may clear the way for some other site-neutral rules adopted by CMS and HHS in 2020 covering additional services. The Biden Administration is backing the change.

There is a clear logic to site-neutral reimbursement. It is important to reining in the high costs of our system as a whole. Hospitals and similar providers have long argued that they deserve to be paid a premium for any facility or service, regardless of location, simply because they own them. For example, because the hospital owns an off-site facility or clinic, it maintains that higher rates should be paid, to support their overall cost structure. In this case, the hospital might be paid twice as much for an ambulatory clinic procedure (that is not even attached to a hospital) compared with the same service offered by an independent clinic, ambulatory center, or physician's office. Hospitals say that these higher reimbursements, regardless of location, are needed to support the critical services of their broader mission.

As a former board member of two hospitals, I am sympathetic to the challenges and financial plight of hospitals. They serve critical functions in the form of emergency care, trauma care, sophisticated surgery, etc. The cost of infrastructure, personnel, technology, and other service provisions are high. Accreditation and regulatory costs are also high. Critical access hospitals perform important functions in rural and other areas. Graduate training and other costs aimed at ensuring America remains an excellent healthcare system are also disproportionately borne by hospitals. All of this should be factored into payment determination to some degree.

But, notwithstanding some of these legitimate costs, many hospitals are inefficient and in some cases dangerous places to be. It's hard to argue that hospital and related provider financing reform is *not* needed. Indeed, the Medicare system tends to set the minimum for what hospitals demand from commercial payers. Further, given how Medicare FFS (and to some extent MA) cost-sharing is structured, not paying providers based on site of service means seniors and the disabled are saddled with much greater costs, depending on the provider that is used.

I do not think we should reimburse hospitals more just because they own a provider or facility at any site of service. In addition, we need to move toward a system that drives service provision to the lowest cost and most appropriate site of service. That is why going down the road of site-neutral payment, as the Trump Administration did, is a good idea.

Not having a site-neutral payment structure essentially inflates costs across the spectrum. Plans and consumers pay more for all sorts of services without really knowing it because of the general lack of transparency in our system. A study underwritten by the Physicians Advocacy Institute found that for three types of services studied (cardiac imaging, colonoscopy, and evaluation and management services), Medicare pays demonstrably more when these services are done in hospital outpatient (even when it is in a hospital "off-campus" setting) compared with those in a physician-owned office.[29-7]

- ○ Cardiac imaging—$5,148 in hospital outpatient and $2,862 in physician's office
- ○ Colonoscopy—$1,784 in hospital outpatient and $1,322 in physician's office
- ○ Evaluation and management services—$525 in hospital outpatient and $406 in physician's office

In Chapter 33, I describe the trend of hospitals purchasing physician groups and practices, and how that leads to more procedures being done in hospital-owned facilities. So, more and more procedures could swing to hospital outpatient and increase overall costs unless site-neutral payments are adopted.

Site neutral payments begin paying reasonable reimbursement by site of service, considering costs for the provision of that service without regard to the organizational entity's other costs—with limited exceptions. Those unique extraordinary costs should be reimbursed related to the actual site of service if justified (for example, inpatient services). As an example, if a hospital owns an off-campus clinic or ambulatory surgery center, it should be paid the same amount—again, within reason—as a free-standing facility or provider. If it is furnishing hospital inpatient or outpatient services, that is where *some* of the unique costs of hospitals may be recognized. Various risk adjustment payment formulas relating to severity of illness have been introduced at various levels and could be combined with site-neutral payment policies. This will help recognize differences in risk among providers even with site-neutral payments.

Site-neutral payments will also better promote the proper use of resources in the health system. While managed care helps drive down over-utilization, it is also true that the current inflated reimbursement structure encourages hospitals and other high-cost providers to extend visits and keep payments coming in, whether it is beneficial to the patient or not.

The move to site-neutral payment could finally make hospitals and other high-cost providers rethink delivery in the modern age. Do we need all the infrastructure and investments we see in hospitals? In many ways, the lack of site-neutral payment policies encourages high-cost providers to build and invest in areas that may not be in the best interest of the healthcare system. As an example, the current reimbursement system helps drive over-specialization and an overabundance of technology. Consequently, compared with other developed nations, we have fewer primary care doctors and too many specialists. This is not to say the other systems are perfect, but simply to note that the current payment system promotes excess.

We must begin to educate consumers and providers about funneling patients to the least costly site of service. Site-neutral payments help in this regard, too. They lower plan payments and cost-sharing by consumers. Hospitals will argue that volume is being moved to cheaper ambulatory surgery settings—owned by hospitals or not. This complicates their ability to support higher-cost services. However, it is hard to rationalize the need to subject anyone to the high costs and sometimes low quality of an outpatient hospital visit when it is cheaper and safer to receive that treatment or service in a different setting (a free-standing ambulatory surgery center or physician's office).

While site-neutral payments are technically FFS transaction payments, their adoption would make it easier to migrate to better reimbursement models. Site-neutral payments could also more easily include quality add-ons in the future. This could begin to shift the focus from pure payment transactions (the trap today) to efficient and quality care delivery.

Do not think of me as too radical. I understand that hospitals need to be reimbursed for some of those costs noted. And there should be reasonable ways to supplement hospital funding, by site of service and other means, without keeping a reimbursement system that drives costs higher and higher each year. Other developed nations have much lower prices and costs and have highly developed health systems with good outcomes. COVID-19 ICU crisis or not, hospitals and other high-cost providers need to be challenged to reform, lower costs, and improve quality. The site-neutral rules are a good step in that direction.

On a related note, major insurers, including United, Anthem, and Cigna, have begun reining in the ability for members to obtain certain testing at expensive settings. For example, they are limiting advanced imaging at hospitals, except in limited circumstances. Of course, hospitals have opposed the move, saying that it interferes with the patient-doctor relationship, impacts choice, and could lead to inferior quality. However, what is the justification for allowing such imaging at high-cost places of service unless there is some medical necessity for the patient to be in such a setting? Such imaging at hospital outpatient sites can be much more expensive than at free-standing facilities or sites. So, plans now are moving beyond just deciding whether services are medically necessary to also determining the right site of service and whether more expensive sites are needed. It is about time. Hospital scare tactics are largely unfounded. Plans can regulate the quality and appropriateness of providers and sites of service. It is a necessity to counter the perverse impacts of provider consolidation and to realign costs in the healthcare system generally.[29-8]

Many plans are also doing something similar with other diagnostic tests and laboratory services, especially limiting these services at hospitals. To save costs as well, plans are now entering into agreements with outside vendors to have specialty medications drop-shipped to physician offices, hospitals, and other facilities to be administered rather than having providers acquiring the drugs at much higher rates. Provider groups are livid and cite quality and access concerns. They are urging federal authorities to bar the practice in government programs. But their objections are largely unfounded.[29-9]

Also, in the final days of the Trump Administration, it enacted another Medicare rule that would phase out services paid only at hospitals. Over 1,700 procedures currently are only paid for when performed in a hospital. The list was to be phased out over a three-year period beginning in 2021. The final outpatient rule would have allowed doctors and patients to determine the most appropriate place of service. Patient safety and evidence-based criteria would have been considered to determine what services will be phased off the list and when. As this book went to print, the Biden administration proposed to keep the Medicare inpatient only list for now as well as halt another Trump rule expanding the services at free-standing ambulatory surgery centers. But Biden may eventually proceed more slowly on both in the future.[29-10]

Hospitals, of course, object to what Trump did and see this as further erosion of their revenue and market concentration. As usual, hospital lobbyists' clarion call again is patient safety. But there is mounting evidence that hospitals can be among the most perilous places for patients. Modern technology allows many services to be administered at other facilities—and even at home—in a safe manner. In-patient only lists have largely gone away in private insurance.

Like site-neutral payments, this move would help drive right site of care (or place of service) and begin to address price issues in our system. Hospitals are at the top of the list in terms of cost. They consume about one-third of the healthcare pie, or over $1 trillion in 2018. Prices in hospitals are uncapped and, even with managed care discounts, mean extraordinary expenses.

Interoperability

Just before the COVID-19 pandemic hit in earnest, HHS announced the finalization of the much-debated interoperability rule with vast implications on health plans and the health system in general. The rule is a major undertaking of the HHS Office of the National Coordinator for Health Information Technology (ONC).

HHS, ONC, and the Centers for Medicare and Medicaid Services (CMS) have been pushing interoperability and the sharing of data for years, but the two new ONC interoperability rules represent a sea change for data transparency. It rivals the passage of the Health Insurance Portability and Accountability Act (HIPAA) for what it can do for the flow of data across payers and throughout the healthcare system in general.

The goal is simple. If you give patients true access to their healthcare data and put them in charge of their health records, they can make more informed decisions and better manage their care. As we know, even today, patients have little insight into their records—a mix of paper files and information buried within electronic medical record (EMR) depositories and health plan systems. And patients have a tough time understanding or synthesizing those explanations of benefit (EOB) statements that arrive in the mail.

CMS has been experimenting with data sharing, by the Medicare Blue Button initiative, since 2018. The new initiative gives Medicare beneficiaries the ability to securely connect their Medicare Part A, Part B, and Part D claims and encounter data to apps and other tools developed in the private sector. Much of the access will occur on smartphones and similar devices, as opposed to conventional computers.

ONC's final rules require the use of secure, standards-based application programming interfaces (APIs) to support the flow of information and patients' access to and control of their electronic health information. Patients can choose the third-party apps and will then be able to obtain their health information—securely and easily—using their smartphone or similar device. These APIs will cover the sharing of both provider EMR information and health plan information. Third-party vendors will need to get permission to retrieve and share the information with the individual.

CMS and the ONC have adopted the Health Level 7 Fast Healthcare Interoperability Resources as the API foundational standard to support data exchanges for the rules.

There may be a number of third parties supporting the initiative, including third-party app providers. There also are a number of entities that will serve as health plan intermediaries to receive the data on behalf of plans, normalize it, reformat it, and ultimately transmit it to the other third parties in the required API. Some of these intermediary entities host and store the data, while others may simply serve as a pass-through entity and transmit the data. Clients may also fulfill these obligations.

Mandates for providers and health plans to share UM and care management data from EMRs and health plan systems rolls out from late 2020 through

2022, but the Biden administration has given some leeway on implementation timeframes. They include:

- ○ Providers sharing hospital admission, hospital discharge, and care transition information
- ○ Providers and health plans sharing various claims, authorization, and care management information
- ○ Health plans making available provider directories and updates to the member apps
- ○ Health plans being required to share claims, authorization, and care management information with other health plans when members move

These rules are initially focused on communications to members from providers and health plans discretely. The electronic standards and framework envisioned will also facilitate deep integration between providers and payers. This lays the foundation for mastering the transfer of primary data from health plans (claims, authorizations, and certain care management) and secondary data (additional diagnoses, clinical notes, and socio-economic factors) from providers, in order to facilitate and improve care and outcomes.

Indeed, in the closing days of his administration, President Trump's healthcare policymakers issued a new electronic prior authorization mandate that adds to these interoperability rules. Currently, it applies only to Medicaid, State Children's Health Insurance (SCHIP), and Exchange plans as well as the Medicaid and SCHIP FFS programs. (Trump policymakers said a related rule for MA plans would be issued, but it was not.) The rule, with implementation effective January 1, 2023, adds the following provisions:[29-11]

- ○ Plans and the FFS programs would be required to include a member's or patient's pending and active prior authorization decisions via APIs.
- ○ Plans would also need to have an API for payer-to-provider data sharing of claims and encounter data (not including cost data), a subset of clinical data, and pending and active prior authorization (PA) decisions. This extends the original provider-to-provider and plan-to-

plan interoperability rule to data-sharing between providers and plans.

- ○ Plans would have to maintain APIs that could be integrated with a provider's electronic health or medical record system (EHR or EMR) to allow providers real-time access to prior authorization requirements for each plan from within the provider's workflow.

- ○ Plans would have to build APIs that allow providers to send PA requests and receive responses within their existing EMR workflow. A specific denial reason would need to be included. PA timeframes would have to be complete in seventy-two hours for urgent requests and seven calendar days for standard requests. This does not impact Exchange plans.

- ○ Public reporting would be required by plans of PA metrics, including timeliness (average time for decision), initial request approval rates, and overturn rates.

As of this writing, while the Biden Administration is supportive of interoperability overall, it was reviewing this last-minute additional rule. My view is the rule will in time take effect, perhaps with longer implementation timeframes, and that it will be extended to MA.

As of May 2021, there was a bipartisan bill in Congress that seeks to mandate electronic PA for medical services in MA as well as fundamentally overhaul the PA process. It could be passed on a bipartisan basis as it is substantially drafted from a 2018 consensus statement of prominent provider and health plan groups. It would do the following:[29-12, 29-13, 29-14]

- ○ Focus on transparency of PA processes, standardizing them, streamlining them, and reducing costs.

- ○ Ensure qualified medical personnel review PA.

- ○ Ensure the use of evidence-based criteria and require that such criteria are shared with members and providers. The evidence-based criteria used in decision-making should be developed in concert with physicians. Modifications to the PA process could occur based on physicians' adherence to the criteria.

- ○ Mandate electronic prior authorization processes for medical services. Retail pharmacy electronic prior authorization is well-established.
- ○ Require real-time approval for certain medical services. The list would be published by the Department of Health and Human Services (HHS) and CMS. This would effectively end prior authorization for these services. This is a big risk in the bill. A liberal HHS/CMS list over time could effectively add demonstrably to spending.
- ○ Mandate reporting of authorization data to HHS/CMS, including timeliness, approvals, denials, and overturn rates on appeals.
- ○ Protect beneficiaries from any disruptions in care due to prior authorization requirements as they transition between MA plans.

Policymakers and lawmakers are hanging their hats on electronic prior authorization based on a 2021 report from the Council for Affordable Quality Healthcare (CAQH). It estimated that $417 million annually could be saved throughout healthcare by automating prior authorization requests.[29-13]

All of these interoperability mandates will take a long time to mature. Providers and plans will struggle with compliance early on. Undoubtedly, patients will have little understanding of the value and there will be a long lead time in the adoption of smartphone apps. There will also be numerous challenges related to data flow, normalization, conflicting terminology, relevance of data, and reconciliation.

However, the interoperability rules are indeed one of the most important events in recent healthcare policy. Over time, it promises to increase transparency in the system as well as promote additional patient responsibility. It will also shift the paradigm from UM to care management by ensuring that vital information is shared timely.

Data interoperability also will open the doors to the maturation of the health information exchanges at a regional, state, and national level, and lay the foundation for real-time data sharing throughout the healthcare ecosystem.

While this will be initially costly, it is a necessity to bend the cost curve, improve primary prevention and care coordination, and move the quality needle in our healthcare system.

Expansion of Healthcare Coverage Access

As I noted in Chapter 27, the Biden Administration strongly supports healthcare coverage expansion and passed enhancements to the Affordable Care Act's (ACA's) premium subsidies on a temporary basis in the COVID-19 Relief bill passed in early 2021. Go back to that chapter for details. While it was adopted on a party-line vote, it was the right thing to do. The bill expanded premium subsidy eligibility and enhanced actual subsidies in the Exchanges. As of this writing, Biden and Democrats were working toward a bill that could make the temporary measures permanent or extend them beyond 2022. We can debate the details, but as I told you, affordable universal access is important to getting rid of our costly uninsured and underinsured crisis. As well, we know that insurance that is too costly for given families means deferred care, which leads only to greater costs down the road.

President Biden also reopened the Exchanges for a special enrollment period due to the COVID-19 pandemic and is investing tens of millions in marketing and outreach. Millions more could enroll in the Exchange over the next few years due to the temporary subsidy expansion, the likelihood of more liberal ongoing enrollment periods, and the outreach and marketing efforts.

A Potential Long-term Care Focus

As part of his early actions, President Biden also proposed a renewed focus on aging in America and long-term care. This is an absolutely positive development. I go into great detail on the aging of America and what we must do in Chapter 35. As of this writing, I did not have many details about Biden's proposal and whether it would pass. But the sheer fact that he has begun to address aging is important. At the time of this writing, press reports indicated that Biden wanted an additional $950 billion for expanded home and community-based services over eight to ten years to avoid nursing home institutionalization. In addition, he would expand the "Money Follows the Person" program, which encourages deinstitutionalization. Actual new dollars will likely be markedly less if passed.[29-15, 29-16, 29-17]

That's it. We have left the gloom of dysfunction in Chapter 28 to the optimism (somewhat) of reform in this chapter. Well, not so fast. We are in the infancy stage, and soon I will be telling you my grand vision to truly turn the tide in favor of true health reform. That comes in Chapter 32.

CHAPTER 30

Various Healthcare Models

During the 2020 presidential election campaign season, many Democratic candidates endorsed Medicare for All. The proposal garnered major headlines. Republicans charged that the effort is an expensive boondoggle that will be unaffordable and essentially endanger the Medicare program as we know it today. Many Democrats saw it as the panacea for the problems that ail the Affordable Care Act (ACA) and for the tens of millions still uninsured despite America's attempts to create universal access.

When described generally, Medicare for All often registered 50% or greater favorability in most polls. When queried about a Medicare buy-in for those over age fifty, and various optional programs that don't disrupt the current system, polls also indicated majority support for the concept.

Digging deeper, however, Americans' support dissipated when certain details on the coverage schemes were provided. As examples, when asked should healthcare costs be financed through taxes and private plans banned, only a minority of Americans then supported Medicare for All.

So, the conclusion, Medicare for All means different things to different people and those details certainly matter.

Review of the Main Healthcare Coverage Constructs

To clear some of the mystery surrounding Medicare for All and other healthcare reform proposals, let's review some of the broad elements of universal coverage and access and where the United States stands today.

In my years of looking at the developed-world healthcare systems, there are three working healthcare system paradigms, although many countries use a blend of more than one of these. Here they are with a little help from *The Economist*:[30-1]

> **Government-run or socialized healthcare**—Under this model, the government takes over the costs of all coverage and provision of healthcare. It funds the health system usually through general government funding financed by taxes on citizens and businesses alike. Everyone is enrolled. Usually, private healthcare does not exist. If it does, it emerges because of inadequacies in the system itself or may offer supplemental or wrap-around services. The government also runs and operates some or all of the healthcare facilities and employs individual medical providers. Some countries run and operate facilities but may contract with individual providers to provide certain coverage in the system.

> **Single-payer health insurance**—In this scheme, the government provides universal health insurance and pays for it, but the vast majority of provision of care is left in private hands. There are one or more government-run and financed health insurance systems. Private health plans usually do not exist, but they could emerge due to the inadequacies of the system, offering wrap-around or supplemental benefits. Everyone is enrolled. The system is paid for by taxes on individuals and businesses. The actual provision of services is usually performed by private facilities and providers. In some cases, governments may operate some facilities.

Universal coverage or access approaches—Here, the government leaves insurance coverage and delivery of care in the private sector, but it provides regulatory oversight and subsidizes as well as mandates coverage for all—via employer and individual mandates. Government is the least involved in the provision of healthcare. Private health insurers cover individuals through various types of products similar to the American Health Maintenance Organization (HMO) and other product types. Private health plans competing for enrollees can be for-profit or not-for-profit insurers or quasi-public entities. They usually are not linked to employers. In most countries, citizens essentially buy their own policies and choose their own health insurer. Private providers and facilities furnish care via contracts with the insurers. Government subsidizes coverage for the poor and lower income citizens. In some countries, children are fully covered by government subsidies. These are financed in various ways, including general taxes, or they may require employers to pay a portion of premiums. In some cases, the government may have a government-sponsored program for certain individuals.

In my years of researching healthcare systems in the developed world, it is clear that some politicians are spreading a big lie. Contrary to popular belief, a truly government-run or socialized healthcare system is not the model for all of Europe and the developed world. Even in the countries with so-called socialized medicine, private insurance may co-exist with the system. Developed countries that do not have socialized medicine include:[30-1]

- ○ France, Canada, and Australia have single-payer systems, with the presence of private insurance; Canada uses provincial governments to run their systems, while France uses non-profit agencies.
- ○ Universal access or coverage predominates in Switzerland, the Netherlands, and economic powerhouse Germany. These countries ensure universal coverage of individuals through government subsidies, but their systems are centered on private insurers and providers. Germany has been using its non-socialized medicine model since—you guessed

it—our friend from Chapter 2, Otto Von Bismarck, chancellor of Germany under Kaiser Wilhelm I.
∘   Even in the United Kingdom's socialized medicine model, private insurers coexist.[30-1]

So, what bucket or category does the United States best fit in from this list? The answer is that we have all of them today.

In the case of the Veteran's Administration (VA), we actually practice a form of socialized medicine. Headlines about the VA healthcare system of late have been terrible, talking about deaths, waiting lists, and outright fraud and inefficiency in the system. The reality, though, is that it is an important safety net for veterans, some of whom struggle economically and medically throughout their lives.

The traditional Medicare fee-for-service (FFS) system is actually a single-payer healthcare system. When you reach age sixty-five or qualify with a disability, you become entitled to Medicare coverage and can go into the FFS system if you choose. In this case, the government pays most of your care—about 75% to 80%—and the rest is paid by you through premiums and cost-sharing. About 57% of Medicare beneficiaries today are in the single-payer FFS system. Medicaid FFS systems in states would also constitute a single-payer model as well.

There are also elements of universal coverage or access in the United States. We see this with the ACA or Obamacare premium and cost-sharing subsidies. The government provides subsidies for the low-income uninsured, but otherwise allows private plans and providers to run the system and furnish care.

If I had to pick one, the United States is largely under the universal coverage or access umbrella, although we don't have complete universal access or coverage. In essence, we have a hodgepodge of coverage programs that help meet insurance needs of Americans, including employer-sponsored coverage that predominates, as well as a series of government programs—Medicare, Medicaid, Children's Health Insurance, Obamacare Exchanges and more—to fill the voids.

While we have stepped toward a universal coverage or access model, we also know the United States continues to have many challenges. As we learned earlier, we spend a much greater percentage of our gross domestic product (GDP) on healthcare—almost 18% compared with demonstrably lower percentages in the rest of the developed world. At the same time, our outcomes are at the bottom on most measures for the developed world. We still have about 32 million people uninsured, about 10% of the population compared with 1% in other developed countries.[30-1, 30-2]

Review of Recent Healthcare Reform Proposals

Politicians are not terribly precise when they speak about their policy proposals. In part, this is on purpose. It shields them from having to give too many details. More importantly, it also allows them to dodge important questions, such as, "How much will it cost?" and "How are you going to pay for it?"

Following are the potential Medicare for All and other related healthcare reform proposals that have been or could be advocated for in the near future. I have deliberately not used the names politicians have used (except for Medicare for All,) given the genuine confusion that these names often cause.

I am not taking positions on these, with two exceptions, except to say that many have their merits and pitfalls. The two exceptions are as follows:

- ○ First, I am not a believer in government-run or socialized systems.
- ○ Second, a true, government-run, single-payer approach, such as Medicare for All that would absolutely eliminate private insurers, would not be well-received and would be problematic. This is the case because most advocates have the traditional Medicare fee-for-service (FFS) system at the core of their proposals. I discuss Medicare for All in the next chapter but, suffice it to say, the traditional FFS system is plagued by fraud, poor quality, and inefficiency. I don't see the quality and reform pilots in this system scoring enough successes to change that. In the end, healthcare in America would be even more expensive and lacking in quality if Medicare for All were adopted.

So, what are the leading healthcare reform proposals out there these days? Most of them are variations of the single-payer model. Aided by the Kaiser Family Foundation (KFF), these come from my assessment and bundling into categories of the various proposals made by the various 2020 presidential candidates as well as proposals in Congress.[30-3, 30-4]

> **Single-payer; No Private Insurance**—Under true, single-payer healthcare, private insurance would be eliminated, and everyone would be forced into a national insurance program. In some proposals, there would be no private alternatives—everyone would likely be part of the Medicare FFS system. In other cases, private insurance might offer wrap-around or supplemental benefits. The program could be extraordinarily rich—with no costs for anyone—or have sliding scale contributions toward premiums and cost-sharing, based on income. The system would be funded largely by taxes, including payroll taxes and perhaps employer taxes or penalties. This is in essence Medicare for All.

> **Single-payer with Contracted Private Plans**—In another option, the above goes into effect and the government might contract with private health plans to provide coverage or have a mix of public and private offerings. This might look a bit like Medicare Advantage (MA) with and without a FFS system.

> **Single-payer with an Opt-out Provision**—In this proposal, single-payer would look like one of the two systems above but private insurance would be maintained, and people could opt out of coverage if they have qualifying coverage—for example, through an employer. Subsidies likely would exist to help with premium affordability and cost-sharing.

> **Medicare Buy-in**—This proposal would keep Medicare as we know it, but also allow people to buy into the program. In some cases, it may only be for people aged fifty and older. In other cases, any uninsured could access the system. Subsidies could be added to help affordability

of premiums and cost-sharing. People could choose either the traditional Medicare program or MA plans.

Medicaid Buy-in—In this type of proposal, a national law would be passed, perhaps with or without state expansion options, to allow the uninsured to buy into Medicaid. Subsidies could be added to help affordability of premiums and cost-sharing. There would be traditional Medicaid FFS for some, but most would be in private Medicaid plans.

Fix Obamacare Exchanges, with or without a Public Option—This is not a single-payer option, but more of a universal access or coverage option. This is what President Biden supports. In this approach, various changes might be made to the Affordable Care Act (ACA) to help stabilize it in about half the states.

One option in this approach would be to create a national public option plan that people could choose, especially in rural and low-plan participation states or counties. This would compete in select areas or throughout the nation with private health plans. This public option would be run by the government and could take on a few different forms:

- ○ People could be enrolled in traditional Medicare.
- ○ People could be enrolled in a new public plan in the Exchanges nationally.
- ○ The government could contract with a private plan on an administrative services-only basis. The private plan would run the public option and the government would pay all the bills.
- ○ The government could contract with one or more private plans that would offer coverage in low-penetration areas. The government would subsidize the plan beyond normal premium and cost-sharing in the ACA.
- ○ In another option, Medicaid expansion might be dictated to grow coverage and lower the uninsured rate in the non-expansion states.

Other, Conservative Options—Some in Washington, notably many in the Republican Party, don't like the single-payer or universal access approaches that were just outlined. Instead, they have recommended the following:[30-5]

- o Repeal most of the ACA, eliminate the Exchanges and Medicaid expansion, and devolve funding to states to create healthcare access programs. Some of these ideas are coupled with block-granting a set amount of money for Medicaid and other healthcare access programs in each state.
- o Facilitate the ability to sell insurance across state borders.
- o Allow for actuarially narrow health benefits to boost affordability.
- o Allow for association health plans, where small employers can band together to purchase insurance.
- o Expand the use of health savings accounts (HSAs) paired with high-deductible health plans (HDHPs) to promote cost-savings and accountability.

This is the path former President Trump took and President Biden is busy unraveling some of the elements above that were put in place.

There are disparate interests in the nation as well as in Washington, D.C. Each is fighting for his piece of the healthcare pie, and there is no solid consensus on the right path forward. So, I don't expect radical change anytime soon.

However, I do hope that the parties come together to at least continue down the path the Centers for Medicare and Medicaid Services (CMS) has taken to bring cost-savings, accountability and quality to all lines of business. I also hope they continue—together—to find ways to reduce the level of uninsured in this nation.

CHAPTER 31

What's Wrong with Medicare for All

T his chapter explores exactly what Medicare for All is, and why I think it would be an utter failure if adopted.

As we discussed briefly in the last chapter, Medicare for All is a single-payer scheme endorsed by a number of Democrats running for the presidency in 2020 and by members of Congress. In its purest form, Medicare for All would look like this.[31-1]

- ○ By and large, it would eliminate all private health insurance for benefits covered by the new Medicare for All program. Theoretically, private insurance could fill in gaps in the benefit—if this were to be allowed.
- ○ Medicaid, Exchanges, and other public programs largely would go away. Medicaid may remain for other social service functions.
- ○ Everyone would be enrolled in one program, beginning at birth and for their entire life.
- ○ The backbone and network of Medicare for All would be the traditional Medicare fee-for-service (FFS) program.

- o   Proponents would basically create a zero-premium, zero-deductible, and zero- or minimal-cost-sharing system.
- o   Benefits would be holistic in nature, including comprehensive benefits for medical, dental, vision, and some long-term care services (with the most expensive custodial care in nursing homes possibly staying with Medicaid).
- o   The government would annually set a global budget for covered healthcare.
- o   The government would negotiate medical and drug pricing and what is included on the program's drug list.

This description sounds good, right? How could it not be? No worries about healthcare. You are auto-enrolled and have it guaranteed for life. No premiums, no deductibles. Limited or no cost-sharing. Comprehensive benefits. What are we waiting for? Sign me up!

Well, not so fast. If something sounds too good to be true, it usually is. Here are the problems that I see with Medicare For All:

Issue 1—The Future Cost Is Unsustainable

The biggest issue impacting American seniors today is the costs within the Medicare FFS system. In general, in the traditional system, the government pays 80% of the costs and beneficiaries pay 20%. There are premiums for Part B each month and large deductibles to deal with before the major 20% cost-sharing kicks in. Those lucky enough to afford Medicare Supplement insurance pay hundreds of dollars to fill the cost-sharing gaps. The Part A program has a huge upfront inpatient deductible and high, per-day co-pays if you exceed sixty days in the hospital or for skilled nursing stays. What's worse, the Part A program's inpatient coverage is effectively capped over your lifetime. Catastrophic stays are not fully covered. This leaves those in the program open to huge financial outlays and medical bankruptcy.

Admittedly, proposed Medicare for All bills would provide financial safeguards during the transition to full Medicare for All and eliminate premiums and ensure minimal cost-sharing once the program is fully implemented. The inpatient cap problem would be solved. But the cost to the government would be phenomenal.

With premiums and substantial cost-sharing, the current Part A hospital and related services portion of the program (funded by payroll taxes) is only able to pay current benefits until 2026.[31-2] Thereafter, there would need to be a combination of more revenue, reduced benefits, or greater cost-sharing to fund this part of traditional Medicare. Part B and Part D are funded by federal program dollars and individual premiums. These parts, too, will eat up tax dollars and require increasing premiums and cost-sharing well into the future given robust inflation—far in excess of economic growth and incomes.

The Medicare for All plan appears to have an actuarial value far in excess of Medicare's current benefit (which, as noted, has huge financial troubles). It is also larger than the Affordable Care Act's (ACA's) Marketplace Exchange benefit. It looks most like Medicaid, where premiums and cost-sharing are usually not levied because low-income persons cannot afford it. Now, all Americans would be given such treatment, although taxes would be raised to fund the system. Proponents fail to understand the important role reasonable premiums and cost-sharing play in encouraging prudent use of health insurance.

To fund Medicare for All, based on articles appearing during the 2020 presidential election, estimates suggest you would need between $33-$52 trillion over the first ten years. Proponents of Medicare for All are quick to retort that their plan could save money overall in terms of total healthcare expenditures over the same horizon. But there are many rosy cost-saving assumptions in the plan, so it is hard to endorse this argument. In addition, the estimates don't count a whole bunch of "filling the holes" that would have to occur to make the system viable, such as provider rate increases, paying for care management and quality performance, greater administrative costs for a retail drug component, and more.

The Centers for Medicare and Medicaid (CMS) actuary projects that Medicare spending growth will average 7.6% from 2019-2028. That is driven in great part by the FFS system. Private health insurance costs are projected to grow at a large but more modest 4.8% annually over the same period.[31-3] Perhaps this is not apples to apples (demographics play a role), but how could America afford a Medicare for All system when it grows 7.6% per year? Further, the aging of America over the next decades has the potential to cripple healthcare financing if an inefficient model becomes its foundation.

Clearly, America is an outlier in terms of costs. It spends about 18% of its gross domestic product (GDP) on its healthcare system. The CMS actuary says our healthcare spending will go from about $3.8 trillion in 2019 to nearly $6.2 trillion by 2028.[31-3] That has to change. But government-run healthcare is not always the answer. Other developed-world countries have adopted a universal access model, leveraging private insurers. They have an efficient framework. For the critics out there, let me concede that not all government-run systems have to be inefficient. The point is that Medicare FFS is tragically so and we are set up for failure from the start.

Issue 2—The Administrative Cost Comparison Is Unfair

Comparing public and private administrative costs is problematic. The track record of the Medicare FFS system may be one of low administrative costs, but it doesn't make it efficient. Indeed, the FFS system doesn't do a lot of the things a healthcare system should do that admittedly add to administrative costs.

While the public system wouldn't have sales spending or a margin as private plans do, consider some of the administrative- or quality-related costs that private plans have. In many instances these are government mandates:

Proper claims payment and fraud, waste, and abuse (FWA) reduction. By contrast, FFS has a largely retroactive process, which is notably fraud-ridden.

Cost controls and quality improvement. In fairness to CMS, the agency has gone down the path of trying to bring quality and cost controls to FFS through a series of pilot programs, including accountable care organizations (ACOs), bundled payments, and more. Similar private plan quality programs will roll out in Medicaid managed care and the Exchanges soon. However, the verdict is out on how effective these reforms are or will be. It is hard to argue that the pilots will ever reach the quality improvement seen in the rigorous Medicare Star quality program in the private, managed care program.

Case and disease management. FFS has very few programs of this type, compared to private plans. (There are some care management pilots with physicians and readmissions penalties and some quality pilots with hospitals.).

Prior authorization and appeals. Medicare for All proponents (also known as anti-private health plan politicians) champion the fact that access to benefits is unfettered in FFS. However, the lack of any prior authorization breeds over- and inappropriate utilization of more expensive places of service. More importantly, CMS now mandates that private health plans use strict, evidence-based criteria for denials of drugs and medical services and requires independent external reviews of denials if desired by the member. CMS audits this area thoroughly. This ensures significant accountability in plan decision-making.

Grievance and complaints processes. FFS does not have a thorough system, while private plans typically do.

Network management and provider credentialing. This is poorly performed by FFS and not governed by national accreditation bodies as private plans are.

Eligibility and member services. This is very rudimentary in FFS.

So, the Medicare FFS system does some of these administrative features, but not all of them. And when it does some, Medicare FFS implements them half-heartedly and very poorly.

So, the 2% (for FFS) versus 10%-plus (for private plans) administrative comparison is simply not fair. A case can be made that the administrative spending will reduce healthcare costs over time. Administrative costs and margin now are effectively capped at 15% due to the 85% minimum medical loss ratio (MLR) requirement in most healthcare programs (80% for the individual market).

Issue 3—A Rotten Traditional Medicare Track Record

The Medicare FFS system is one of the most inefficient systems out there. It is fraud-ridden, fragmented, lacks appropriate oversight, lacks quality, and is quite expensive. It is hardly the model we need to adopt if we are to bend the cost curve.

Supporters argue simply that government will do it better. But this ignores the glaring inadequacies of the current Medicare FFS system. Indeed, both the government-run Medicare and Medicaid FFS systems have shown that simply giving enrollees access to a healthcare system, even with minimal or no cost-sharing (as is the case in Medicaid), doesn't mean quality or even true access.

The current system offers little or no care management or care coordination. People, especially the elderly and those with social barriers, are left on their own to navigate the labyrinthine system. Horror stories abound related to poor care and missed, life-saving opportunities. Creating a care management structure in the FFS world would cost billions. Providers have lower rates in public programs and won't magically become exceedingly altruistic and provide free care coordination or management. The Hippocratic oath goes only so far.

The Obama Administration tried to reinvent these FFS delivery systems in both Medicare and Medicaid through myriad quality-based reforms. The Trump Administration continued these efforts. CMS says that about 61% of all payments in Medicare FFS are now tied to alternative payment schemes—other than traditional FFS payments.[31-4] But, while I support such experimentation, thus far savings and quality outcomes have been suspect. This is driven in part by the underlying individual-transaction-based system and the lack of sophistication of most providers to understand, invest in, and make these alternative incentive-based payment schemes a significant game-changer in the inefficient traditional system. In the end, it is hard to fundamentally change a system that has so many built-in disincentives.

Issue 4—Challenging Networks and Access

Medicaid FFS networks are notoriously narrow. Providers were scared away by low reimbursement rates. While provider losses in the Medicare world have slowed down, Medicare providers are still leaving the program due to low reimbursement as well. Medicare has its network and access challenges, too.

Eliminating private insurance may give the medical profession little choice but to join the government system, but the reality is that government lacks the innovation capability of the private sector to offer robust networks. This includes growing alternative payment schemes and leveraging commercial relationships. Indeed, the best thing to happen in the Medicaid and Medicare worlds was for private health plans to leverage providers to join all their lines, thereby giving Medicaid and Medicare enrollees access to the same private doctors that half the nation has.

There are underpayments in the public program world, made up by a cost shift to the commercial world. Half the nation pays higher costs of insurance because Medicaid and to some degree Medicare do not pay enough. This problem does not magically go away with Medicare for All. If current Medicare provider rates, especially for primary care, were not increased, access would be an issue in the already narrower system, when compared with commercial plans.

So, Medicare for All would have to spend tens of billions in higher payments to replicate the robustness of private networks. Hospitals can be among the most inefficient and wasteful providers, and the financial accounting for their so-called "under-reimbursement" is dubious. However, some estimates suggest that Medicare and Medicaid under-reimbursement and other uncompensated care is over $100 billion annually for hospitals—an additional $1 trillion in costs in the first ten years of Medicare for All.[31-5]

Medicare for All proponents' other problem is that retail drug provision is totally private in Medicare. So, tens of thousands more providers would have to be contracted with to complete the grand vision of government-run healthcare.

Issue 5—Medicare for All Is About Going Back in Time

Medicare for All supporters want to go back in time to the early days of healthcare policy and endorse the indemnity, transaction-based model of healthcare as opposed to more progressive managed-care concepts. For them, managed care is diabolical and an invention of the self-interested private sector.

The history of healthcare in America shows the indemnity/FFS/transaction system to be expensive, inefficient, and not quality centered. Is there a Medicare for All tenet to incorporate managed care principles relating to care management and quality into their archaic delivery system? Simply put, except for some of the pilots, the answer is no.

Instead, Medicare for All would return to your Dad's or Grandpa's FFS healthcare system and make it even worse. Consider the following:

- With limited cost-sharing, utilization of services and costs will soar.
- The overly generous, one-size-fits-all philosophy behind the program will also drive up costs.
- By zeroing out the 20% consumer share, there is no reasonable skin in the game for enrollees and personal responsibility will go out the window. Financial incentives or penalties—as long as they are affordable—encourage consumers to think before they act. I favor affordable access to healthcare. But, as our parents have taught us, there often can be too much of a good thing. Prudent use of the healthcare system is key, and premiums and cost-sharing play an important role. Entitlements create entitlement.

Medicare for All creates a system where benefits are too rich and lives within an anachronistic delivery system—it is the worst of both worlds. And as noted, it will be unaffordable.

How will government try to afford the entitlement? It will act as it usually does in Medicare and Medicaid when spending gets tight. Provider rates will be cut, impacting access. Wait times will balloon as the government seeks to defer costs. Benefits may be rationed, initially through cloak-and-dagger methods and later outright. You say this is just speculation, but this is what we see today in many of the nationalized systems and single-payer systems around the world. Private insurance pops up because of those waiting lists and wait times. Or if they can afford it, people come to America for care.

Issue 6—Medicare for All Stops Progress

As a corollary to the previous argument, America has made progress toward accountability, cost limitations, and quality over the last several years. Much of this has been done in the private commercial world and the private health plan portions of Medicaid and Medicare.

CMS has created a vigorous compliance regime and a Star quality program that are first-rate in Medicare, and which will inevitably be passed to the Medicaid and commercial worlds over time. It will take years for all benefits to come to fruition, but these are important in changing the healthcare paradigm. The reforms constitute an emerging public (regulator) versus private (delivery innovator) model.

By the way, health plans and insurers often foolishly rally against the compliance and quality dictates. While sometimes CMS can go too far on given items, what they have created is a reasonable compliance and quality regime. It allows everyone to have faith in healthcare delivery. What plans often fail to realize is that the compliance and quality regime has neutralized many of managed care's detractors and created a system that is humming along nicely for them. The negative noise of the past is basically gone. Health plans can now argue that they are fully accountable entities and that members are feeling relatively good about their plans.

Issue 7—Medicare for All Ignores Where Americans Flock

Medicare for All proponents ignore the fact that private insurance has been good for the healthcare system and is where Americans flock. About half of the nation continues to have private health coverage, and the vast majority are satisfied. Seventy-five percent of Medicaid recipients today are in private Medicaid managed care plans because states realized that holding private plans accountable is better than continuing to run a decrepit FFS system. Quality outcomes were just so embarrassingly low—something that private plans are beginning to change.

Seniors and the disabled are enrolling in private Medicare Advantage (MA) plans due to the value proposition and the unprecedented quality. Seniors and the disabled in America have become such savvy consumers that almost 80% of them have enrolled in the highest-rated private MA plans for 2021. As a result, MA has grown to over 43% of beneficiaries in the last twenty years (up from about 15%). Today, MA covers a majority of enrollees in many major urban markets. By 2025, private estimates suggest MA will hit 50% of enrollees nationwide as the popular PPO product expands into suburban and more affluent markets and the HMO product continues to penetrate urban markets. And 70% of Medicare beneficiaries could be in MA between 2030 and 2040.[31-6]

Medicare for All proponents are right to say that Medicare is popular. It is a government program covering the broad masses and it allows access to anyone you want to be in the network. What's not to like, theoretically? But more and more, seniors are viewing MA—not traditional Medicare—as exciting because it responds to their needs. Early Baby Boomers liked the open Medicare networks. After all, they came into healthcare coverage under the old indemnity models of the 1940s to the 1970s. Later Baby Boomers—those who have recently aged into Medicare or will do so over the next decade—acclimated to managed care that began in the 1970s and took root during their working years. They understand the give-and-take of managed care. They also are more attuned to recent higher costs.

What is that great value proposition that MA plans have built? For roughly the same price as Medicare FFS, private plans do several important things. They provide base Medicare benefits at huge savings. Then they roll the difference into major benefit add-ons, including reduced or eliminated premiums and reduced cost-sharing. They also add inpatient days to prevent bankruptcy or altogether eliminate the day cap, as well as provide myriad services not covered or poorly covered in traditional Medicare, such as dental, vision, hearing, and more. This saves the average American hundreds if not thousands of dollars each year compared with what they would pay in traditional Medicare. For low-income folks, it is a godsend—basically, an alternative social welfare program at no cost or minimal cost to the taxpayer.

Private MA plans also improve quality through a wonderfully crafted Star bonus program. Typically, they reduce waste, fraud, and abuse as well as overall costs and the future cost curve by setting up accountable networks and prior authorization for medical and drug services, using evidence-based criteria.

Such plans invest in care management activities that are beginning to emphasize prevention, disease management, and care coordination. This is often done through incentive payments and bonuses to providers. Shifting from utilization management (UM) to care management is critical to bend the cost curve and bring about quality. The Medicare FFS system neither controls utilization nor performs care management. MA plans are working with CMS to change the paradigm.

In addition, MA plans serve the dual eligible populations, who are both elderly or disabled and low income. These populations consume a disproportionate share of the healthcare dollar in Medicare and Medicaid. MA plans work on both the medical and social determinant aspects of these members to reduce costs and improve quality.

Finally, private MA plans work with CMS to experiment on combining Medicare and Medicaid clinical pathways and finance. While Medicare for All bills have been amended to add certain chronic home and community-based services, Medicare for All would not create linkages between acute medical care and Medicaid long-term care as many Medicare and Medicaid managed care plans are doing. The coordination is essential as America ages.

In summary, private MA plans add to benefits by being efficient, saving Americans millions of dollars, reducing medical bankruptcies, and creating better quality outcomes. This is especially true for low-income, urban markets.

Critics argue that plans can do all this in part because of the beneficial selection (the healthier population they attract) in MA and some risk adjustment maximization performed by plans. But the reality is that the value is there in MA. Such plans can provide basic benefits far more cheaply, add benefits, and still make a profit. This proves the FFS system's inherent inefficiency.

It is hard to find a lawmaker, except for the Medicare for All proponents (some of whom even equivocate) who would get rid of MA. Largely, each side of the political aisle has championed the private alternative program's growth because of what it does for seniors and the disabled.

But to the Medicare for All proponents, Big Brother seems to know best. They want the political win of telling everyone they have free healthcare. Of course, there is a massive tax increase and a lackluster system in the best-case scenario. They would rather sing from the political hymnal than work toward a public-private model. Such an approach would be driven by private-sector innovation—and some government oversight—that may actually pay the most dividends and, over time, have the best shot at righting the healthcare ship of state.

Endorsing Medicare for All and the dilapidated FFS system means championing tired, old ideas and a system that is worn out and a relic of the past. On its face, Medicare for All would mean no hope of transforming our healthcare system by reducing cost and improving quality.

CHAPTER 32

The Right Healthcare Reform Solution

"Of all the questions which can come before this nation, short of the actual preservation of its existence in a great war, there is none which compares in importance with the great central task of leaving this land even a better land for our descendants than it is for us and training them into a better race to inhabit the land and pass it on. Conservation is a great moral issue, for it involves the patriotic duty of insuring the safety and continuance of the nation. Let me add that the health and vitality of our people are at least as well worth conserving as their forests, waters, lands, and minerals, and in this great work the national government must bear a most important part."

Teddy Roosevelt, The New Nationalism Speech, August 31, 1910. Roosevelt left the White House in 1909 and failed to regain the presidency in 1912 running on the Progressive "Bull Moose" Party ticket.

> "As a matter of national policy, and to the extent that a nation's
> health system can make it possible, should the child of a poor
> American family have the same chance of avoiding preventable
> illness or being cured from a given illness as does the child of a
> rich American family?"
> *Uwe Reinhardt, originally in "Wanted: A Clearly Articulated*
> *Social Ethic for American Healthcare,"* Journal of the American
> Medical Association, *1997, restated in his book* Priced Out.

We have arrived at that all-critical point in the book—where do we go from here to improve a dysfunctional system, and how do we build on some of the small advances we have made? You now know about all the healthcare system types and why I think a single-payer system would not be good. Now, educated on our system, you will ultimately arrive at your own conclusions, but here is my take on moving forward to bend the cost curve and improve quality in America's healthcare system.

The system type I favor is affordable universal access. Here are my reasons:

First, I am a pragmatist. I don't believe America is ready to give up private healthcare. In many ways, it is not what we stand for. I don't believe America wants socialized medicine or even a universal, single-payer system.

Second, we are also not ready to abandon employer-sponsored coverage as the displacement could be huge in any conversion. Sticking with the status quo will mean that employers bear a burden that businesses in other countries do not. However, if we do this right, then American businesses won't be uncompetitive. Reform will help lessen the burden on employers.

Third, statistics show that all three healthcare system types can mean quality and lower overall costs. It does not mean one is better than another. They all can be efficient and drive positive outcomes.

Finally, despite tremendous overlap and duplication, we are closest to the universal access model in America. We should build on this.

One admonition: Affordable universal access will mean some additional, short-term spending. Critics will argue that more money will mean Big Government is further down the road of taking over healthcare. My answer is that somewhere between one-half and two-thirds of all healthcare expenditures in America are already paid by Uncle Sam. Reinhardt notes in chapter 4 of his book, *Priced Out*, that the employer deductibility of health insurance premiums significantly dwarfs the subsidies doled out in the much-maligned Marketplace Exchanges. Employer subsidies are 2.5-3 times higher.[32-1] So, what is the aversion to a responsible and simple way of ensuring everyone has access to quality healthcare coverage? Think of the trillions of dollars that could be saved annually if the system is rationalized with some investment now. Consistent access would finally bring wellness, prevention, and quality to the fore. Federal spending and healthcare's proportion of GDP might actually be *reduced* over time.

So, what are the critical features to further reforming America's healthcare system? Let's name them, although some were captured earlier in Chapter 29 as emerging reforms. In addition, I highly recommend reading *Priced Out* by Uwe Reinhardt. Rather than citing the book each time, I will use Reinhardt's name and, where important, cite a specific chapter for your reference.[32-1]

The Social Good Concept Must Take Hold in America

At the beginning of the chapter, you read Reinhardt's provocative quote about whether a poor child deserves as much of a chance to live a healthy life as a rich one. The answer, of course, is yes. Sadly, however, the United States has not come to consensus on this. Let me refine my thought here: I believe that the vast majority of the American public believe that poor children should have that chance, but that many elected lawmakers may not. This has stymied efforts to enact healthcare policies that live up to this dream. Many would argue that we have Medicaid and other social safety nets. But this misses the broader point. There is vast inequality between rich and poor as well as between whites and minorities when it comes to healthcare affordability, access, and outcomes. Poor and minority communities are the biggest losers in the dysfunctional healthcare system we now have.

Some in my party would say I am some sort of a Republican in Name Only (RINO), having abandoned the core principles of the Grand Old Party and embraced socialism. But, as Reinhardt notes in chapters 6 and 8 of *Priced Out*,

America is the only developed country without a consensus that affordable universal access is a social good. This is a stain on our nation. Every other major party across the political spectrum in developed nations cannot be totally wrong. Thus, I believe we must build a consensus in this nation that affordable universal access is a worthy pursuit. As Reinhardt notes:

- We need an ethical vision of healthcare in America.
- We must overcome the practice of "distributive ethics," where a rich country like the United States subjects some of its most vulnerable citizens to poor health and disease.
- Due to high costs and lack of consensus on healthcare's social good in America, we ration healthcare by income class.

This is not an attack on the free market; it is something I strongly believe in. I also have concluded over the years, though, that if healthcare is not an absolute right, then it is close to it. As a developed nation, we owe it to our citizens to have a chance at good health. And, as I have pointed out in a previous chapter, there are well-founded economic reasons to go down this path. Ultimately, it saves money and makes us more competitive economically. What could be more Republican than that!

What will it take to get to such a consensus? Sometimes, it seems like the gap is overwhelming and irreconcilable. Certain parts of the Democratic Party have radical views on healthcare, which creates a reluctance among other political players to embrace the good of universal access. It becomes a leap too far for them. What might such an endorsement mean to America, they ask? On the flip side, certain elements of the Republican Party view healthcare as some sort of Wild West, "pull yourself up by your own bootstraps" commodity that you may enjoy if you can afford it. Where is the compassion and mercy? So, getting to a middle ground will be difficult, but it does exist. Affordable universal access and personal responsibility can help drive transformation from a system more focused on emergency room chaos to one centered on wellness and prevention. But we do need an appetite for change and the right leaders in our country to implement it.

In many ways, if we cannot come to this consensus, we really cannot move healthcare reform forward in a meaningful way. It is the logical first step.

Further Build Public-Private Partnership Accountability and Compliance Infrastructure

As noted in Chapter 29, the Department of Health and Human Services (HHS), the Centers for Medicare and Medicaid Services (CMS), and other federal and state authorities are building a public-private partnership with private health plans. In this model, government plays the role of broad policymaker, setting accountability and quality standards. Private health plans use innovation to bring efficiency and quality forward. Further extending such progress in Medicare and bringing it fully to Medicaid and commercial lines of business is important to drive consistency and remove undue administrative costs and inefficiency.

Come to a Consensus on Healthcare Funding for the Long Haul

This is similar to the notion of a social good described previously. The nation, too, must grapple with what its healthcare commitments and spending will be moving forward. When it comes to fashioning long-term healthcare policies, with concomitant financial reforms, no party has ever had the courage to deal with the looming issue. It has always been "kick the can down the road" given the political sensitivity of the issue. As such, any real progress toward reforming healthcare has been held hostage.

What do we know about the status of our healthcare programs? Medicare's Part A Trust Fund will be insolvent by 2026.[32-2] All parts of Medicare are greatly impacted by inflation, driven by the archaic and inefficient fee-for-service (FFS) system. Despite having low rates, Medicaid is taking up ever-increasing portions of federal and state budgets.

At the same time, we know that both programs, along with many others, are critical to our healthcare future. Medicaid will be relied on as America ages and to reduce the number of uninsured. Both programs must be put on a solid financial footing for the future.

Let's take the Medicare solvency issue. A presidential candidate immediately would be pilloried if he or she dreamed of recognizing the issue or recommending ways to keep the program afloat. Thus, neither presidential candidate dared mention any meaningful change that may be needed in Medicare. Indeed, President Biden has recommended lowering the Medicare eligibility age from sixty-five to sixty, which could add considerably to overall costs. In his budget proposal for federal fiscal year 2022, Biden made vague references to the pending insolvency, offering few details about how the funding gaps will be closed.

There are myriad ideas that Congress and policymakers can take to address long-term sustainability of Medicare. To do so will require give-and-take on each side of the aisle. These include:

- Means testing the program or having wealthier folks pay more for premiums and perhaps cost-sharing
- Potentially looking at the eligibility age
- Further refining the Medicare payment system for medical services and drugs
- Re-examining the benefit structure. It could mean augmenting in some areas and deprioritizing other areas
- Reining in fraud, waste, and abuse (FWA)
- Reining in myriad reform pilots in traditional Medicare in hopes of gaining traction on lowering costs and improving quality
- Fostering additional growth in MA as well as a delinking of the rate structure from traditional FFS
- Further enhancing how dual eligible populations are overseen, especially integrating medical and long-term care between Medicare and Medicaid
- Allowing people to opt out of Medicare with a premium subsidy from the federal government that they could take somewhere else to obtain coverage

Medicaid's financing structure must be responsibly addressed, including the rich benefit, entitlement nature, and onerous mandates. We must look at a generous and flexible per-capita cap program, instead of the current entitlement or a strict block grant. On the flip side, we do need to grapple with low provider reimbursement so as to improve network access and quality.

Move to a Care Management and Population Health Focus to Drive Quality; Reform Payments and Price

As noted in Chapter 29, pivoting to a care management, wellness, and prevention focus is critical. Plans should become extremely efficient on how they administer prior authorization and utilization management (UM), while reallocating resources to various wellness, prevention, and care management programs.

As a nation we must ensure that every American has a primary care physician and medical home. In 2021, the National Academies of Sciences, Engineering and Medicine came out with a strong message that we must connect people with a primary source of care and bolster primary care. We must move dollars from higher cost of care sites, including specialists, to primary care. Further, we must enter into reimbursement structures with primary care physicians (PCPs) that emphasize wellness, prevention, and chronic condition management, as well as shifts from transaction payments.[32-3]

Plans must build population health initiatives to identify risks and care gaps in members and proactively engage members and providers to address them and drive quality. This includes technology to promote interoperability, sharing data between providers and payers in real time. They must ensure that every member has some form of a model of care to drive outcomes. They must also invest in care management and care coordination to prevent admissions, reduce readmissions, and manage disease states.

Significantly, plans must prioritize both clinical conditions and social determinants of health (socio-economic barriers). A number of studies indicate that socioeconomic status or barriers can be a greater predictor of health than underlying disease states. Addressing things like health literacy, housing, food security, transportation, loneliness, and socialization all can pay huge dividends for outcomes and costs. A number of programs have been launched at the state and federal level for both Medicare and Medicaid (in the FFS system and private plans). Health literacy and education is key to driving people to the most appropriate site of care.[32-4]

Finally, employers need to continue to push the envelope and demand a focus on employee wellness and outcomes.

All this should help lower costs for the most expensive patients, whom I noted consume the lion's share of costs in the healthcare system.

America must abandon the old FFS reimbursement system—pushing forward to the next generation of managed care and value-based payment. We must retire the old FFS reimbursement that drives over-utilization and neglects quality. This is a leading driver of the fraud, waste, and abuse (FWA) we have in our system. Initiatives must include:

- **Deepening global and partial risk capitation** to incentivize provider groups to control costs and improve quality.
- **Driving capitation and quality incentives for primary care physicians (PCPs)** to help improve quality.
- **Moving from inpatient per diems and percentage-of-cost reimbursement to episodic or bundled payments tied to quality outcomes.** These initiatives should include physicians and other post-discharge providers to ensure coordination of care.
- **Driving value-based and outcome reimbursement and pay-for-performance models throughout the system,** including hospitals and drug payments.

Most controversially, we must get our arms around price in the system. A refocus on care management will naturally bring some costs down by diverting care to lower cost places of service. But America must grapple with the fact that prices throughout the system are exorbitant when compared with other developed nations. In Chapter 28, I discussed the huge difference in prices between America and other developed nations. In a coming chapter, I will address drug price reform and changes needed in the system.

I am not a fan of the concept known as "any willing provider" rules. This is where a provider willing to accept a given reimbursement rate can be in a plan or government program's network. Private plans should be free to negotiate rates with providers and create their own networks to ensure quality, efficiency, and alignment with the plan. But a case can be made that uniform rates could be established by state or region to address the effect of hospital monopolies, exorbitant price masters, and high rates in general. This would bring better price transparency, stop surprise billing, and more. Each plan could utilize this uniform rate structure, negotiate from there, and require providers to ensure efficiency and quality. In addition, this could also significantly standardize and simplify contracting, which alone could save huge amounts in the system overall.

In Chapter 3 of his book, Reinhardt notes that an all-payer rate system with uniform fee schedules might be a reasonable option—as practiced in the rest of the developed world (socialized medicine, single-payer, and even most universal access countries). This is not unlike what is done in Medicare FFS, which helps private plans drive better overall rates in the system, both in Medicare and to some degree the commercial world. Some Medicaid states have experimented with provisions that require good-faith negotiations to occur between health plans and providers. If such talks fail, a rate tied to prevailing reimbursement or a low Medicaid FFS system rate is automatically adopted. The Bipartisan Policy Center (BPC) suggests that exorbitant hospital rates in uncompetitive areas could be tackled by pegging maximum rates to either the average Medicare Advantage (MA) rate in a given market or the commercial payment in a competitive market. The BPC would also bar anti-competitive contracting standards (contracting with every provider owned by a hospital or system rather than specific providers the plan needs).[32-5]

I am not a fan of creating a government-sponsored or -administered public option in the Exchanges. I will discuss this later in the chapter and lay out better alternatives. However, the Urban Institute recently did a study on the effects of the uninsured rate and costs if a public option were to be created in the nation and used rates that were pegged to Medicare rates (or just above it in some scenarios). While having a public option for just the non-group markets did little to reduce costs or the uninsured rates, it did save substantial sums if group market employers chose the public option for employees.[32-6]

- ○ If some employers took advantage of the opportunity, the uninsured rate could drop by up to 1.7 million and employers would save up to $143 billion per year.[32-6]
- ○ If all employers were in a public option plan, the uninsured rate would drop by up to 1.6 million and employers would save up to $224 billion per year (all employer scenarios had add-ons only to the Medicare rates).[32-6]

A RAND study found that setting prices for all commercial healthcare payers could reduce hospital spending by between $62 billion and $237 billion annually if the rates were set as high as 150% to as low as 100% of the traditional Medicare program. This could cut overall health spending by between 1.7% and 6.5%.[32-7]

A Kaiser Family Foundation (KFF) study found that total healthcare spending for the privately insured population would be $352 billion lower in 2021 if employers and other insurers reimbursed at traditional Medicare rates.[32-8]

Again, my reason for citing these studies is not because I think a public option is a good idea, but to show how Reinhardt's all-payer rate system with uniform fee schedules would save a great deal.

I would note that the "1% Steps for Health Care Reform," a project that includes leading healthcare academics, is busy publishing ideas to incrementally reduce healthcare costs and reform the system. One main focus is on introducing reasonable provider price and growth gaps. Their work will grow over time and be very important.[32-9]

Vast conflicts of interest and kickbacks also dominate healthcare, despite laws that theoretically bar this. All the safe harbors that exist in these anti-kickback or conflict-of-interest statutes and rules should be withdrawn. This would reduce costs, as well as rationalize and bring transparency to the system.

I am a fan of creating value-based networks within health plans. High-value providers can help reduce health plan premiums to consumers. If the providers are truly high value, then consumers should be delighted. It does not have to be limited to the old narrow networks of several decades ago, when it was all about cost and not quality. A number of health plans are now teaming up with top-rate providers (such as premier hospitals that own various facilities and physicians) to offer these next generation of managed care plans.

Promote Personal Responsibility with Reasonable Skin in the Game

I am a big believer in personal responsibility. Reinhardt notes that this is a difficult proposition in today's healthcare world. But personal responsibility does belong as a tenet of the system. People should be accountable for where they access care and pay more for receiving services at a site that is not appropriate, such as an emergency room in lieu of a primary care physician or urgent care. People should also be penalized if they don't seek care or preventive services and their conditions exacerbate. What should these penalties be? They can be monetary (greater out-of-pocket costs or premiums, for example) or loss of certain benefits (such as better cost-sharing for certain services).

At the same time, I am not a proponent of product offerings that serve as a disincentive to seeking care. Consumer-directed health plans (CDHPs) or high-deductible health plans (HDHPs) with health savings accounts (HSAs) may have some role with younger populations, where we are seeking to keep costs low and encourage coverage. However, generally speaking, while preventive services may be included for most of these plans, high deductibles and other cost-sharing can serve as a barrier for lower-to-middle-income citizens to obtain consistent care. In other words, they become a barrier to personal responsibility.

Comprehensive, affordable coverage will help individuals to be responsible, make the right healthcare decisions, and not forego care. In the end, this strategy is sure to save money in the future by helping people access care earlier and managing disease states. Admittedly, the penalties and comprehensiveness will be a balancing act.

All this said, it is not unreasonable to ask whether the actuarial value of benefits are too high. Militating against a reduction in benefits at this time is the sheer cost in the system. As long as costs are so high, a marked erosion of comprehensiveness could lead to people foregoing care. But as costs come down over time, it may not be unreasonable to ask some citizens to pay a greater percentage share of their healthcare.

Drive Price Transparency, Data Interoperability, and the Right Site of Care; Eliminate Aberrant Provider Practice Patterns

Related to personal responsibility, we need to leverage technology to give both providers and members the information they need to demystify price in the healthcare system and make the right decision as to the most appropriate site of care for treatment.

In Chapter 29, I talked about the need for additional price transparency. As Reinhardt notes, American health consumers are essentially blindfolded shoppers in our incredibly opaque system. He describes it as "exceedingly complex" and "almost beyond human comprehension." He says that consumerism is not about to work in the current system. It will take time, but the reforms that have started are a good first step. Technology affords the ability to get there over time as well. I hope for a time when price transparency does increase consumerism in healthcare. Indeed, Americans make deliberate, well-educated decisions in most areas of the economy every day. They balance cost and quality. So, why not do so when it comes to healthcare?

Similarly, driving the sharing of data between plans and providers (in a safe and secure manner while protecting privacy) is essential to ensuring that we transform our system and focus on care management and coordination as well as reduce administrative expense related to prior authorizations. This includes remote monitoring and biometric devices that can instantaneously inform a plan care manager of critical data, such as:

- ○ Blood sugar test results for diabetic patients
- ○ Breathing test results for those with asthma and other pulmonary disorders
- ○ Blood pressure readings for those with hypertension
- ○ Weight gain for those with chronic heart failure

America must focus on ensuring that people have the information they need to make informed decisions. Access to their clinical information is key. Health plans and providers sharing data is also key. Then, plans should also assemble important network and provider performance to help consumers make the best, most informed decision about where to seek care.

Plans as well as the government need to tackle the problem of aberrant provider practice patterns. This touches hospitals as well as physicians. The Dartmouth Atlas Project looked at Medicare FFS medical service patterns around the nation for decades and has benchmarked regions. Patterns can differ markedly between regions and within regions. Dartmouth made several conclusions:[32-10]

- ○ The most recent assessment shows a wide disparity in spending throughout the nation. New York City and Miami per-capita Medicare spending is almost twice as high as spending in Salem, Oregon.
- ○ High-spending areas can be both large metropolitan areas like Miami, but also much smaller regions of the country.
- ○ Price or Medicare reimbursement between regions is not the real driver of spending differences—utilization is.
- ○ The supply of hospital beds, as well as specialists and physician practice patterns, drive utilization and the aberrant practices. Thus, an overabundance of availability or supply arguably creates artificial demand in healthcare.
- ○ Aberrant practices are a big part of up to 30% of wasteful, abusive, or fraudulent spending.
- ○ More care is not better. Death rates and outcomes are not better for high-utilization regions. In fact, it is associated with higher mortality.

Plans should be able to extend this type of benchmarking to its own network and create comprehensive analyses, in part using evidenced-based criteria, regarding aberrant practices or providers. This can be used subsequently for provider education or network termination. In many ways, this is one of the most important avenues to drive an efficient system with quality.

One of the leading authorities these days on aberrant provider practice patterns and excessive costs is Dr. Marty Makary, M.D., a renowned Johns Hopkins University professor and surgeon. He has written two books, *Unaccountable* and *The Price We Pay*. While both are great reads, I highly recommend *The Price We Pay*. Among other key reform discussions, Dr. Makary describes how doctors test far too much, undertake unneeded services, and drive over-treatment. In some cases this is driven by greed and fear of lawsuits. But, in many cases, it is driven by sheer ignorance and lack of time among physicians. He also shows how excessive costs, especially at hospitals, devastates lives. He has personally intervened to save many people from greedy hospitals and has helped drive passage of bills for price transparency and surprise billing. His Improving Wisely initiative, which aims to educate on aberrant practice patterns, promises to do as much for healthcare reform as many of the proposals in this book.

Americans must also begin to seek services at the right site of care. The system can no longer sustain provision of services at expensive settings. Part of this is encouraging health and wellness by having members seek care at primary care sites. But it also entails training both patients and providers regarding the right site of care or place of service, taking into consideration the current health status of an individual. Increasingly, patients can seek care at physicians' offices, at home, and in ambulatory settings—safely and often with better quality than when these services are furnished at expensive hospital inpatient and outpatient settings.

We want to maintain reasonable cost-sharing, so as not to create barriers to care. It is also not unreasonable to create a system where a low-cost, quality provider or drug is covered with reasonably modest cost-sharing. However, choosing another provider within a place of service or a more expensive setting might mean you pay 100% (or a large portion) of the difference in cost. This is what is referred to as reference pricing, an upper limit a payer will reimburse at, with the consumer covering the additional amount. In addition, site-neutral payments by government programs and health plans are key to ensuring that we ratchet down costs.

The COVID-19 pandemic has also shown us how technology can be leveraged in the form of telehealth or virtual care. The price is clearly right. While more needs to be known about the quality of care, its ongoing use is surely something to embrace for many services.

End Surprising Billing

There is a need to end surprise billing in this nation. I have already discussed the forms of surprise billing. In many cases, you could do everything exactly right (for example, go to an in-network facility) and yet be saddled with a bill for thousands, tens of thousands, or even hundreds of thousands of dollars. A majority of states have passed bans or restrictions on this practice, but in many cases they have not done enough. A new federal law will go into effect on January 1, 2022, eliminating surprise bills related to emergency care and air ambulance service. In addition, most bills from out-of-network providers who render services at in-network facilities will also go away. However, not all surprise bills are banned. Instead of paying such bills simply based on regional, median in-network rates, an arbitration dispute resolution process has been adopted. This will lead to confusion and continued high costs. Provider groups have flexed their powerful Capitol Hill muscles at the expense of the country. Further reforms are needed; all it takes is some political courage. What's more, adopting some form of a national, state, or regional price master and establishing uniform rates could eliminate the issue altogether.[32-11]

Develop a National Long-term Care Policy

In Chapter 35, I tackle the aging-of-America issue. I will leave much of the statistics and discussion for that chapter. But there is a clear need for America to develop a national, long-term care policy. As the nation ages, costs will increase dramatically. This will be the case for both acute medical care and chronic, long-term care. As with acute medical care, many lower- and middle-income families are priced out of alternatives to nursing home institutionalization. This puts a huge burden on families as they struggle to take care of elderly parents and these individuals end up in expensive nursing homes when they could be maintained much more cheaply and humanely in the community.

The long-term care policy must address how all Americans buy into long-term care coverage, both privately and through the government. Affordable universal access must, by its nature, address both acute medical and long-term care needs. The policy must get the relatively young to think about long-term care insurance much like auto, home, life, and health coverage.

Endorse Private Managed Care as the Solution for Medicare and Medicaid

I have gone out of my way to talk about why I think private sector innovation, in tandem with government accountability and oversight, is the best course for America's health system. I think this is especially true for the Medicare and Medicaid programs. The alternative is continuing to rely on the dilapidated traditional fee-for-service (FFS) systems in each program. I see no way of reforming those systems. And the fact that people are flocking to Medicare Advantage (MA) and states are moving more and more populations into Medicaid managed care proves the point.

Thus, for the long-term viability of both programs, policymakers should work with private health plans on ways to bring MA and Medicaid managed care to all corners of America for each program.

We need to encourage further creation of MA throughout the nation, especially in rural and suburban areas. This will take creativity and perhaps incentives to enter rural areas. Private plans offer the greatest chance to save and improve quality. Private plans can focus on the conversion from a UM focus to an upfront care management focus.

Earlier, I told you that I reject the Medicare Payment Advisory Commission's (MedPAC, the congressional advisory panel) view that MA does not save. It clearly does. I also reject the idea that we should radically and too swiftly change reimbursement structures as it will impact the important social safety net that MA is for poor and lower-income Americans. But, without upsetting the innovation of MA, over time we should begin the process of delinking MA rates from FFS costs to derive greater savings. MA cannot forever live off the inefficient system. And the nation cannot afford it. MA has gone through other rate realignment before. It survived and thrived.

Protect the Affordable Care Act (ACA) and Continue Investments

As we have discussed at length, the uninsured rate in America remains over 30 million, or about 10% of the population. This is a stain on our country, especially since most developed nations have uninsured rates of about 1%. The ACA has reduced the number of uninsured considerably and has been a godsend to at least 30 million Americans. What's more, the framework is good in the short term. It is all about implementing a few reforms to further drive down the uninsured rate. According to a Congressional Budget Office (CBO) analysis:[32-12]

- ○ Almost 11 million of the uninsured are currently eligible for sub-sidized Medicaid, State Children's Health Insurance program (SCHIP), or Exchange Marketplace coverage. Eligibility is roughly split between Medicaid/SCHIP and the Exchanges.
- ○ Another over 3 million would be eligible for Medicaid if remaining states expanded Medicaid as allowed in the ACA.
- ○ Another over 9 million are eligible for employer coverage and they could obtain affordable coverage if we tweaked some aspects of the ACA.

At least 28 million have benefited from the ACA Medicaid expansion and Exchanges, with almost as many noted above eligible for coverage but not enrolled. So, taking away the ACA would be detrimental.

We need to protect and expand the ACA. By doing so, U.S. healthcare policy would:

Ensure that it preserves the various reforms dictated by the act, including barring the denial of insurance coverage for those with pre-existing conditions. It would also preserve the elimination of waiting periods or denial of benefits for pre-existing conditions, as well as higher premiums due to health conditions and annual and lifetime limits in most benefit areas.

Further, protecting the ACA would preserve coverage for children up to twenty-six years of age on their parents' insurance. It would also preserve community rating in lieu of underwriting in the individual market. Many Republicans cry foul as it relates to retaining community rating, where, except for age and sex, everyone is given the same rate. But as Reinhardt notes, this is the exact methodology used by employer-based coverage, in MA, and throughout the developed world. Why should this be controversial? It also ensures that those with pre-existing conditions or disease states get coverage and have access to upfront care instead of using the most expensive settings because they are uninsured.

Keep the employer mandate and small business tax credits, but restore the individual mandate penalty. As Reinhardt notes in chapters 7 and 9 of his book, an explicit penalty is an important factor in community rating, lest healthier people "free ride" the system until they need it. There are but two alternatives. The first is to have a penalty big enough to force someone to accept the social responsibility of getting covered. The second is to let them be uninsured as long as they don't get access to the community-rated product when they need it. Instead, they might receive a medically underwritten rate or be barred from the community rating for a number of years (perhaps as long as he or she eschewed coverage). They might also have to face a waiting period to get in, although this might be counterproductive. Another alternative is that they might face additional penalties based on the time they lacked coverage—something practiced in Medicare.

I tend to favor the simplicity of an upfront penalty, but I am open to any sane plan to get people to understand the need for coverage. This could include the following ideas.

Find ways to further expand Medicaid coverage. Today, just twelve states have not yet adopted expansion of Medicaid under Obamacare. It is clearly the most cost-effective and stable way to cover the uninsured. Although stabilized, the Marketplace Exchanges are volatile in many states. High premiums, low plan participation, and low provider access are issues in these states. Millions could be covered if these remaining states expanded Medicaid coverage. CMS should consider partial expansion to say 100% of the federal poverty limit (FPL) to convince recalcitrant states to join the national experiment. These states worry about the rising share of Medicaid in state budgets and the potential for woodworking (when people already eligible sign up as well—they come out of the "woodwork" so to speak). Both the Obama and Trump Administrations turned down previous efforts to do so (for different nonetheless petty political reasons). Partial expansions would ensure everyone has the opportunity to be covered—in Medicaid if your income is up to 100% of FPL and in the Marketplace Exchanges if it is over. Currently, in non-expansion states, people are in a no-man's world: they are too poor to obtain Marketplace coverage because they are not at 100% of FPL, yet their states have not expanded Medicaid. If all states adopted at least the 100% of FPL standard, perhaps over 3 million would be eligible to enroll.[32-12]

Fund and work with states to raise awareness of Medicaid and SCHIP eligibility rules and availability. When I was Connecticut's State Budget Director and we initially created our SCHIP program, we went on a marketing campaign to raise awareness of eligibility for both Medicaid and SCHIP for children. It bore huge dividends. Thousands eligible for Medicaid came forward and enrolled, along with those who enrolled in the new SCHIP program. A similar national program is occurring in 2021 to raise awareness and get over 5 million adults and children already eligible for Medicaid or SCHIP to enroll.[32-12]

Experiments with auto-enrollment or passive enrollment could be attempted. Vast public data exist for other programs that can identify individuals currently eligible for Medicaid but who have not enrolled for any number of reasons (such as a lack of knowledge or the social stigma). Passively enrolling them and their children may be the impetus they need to come around and recognize the value of healthcare in their lives. They can always opt back out.

I am not a proponent of Medicare at sixty years of age or a public option for the Marketplace Exchanges. Medicare at sixty has numerous implications for both the Medicare and employer markets. Private plans could be disadvantaged in a public option, premiums could increase, and coverage choices could decrease. However, I do think that several reforms should be undertaken to further stabilize the Exchange offering in states that continue to see low plan and provider participation. This could include the following:

Create financial incentives for plans to enter the market and expand provider participation. This could include a return to the risk corridor and reinsurance programs, adequately and fully funded, of course. Exchange plan premiums were 50% higher, on average, in areas with only one plan compared with those with more than two insurers. This also could mean extending Medicare pricing (or just above it) to plans that participate in certain regions that are underserved or throughout the Exchanges.[32-5, 32-6, 32-13]

Look at auto-enrolling or passively enrolling subsidy-eligible people in the Marketplace Exchanges. This would ensure consistent coverage for those already eligible for subsidized coverage.[32-5] I would also note that if holdout states do not expand Medicaid, those too poor for Exchange coverage but above Medicaid income standards should be made eligible for Exchange coverage with the most generous subsidies. Some Democrats want to set up a whole new program nationally just for these individuals. This would be duplicative and wasteful.

As President Biden is now doing, roll back the marketing and outreach funding reductions as well as the enrollment and administrative barriers that were put in place by the Trump Administration. This could help over 5 million people obtain coverage with the most generous subsidies.[32-5, 32-12]

Consider making subsidies more generous for middle income earners (for example, 300-400% of FPL) and expand subsidies beyond 400% of FPL. Currently, premiums in many states simply are not affordable, and a high number of middle-income earners remain uninsured because subsidies are too small or non-existent. President Biden led efforts to lift the premium subsidy cap and enhance premium subsidies. This is temporary for 2021 and 2022. As of this writing, Biden and Democrats were looking for ways to make this permanent or extend them. America could also experiment with a fixed subsidy approach, where everyone in need of coverage is given a fixed amount to purchase insurance based on family size. This could be used in the employer market, Exchanges, or even to buy into Medicaid. This could also be used in combination with an income-based approach as is in law now.[32-5]

Enact an appropriation for the cost-sharing reduction (CSR) subsidies to return to the original intent of the law. The Trump Administration removed the subsidies. Plans had to continue to offer low-income CSR plans and instead inflated premiums, which caused massive lack of premium affordability for those out of reach of premium subsidies. This resulted in increased premiums of 10% and will mean increases of up to 20%, with the government picking up more costs than it otherwise would have through the premium subsidies. CSR subsidies should be permanently funded and perhaps enhanced as well to greater numbers of people. As of early 2021, a Democratic bill in the Senate would do both. The bill may be too generous in terms of CSR subsidy enhancements but should be considered.[32-5]

While comprehensiveness of benefits is important, as costs come down in the system, we must revisit the scope and breadth of the mandated ACA benefits. While the vast majority of increases in ACA premiums over the years was tied to actions taken by both the Obama and Trump Administrations that destabilized the program (e.g., not funding the risk corridor and reinsurance programs fully and removing CSR payments to plans), there is no question, too, that premiums rose pre-ACA to post ACA due to major changes in mandated benefits.

Work with employers to promote coverage and pass legislation as necessary. President Biden could work closely with employers—largely small ones—to promote better affordability. The following should be considered and could help up to 10 million Americans obtain coverage:[32-12]

- ○ Expand small business tax credits.
- ○ Retool the small business Marketplace option.
- ○ Expand the ability of low-income earners to enroll in the Marketplace, in lieu of employer coverage, even if offered. This includes fixing the so-called family glitch, which keeps dependents from accessing the Exchange subsidies because of a quirk in the law related to affordability of single coverage (but not dependent coverage).
- ○ Potentially look at additional premium tax credits for certain low-income workers (perhaps refundable) to help them better afford employer coverage. This could be packaged with increased marketplace subsidies in Congress.

When the national COVID-19 public health emergency comes to an end, we must ensure that people do not fall through the cracks and rejoin the ranks of the uninsured. The Biden administration has said that states will have up to 12 months after the declared emergency ends to remove people from the Medicaid rolls (this is up by 6 months from the Trump administration policy). Ongoing eligibility requirements were waived during the COVID-19 pandemic, which has led to record Medicaid enrollment. The Biden administration has also announced additional transition protections, including a required redetermination before someone is removed from Medicaid. This timeframe and the protections may not be enough. States and the federal government need to work together to ensure adequate funding and time for people to transition from Medicaid to the Exchanges or employer coverage. Having the remaining states expand Medicaid eligibility would also help. Between 15 and 25 million could lose coverage if this is not approached judiciously.

A Nixonian Solution: America's Future Health System

While I am a proponent of keeping the Marketplace and Medicaid as part of the ACA, I believe there is a better alternative for the future. It is one that will reduce administrative costs and duplication, rationalize the system, and mean truly affordable universal access.

Let's first look at some recommendations from the Bipartisan Policy Center, a thoughtful group of former lawmakers, CMS administrators, and policymakers, led by former Senators Tom Daschle (D) and Bill Frist (R). In early 2020, the center issued a report, "Bipartisan Rx for America's Healthcare: A Practical Path To Reform." Its main principles are the following, copied directly from their preamble to the report:[32-5]

> 1. **All individuals should have meaningful and affordable public or private health insurance.**
>
>   We acknowledge a continuing role for both private and publicly financed insurance. Regardless of the source of coverage, benefits should be evidence-based, and sufficient to ensure access to

needed care, while avoiding poorly designed financial incentives that lead to either over- or under-use of care. Low- and moderate-income households need to be adequately subsidized so that they can enroll in insurance plans that provide them with ready access to quality, affordable care when they need it.

2. **Health reform should be designed to avoid major disruption because many patients rely on today's long-standing arrangements to get needed care.**

   Reform should provide incentives for existing systems (employer-sponsored, individual markets, Medicare, Medicaid) to better align, become more efficient, and improve quality and care relationships. Reform should expand, rather than reduce, the options individuals have to improve upon their existing coverage.

3. **Insurance markets should be stable, not endangered by premium increases due to adverse selection or insufficient pooling of risks.**

   This will require coping with extraordinarily expensive outlier health conditions through options such as adequately financed and administered reinsurance, alternative tax credit structures and adequately financed and structured high-risk pools. Reform proposals should ensure broad-based participation in private insurance markets to ensure pre-existing condition protections and market affordability and stability.

4. **Health reform should reduce excessive and unnecessary healthcare cost growth.**

   This will require policies that are designed to achieve more effective competition among insurers and providers of medical services; promote more and clearer choices for consumers; encourage payment reforms that promote improvements in care; achieve more efficient delivery of care in all settings; and encourage preventive interventions that improve health status and outcomes.

5. Reform policies must be politically and financially sustainable over the long-term.

Bipartisan solutions are more likely than approaches supported primarily by one party to produce policies that can be sustained over many years and election cycles. The hard work of developing and securing bipartisan agreements in these areas will pay dividends in terms of greater stability and certainty for patients and their families, employers, providers, plans, governments, and taxpayers.

I have noted many of these points, but the preamble is worthy of comment. Note the bipartisan commitment to healthcare as a social good and subsidies for lower income Americans. Note also the comments on the need for comprehensive coverage, the need to stay away from financial disincentives to seeking care, and the preservation of the employer-based system for fear of major disruption.

While I don't think high-risk pools are viable, note the report authors' commitment to coverage for everyone, regardless of pre-existing conditions, and a stable financing system. The authors focus on getting rid of excessive spending through private insurers, competition among payers and providers, transparency, choice for consumers, wellness and prevention, and payment reform promoting more efficient delivery and quality of care. Finally, note the focus on policy planning and financial sustainability, including a focus on bipartisan solutions.

The report goes on to outline reforms for the Marketplace Exchanges, some of which I have noted previously, as well as employer coverage reforms and lowering hospital and physician costs. It also addresses reducing drug costs, which I will discuss in Chapter 34. Finally, it addresses surprise billing, Medicare costs, including reforms for medical drug payments, and Medicaid reforms.

So, what is my plan?

I don't believe we should mimic the universal access systems in the developed world. In these systems, insurance is largely divorced from employment, although private health plans do compete to enroll individuals in coverage. Doing so would take away the duplication and fracture we see in the United States, but I believe it could massively disrupt our system and the progress already being made.

Instead, I believe that an employer-sponsored system, along with a master social safety net program, is the best course for the United States. How would it work? Well, we have much of the policy in place already.

- The current, employer-sponsored system, served by private plans and networks, would be the backbone of our healthcare system, with the vast majority of Americans covered in it.
- It would include an employer mandate as exists today with required sharing of premiums with employees. Existing small business tax credits would remain in effect and could be expanded to incentivize small and even larger enterprises to provide coverage.
- An individual mandate with substantial penalty would be in effect.
- Those with low incomes could receive a refundable tax credit to help better afford employer coverage.
- Medicare would continue to serve seniors and the disabled. Private plans would be a growing piece of that program as well.
- For citizens whose nexus to employment is weak or who are low-income and cannot afford traditional employer coverage, America would have one social-safety-net healthcare program. This could come in one of two forms—either the current Medicaid system run in each state or a national Medicaid-like program.
- The healthcare social-safety-net program would have a sliding-scale premium and cost-sharing subsidy program based on income. This is similar to the ACA Exchanges today. It would cover both acute and long-term care and those with employer coverage could access long-

term care on a similar sliding scale. Private health plans exclusively would provide the care. There would be no antiquated FFS program.

o   All other ACA policy changes would remain in effect.

What might the premium subsidy look like? As in Medicaid today, the lowest income individuals might have no premium and no or limited cost-sharing. For those earning higher wages, we know that the current Marketplace Exchange premiums require some middle-income American families to kick in as much as 10% of income before receiving a premium subsidy. Given the huge costs in the American system—at least 50% more and perhaps greater than double other developed nations—paying this amount is too much. In the short term, the amount of income a family has to contribute toward healthcare premiums should be well below the 10% of income threshold.

Indeed, even though costs are already substantially lower in other developed nations, many European countries subsidize or cap premiums at relatively low income levels. For example, the Swiss cantons (effectively like states in the United States) begin subsidizing premiums at about 8% of income, with 35-40% getting some form of subsidy. In Germany, citizens pay no more than 7.3% of income for premiums for government scheme insurance, with another 7.3% paid by employers.[32-14, 32-15] As costs come down and money frees up, we could also choose to fund more generously the cost of care for all low- and moderate-income children (or even later all children) to ensure a healthy start in life.

This proposal is substantially similar to a proposal by former President Richard Nixon, a Republican, in 1974. Nixon would have replaced Medicaid with a national program.[32-16, 32-17]

An advocate of limited government, Nixon did understand the moral and financial rationale for affordable universal access. Quite simply, he wanted every American to have "financial access to high-quality healthcare."

Consider some of what Nixon said at the time in his message to Congress proposing the sweeping program:[32-17]

"Without adequate healthcare, no one can make full use of his or her talents and opportunities. It is thus just as important that economic, racial, and social barriers not stand in the way of good healthcare as it is to eliminate those barriers to a good education and a good job.

"For the average family, it is clear that without adequate insurance, even normal care can be a financial burden while a catastrophic illness can mean catastrophic debt.

"Beyond the question of the prices of healthcare, our present system of healthcare insurance suffers from two major flaws: First, even though more Americans carry health insurance than ever before, the 25 million Americans who remain uninsured often need it the most and are most unlikely to obtain it. They include many who work in seasonal or transient occupations, high-risk cases, and those who are ineligible for Medicaid despite low incomes. Second, those Americans who do carry health insurance often lack coverage, which is balanced, comprehensive, and fully protective...

"These gaps in health protection can have tragic consequences. They can cause people to delay seeking medical attention until it is too late. Then a medical crisis ensues, followed by huge medical bills—or worse. Delays in treatment can end in death or lifelong disability.

"Every American participating in the program would be insured for catastrophic illnesses that can eat away savings and plunge individuals and families into hopeless debt for years. No family would ever have annual out-of-pocket expenses for covered health services in excess of $1,500, and low-income families would face substantially smaller expenses.

"This Comprehensive Health Insurance Plan has been designed so that everyone involved would have both a stake in making it work and a role to play in the process—consumer, provider, health insurance carrier, the states, and the federal government. It is a partnership program in every sense.

"Comprehensive health insurance is an idea whose time has come in America."

Throughout this book, I have echoed much of what Nixon did back in 1974, before the Watergate scandal killed any hope of the concept passing and sent him from office. But truer words have never been written.

Even in 1974, Richard Nixon knew that the average American was being priced out of quality and affordable healthcare. He knew it was a social good to have affordable universal access. Reinhardt made this same point in 1997.

In 1974, Nixon knew that the uninsured crisis was leading to huge costs for America and tragedy. He knew that the best approach was to leverage government, private insurers, providers, and consumers in partnership.

As Nixon stated, and it is even more true today, healthcare reform is an idea whose time has come in America.

Will Congress wake up and drive toward compromise?

CHAPTER 33

The Healthcare Consolidation Craze

This chapter will look at some major consolidation and market force trends in healthcare. Let's first look at some fundamental terminology. A few terms are especially important when thinking about business growth.

First there is organic and inorganic growth. Organic growth is expanding a company's revenue or profit margin by engaging in activities internal to its organization. Examples include focusing on new sales, expanding output, or expanding product portfolios to derive additional revenue. Inorganic growth occurs through acquisitions, joint ventures, or mergers.

In the area of inorganic growth, there can be both horizontal and vertical integration. Horizontal integration is acquisition or merger of a similar or like company in a given industry—often a competitor. A good example might be two hospitals merging or a health plan acquiring another health plan. In this case, the two companies—now one—were on the same *horizontal* line of business.

Vertical integration is when a company acquires or merges with another company in the same industry but one that performs different functions in a given supply chain. We don't really think about supply chains very much in terms of healthcare, but they are particularly important to manufacturing. A vertical integration acquisition in manufacturing might be an automobile producer acquiring a parts manufacturer to reduce costs and streamline delivery timeframes.

In healthcare, a good example of vertical integration would be a health plan acquiring a physician group. In this case, a health plan contracts with providers to deliver services. Thus, providers are in a health plan's supply chain. Another example might be a hospital or integrated delivery system acquiring a health plan to be able to get them into the health insurance business. In both of these healthcare cases, the different functions in the same healthcare *vertical* line are the provision of health services (done by hospitals and physicians) and administering healthcare benefits (done by a plan).

The fact is that businesses generally have organic growth year over year and from time to time engage in inorganic growth. When they do, often it is horizontal integration of a like business (perhaps a competitor). However, vertical integration is becoming more and more popular in healthcare as well.

Provider Integration and Consolidation

Provider integration in healthcare is increasingly popular. Provider entities are consolidating for a number of reasons: [33-1, 33-2, 33-3]

- They may desire the ability to gain more leverage and share in the market with health plans.
- They may be facing financial pressures, negative credit outlooks, and capital constraints or seeking greater access to capital.
- They may need the ability to economize with scale and improve financial performance.
- Providers may be facing large demands for expensive infrastructure and technology.
- They may want the ability to distinguish themselves in key revenue-producing specialty areas as centers of excellence.

- ○ They may be seeking changes to more sophisticated payment structures, including a focus on cost-efficiency and quality.
- ○ This may involve experimenting or performing well in new payment schemes, such as bundled payments or performance initiatives.
- ○ They may also be seeking to form integrated delivery systems to deliver more coordinated care and quality-oriented care, or to improve quality overall.
- ○ Providers also may be seeking to form these integrated delivery systems to compete against health plans via accountable care organizations (ACOs) or provider sponsored networks (PSNs).

In these cases, hospitals and physicians may engage with health plans in the following four ways:

A large physician group may become a fully or partially delegated entity, taking on risk from the health plan—upside risk (a financial reward for cost-savings against the providers' assigned panels), downside risk (penalties for cost overruns), or both.

A large physician group may become the backbone of an independent practice association (IPA) (including other providers) created to negotiate with health plans.

A large physician group may become a management services organization (MSO) to serve its own doctors as well as others. The MSO may perform various clinical and administrative functions as well as be an IPA.

A large hospital system or integrated delivery system may become a physician-hospital organization (PHO) that contracts with health plans, accepts delegated risk, and performs various clinical and administrative functions for its providers.

Major provider consolidation and market forces include the following trends. Provider entities are attracting significant private equity investment. Hospitals are acquiring other hospitals and consolidating in great numbers. This has especially been the case since 2010.[33-1] Provider practices are consolidating in the specialist arena and, to a lesser degree, for primary care physicians (PCPs). Hospitals are taking over physician practices, both PCPs and specialists, as well as skilled nursing and related facilities and home health entities. Other entities in the healthcare arena are consolidating as well, including home health, hospice, allied health, skilled nursing facilities, and others.

Two Deloitte studies show the significance of hospital consolidation. A Deloitte 2014 report states that hospital consolidation volume increased 14% annually from 2009 to 2013. The firm says that hospitals and delivery systems are in a rapid consolidation phase. Large systems and national chains are getting bigger. Market share of the top twenty health systems grew from 21% in 2007 to 25% in 2012. Mid-tier health systems have been acquiring independent health systems in their local markets as well. In the 2014 report, Deloitte estimated that only 50% of current health systems were expected to remain within a decade. A 2017 Deloitte study says that from 2008 to 2014, more than 750 mergers or consolidations occurred.[33-1, 33-2]

Consolidation continued through the end of the decade. Hospital mergers and acquisitions were down in 2020 due to the COVID-19 pandemic, but they seem to be rebounding. There were only seventy-nine announced deals in 2020, down 25% from the ten-year average. But, twenty-eight deals were announced in the last quarter of 2020 and twenty-seven more transactions were announced in the first half of 2021.[33-4, 33-5]

The American Hospital Association and related groups tout their studies showing that hospital mergers save on costs and improve quality. While some hospital mergers may bring efficiency and quality, multiple studies have also shown that hospital mergers lead to higher prices. In the twenty-five metropolitan areas with the highest rates of consolidation as measured by the Federal Trade Commission (FTC), prices increased by 11-54% following mergers. A 2018 Harvard and Columbia study found that prices increase 7%

to 10% when hospitals that are between 30 minutes and 90 minutes apart merge. Hospital costs are not just an issue in highly consolidated areas.[33-3, 33-5]

Physician group investment and consolidation was a major area of interest for private equity investors in 2019. One study found that activity in the physician area would reach 250-300 deals in 2020.[33-6] The COVID-19 pandemic has shown the huge risk of having a private, small group practice and actually spurred greater consolidation as physicians abandoned private practice for employed status with hospitals, other entities, or provider groups.

Hospitals and health systems, too, are acquiring physician practices to have greater leverage in the market. From July 2012 through January 2018, there was a significant nationwide trend of physicians leaving private practice in favor of working for hospitals or health systems. From July 2016 to January 2018, 14,000 more physicians were employed by hospitals, an increase of 6%. This is up more than 70% since July 2012. About 8,000 physician practices were acquired by hospitals between July 2016 and January 2018, an increase of 5%. By January 2018, hospitals owned more than 31% of physician practices nationwide. By early 2018, almost half of all physicians (44%) were employed by hospitals or large healthcare systems. This is up from about a quarter in July 2012. [33-3, 33-7]

All told, due to the COVID-19 pandemic fallout, as of 2021 almost 50% of all physician practices were owned by either hospital systems or private corporations. Physicians employed by either hospitals or private corporations hit 70% in 2021.[33-8, 33-9]

This trend will result in increasing costs, especially for Medicare. One of the studies underwritten by the Physicians Advocacy Institute (PAI) notes that hospital-employed physicians perform more services at hospital outpatient facilities than in physician offices or other locations, which means much higher costs. As an example, for three types of services studied (cardiac imaging, colonoscopy, and evaluation and management services), Medicare pays demonstrably more when these services are done in hospital outpatient facilities (even when it is in a hospital "off-campus" setting) compared with those in a physician-owned office.[33-7]

○ Cardiac imaging—$5,148 in hospital outpatient and $2,862 in physician's office

○ Colonoscopy—$1,784 in hospital outpatient and $1,322 in physician's office

○ Evaluation and management services—$525 in hospital outpatient and $406 in physician's office

A November 2017 PAI-sponsored study found something similar for four specific services in the areas of cardiology, orthopedic, and gastroenterology services over a three-year period. It found that the physician-hospital integration trend meant $3.1 billion in increased costs from 2012-2015. Medicare paid $2.7 billion more, while beneficiaries picked up about $400 million in cost-sharing for these services.[33-7]

In general, consolidation of provider services tends to increase overall costs. As I have discussed, growth in private insurance has primarily been driven by provider costs. Between 2007 and 2014, hospital inpatient prices grew 42%, and physician inpatient prices grew 18%. This is due in part to the consolidations noted previously and the control that hospitals and systems have on pricing in the primary care, specialist, outpatient, and hospital inpatient worlds. The Bipartisan Policy Center suggest several ways to alleviate the effect of these consolidations on cost, including anti-trust investigations, more scrutiny of mergers, and pricing-benchmark and related reforms.[33-3] The Biden administration did announce its intent to review and revise merger guidelines as well as strengthen federal oversight.

Health Plan Integration and Consolidation

Health plans have been busy growing inorganically, through mergers and acquisitions. As with provider activity, it is done for a number of reasons, such as growing membership, reducing administrative costs (by spreading over a greater number of overall members), or the desire to enter a new line of business (Medicare, Medicaid, or commercial). Inorganic growth is also fueled by the need to enter new geographies, as well as the need to meet demands by shareholders and markets for return on stock investments.

In the Medicaid world, mergers and acquisitions may be used to expand physician access.[33-10]

Health plans also need to directly control a pharmacy benefits manager (PBM) to reduce drug costs. You will see below how health plans acquire PBMs to do just that.

Such action is also taken to acquire specific provider entities or types, in order to have more control over provider costs and quality of care. It may also build more integrated delivery system—given demands by regulators for quality achievement and enhancing primary care.[33-10]

Acquisition of provider groups by health plans is in reaction to the significant acquisition of physicians by hospitals.[33-10] With the imposition of minimum medical loss ratio (MLRs), margins within health plans are effectively capped. Acquiring provider entities gives plans the ability to downstream risk and funds to owned provider entities. To avoid any fraud accusations, however, it needs to ensure that financial arrangements with owned entities are arms-length and market competitive.

Health plan acquisitions tend to come in a few forms. Health plans may merge with or be acquired by another health plan. Health plans may purchase physician groups and related providers. Health plans may acquire unique provider entities, such as long-term care providers and other assets, given significant trends in health transformation.

Here are some major failed or successful health-plan consolidations and other vertical health plan activities I have tracked over the past several years. Dates are when the proposed acquisitions were announced, with formal takeover taking a year or more:

- ○ 2015 horizontal—acquisition of long-term care pharmacy Omnicare by CVS Health
- ○ 2015 horizontal—acquisition of Catamaran PBM by Optum (United's services subsidiary)
- ○ 2015 horizontal—acquisition of Group Health Cooperative by Kaiser Permanente

- ○ 2015 horizontal—acquisition of Health Net by Centene
- ○ 2015 horizontal—acquisition of Humana by Aetna failed on antitrust grounds
- ○ 2015 horizontal—acquisition of Cigna by Anthem failed on antitrust grounds
- ○ 2017 vertical—Anthem and CVS announced they would collaborate on an Anthem-owned, in-house PBM; launched in 2019
- ○ 2017 vertical—acquisition of Aetna by CVS Health (which owns PBM Caremark)
- ○ 2018 vertical—acquisition of PBM Express Scripts by Cigna
- ○ 2019 horizontal—acquisition of WellCare by Centene
- ○ 2019 horizontal—merger of Tufts Health Plan and Harvard Pilgrim
- ○ 2020 vertical—acquisition of Beacon Health Options, a behavioral health managed care company, by Anthem
- ○ 2021 vertical—acquisition of Magellan Health, a PBM and specialty service company, by Centene

The following large health plans are investing significantly in provider-group acquisition:[33-10]

- ○ United, through its Optum subsidiary
- ○ Anthem
- ○ Cigna
- ○ Centene
- ○ Humana
- ○ Kaiser Permanente through affiliated companies

Here are a few interesting notes about some plans' physician acquisition:

UnitedHealth's Optum division bought dialysis provider DaVita's medical group. The medical group employs more than 750 primary care physicians (PCPs), directly or through associated groups. It contracts with thousands more.[33-10]

Humana has concentrated on acquisition of closely aligned, large-scale physician practices in its Medicare business in lucrative markets, such as Florida.

It should be noted that health plan ownership of physician groups is relatively tiny, especially compared with hospitals and hospital systems. The American Medical Association (AMA) found only 2% of all physicians in 2016 were employed by a health plan or a health-plan-owned entity. The American Academy of Family Physicians also said the number has been at about 2% in recent years.[33-10]

As I mentioned, health plans are going beyond acquiring health plans, PBMs, and physician groups. Here are a few additional novel acquisitions by health plans that relate to some of the populations or services health plans cover:[33-10]

Humana and two private equity firms bought post-acute provider Kindred Healthcare. Humana got a minority stake in the company's home health, hospice, and community-care division. The division employs physicians and 40,000 caregivers.

Humana and the same private equity firms bought hospice operator Curo Health Services to combine it with Kindred.

Anthem is buying Aspire Health, a non-hospice palliative-care entity, including physicians and other clinicians.

In the end, both providers and health plans are jockeying for the best position possible in the healthcare arena. Providers have been very much on the offensive in consolidating to boost market share and negotiating power. On the provider acquisition front, health plans are acquiring provider groups more as a defensive move. On the offensive side, health plans and other assets are combining again to have the greatest leverage possible in the healthcare system as well as to lower administrative costs.

CHAPTER 34

The Big Drug Debate

ealth plans view prescription drugs as both a curse and as a salvation. Done right, the use of prescription drugs helps avoid other, more expensive forms of care. Also, generic drugs today are extremely economical. At the same time, however, prescription drugs represent a fast-growing piece of the healthcare pie. While there has been some price-increase moderation lately, drugs generally represent one of the highest inflationary sectors of healthcare, competing with hospital costs.

Let's review some of what we have learned about prescription drugs:

There are **retail prescription drugs** largely obtained at our local pharmacies. There are also **medical drugs**, usually administered or infused at physician offices or other outpatient locations.

There are **brand and generic drugs**. Brand drugs are those that are usually still under patent protection. While there may be other drugs in the same or similar therapeutic class (namely other drugs that can be used to treat the same disease state or condition), a given brand drug is the only one sold with that exact chemical composition. In contrast, generic drugs are generally not subject to patent and therefore any manufacturer is free to create the drug with the same chemical composition and sell it.

Generally, brand drugs are much more expensive: in the hundreds of dollars—sometime thousands—for a thirty-day supply. The average brand cost is about $567 for a thirty-day supply. Generics are typically low cost. Over 90% are twenty dollars per month or less and the average price is about thirty dollars per month. Plans encourage the use of generic drugs whenever possible unless a brand drug is absolutely needed for a disease state or condition.[34-1, 34-2]

Drugs can be reimbursed through a variety of means. Three of the most popular are based on:

- A discount to the average wholesale price (AWP)—usually for brand drugs.
- A maximum allowable cost (MAC) list created by a pharmacy benefits manager (PBM) or health plan—usually for generic drugs.
- The average sales price (ASP) plus a percentage for medical drugs. There are also other emerging payment methodologies for medical drug payment.

In 2019, retail prescription drugs (not including over-the-counter drugs) and certain diagnostic equipment and supplies that need a prescription (e.g., diabetic supplies and test strips) accounted for about 10% of total health-care spending. That was about $380 billion. These numbers do not include so-called medical drugs that are administered in inpatient, outpatient, or in physician offices. These are captured in other categories of health spending, including inpatient and various outpatient categories. The Kaiser Family Foundation (KFF) also compiled various data to determine that all retail and medical drugs spending across all lines of business in the United States was about $591 million in 2019. This puts overall drug spending closer to 16%.[34-3, 34-4]

Medicare tends to drive drug spending. Medicare's share of the nation's retail prescription drug spending increased from 18% in 2006 to 30% in 2017. In large measure, this is due to the creation of the Medicare Part D program.

Also, prescription drugs covered under both Part B and Part D accounted for 19% of all Medicare spending in 2016, higher than the 16% overall line of business spending.[34-5]

Drug Trends Past and Future

Here are a few quick facts on past and expected drug trends. In general, we have been in a relative drug cost increase lull over the past five years. Inflation was robust some time ago and is expected to rise again. However, this does not take away from the fact that Americans have real issues paying for needed drugs.[34-6, 34-7, 34-8, 34-9, 34-10]

- On a per capita basis, inflation-adjusted retail prescription drug spending increased from $90 in 1960 to $1,025 in 2017.
- The United States saw drug spending and inflation begin to shoot through the roof in the late 1990s, throughout the 2000s, and until about 2015. Retail prescription drug spending growth for private health insurance peaked in 2014 and 2015. High-cost hepatitis C treatment drugs were a big factor in the increased overall costs.
- Between 2016 to 2019, inflation was extremely modest or negative. Beginning in 2020, annual inflation was expected to rise from 3.2% to the mid-to-high 5% range. This will be due to the introduction of new drugs, primarily specialty drugs—those used for complex, extremely chronic, or rare conditions. Included in this category are so-called biologics. Of the almost 300 drugs to be released between 2019 and 2021, about two-thirds will be specialty drugs. Between 2010 and 2016, specialty drugs moved from 19% to 42% of retail drug spending. By 2020, 55% of all retail and medical drug spending will be specialty drugs.
- By 2015, retail drug spending per capita was over $1,000 per person. Prices for common generic drugs have dropped by 37% since 2014, while we have seen an increase of over 60% for brand drugs.
- Another study said that brand-name prescription drug prices in the United States have increased nearly 100% in the past six years.

- ○ Through 2027, retail drug costs will represent the same rough percentage of healthcare expenditures—just below 10%. This is due to overall high growth in costs across the healthcare sectors.

- ○ Medical drugs are driving overall healthcare costs up considerably. From 2014 to 2018, medical drug costs grew by 65% and 40% in commercial and Medicare, respectively.

- ○ In the commercial world, the ten most expensive medical drugs averaged about $522,000 per patient in in 2019. In Medicare and Medicaid, it was about $301,000.

- ○ The newly approved and controversial Alzheimer's drug Aduhelm threatens to further blow the roof off of medical drug costs in the future.

To summarize, a study by GoodRx found that retail prescription drugs indeed do have the highest inflationary factors in healthcare lately. Since 2014, they have increased by 33%. Inpatient hospital services, nursing home care, and dental services have increased by 30%, 23%, and 19%, respectively. Overall, GoodRx found that medical services costs increased by 17% over the timeframe.[34-11]

How Do We Compare in Terms of Cost and Price?

Estimates of drug costs in the United States versus other developed world countries can differ markedly, but it still amounts to a huge difference. Here are some statistics from various sources.[34-6, 34-8, 34-10, 34-12, 34-13]

A Commonwealth Fund review of ten developed world nations (including the United States) found that the U.S. per capita retail drug spend was $1,011. That of other developed nations ranged from a low of $351 in Sweden to a high of $783 in Switzerland. Due to this, 14% of U.S. insureds and 33% of uninsured people reported skipping prescriptions. This compares with 2-10% in other developed nations.

In one study, individuals globally saved 56% compared with Americans on select retail drugs. That means Americans pay more than double for those same drugs. Just north of us, Canadians paid $772 compared to Americans' $1,112, a 31% difference.

A U.S. House of Representatives Ways and Means Committee report said that costs are actually orders of magnitude higher. It found that prices are almost four times higher than the average in eleven similar countries. The committee analyzed 2018 pricing data of seventy-nine drugs sold in the United States, the United Kingdom, Japan, Canada (Ontario), Australia, Portugal, France, the Netherlands, Germany, Denmark, Sweden, and Switzerland. Average per capita spending in the eleven countries was $626 compared with $1,220 in the United States.

It is interesting to look at some specific costs of commonly used drugs. This gives us a chance to see what the burden is not only on the system in general, but on the out-of-pocket costs people pay:

- Humira is a biologic drug used for a number of different diseases, including Crohn's disease, ulcerative colitis, rheumatoid arthritis, psoriatic arthritis, and plaque psoriasis. In 2014, the average price of Humira in the United States was $2,699 per month, or over $32,000 per year. In the United Kingdom it was $1,362, and in Switzerland $822. That is a range of 96-225% higher. (What is interesting here is that the United Kingdom has socialized medicine, but Switzerland has a universal access model.)
- Xarelto, a drug used to prevent or treat blood clots, was more than twice the cost in the United States than in the United Kingdom or Switzerland in 2014.
- Harvoni, a high-cost specialty drug used to essentially free someone from a lifetime with Hepatitis C, was 42% higher in the United States in 2014 than in the United Kingdom and 90% higher than in Switzerland.
- Truvada, used to treat HIV/AIDS, was 44% higher in the United States than in Switzerland, and 89% higher than in the United Kingdom.

- Avastin is used to treat some cancers. It was 124% higher in Switzerland in 2014 and 125% higher than in the United Kingdom.
- In 2015, another study found something similar for drug prices:
  - Crestor for high cholesterol: U.S. $86; other surveyed nations $4 to $41
  - Advair for asthma and pulmonary disease: U.S. $155; other surveyed nations $10 to $74
  - Januvia for diabetes: U.S. $169; other surveyed nations $14 to $68
  - Lantus for diabetes: U.S. $186; other surveyed nations $42 to $139
  - Humira for various chronic diseases: U.S. $2,505; other surveyed nations $570 to $1,750
  - Herceptin for breast cancer infusion: U.S. $4,755 every three weeks; other surveyed nations $1,557 to $3,547

By the way, the prices given above are post drug rebates that manufacturers have given to health plans and PBMs after the drug transaction. So, the cost comparisons are apples to apples.

Why Are We So Expensive?

Except in some very narrow cases, America has no price controls on drugs. Drugmakers (in the case of brand manufacturers, represented by the Pharmaceutical Research and Manufacturers of America or PhRMA) are able to set their prices and change them annually, receiving increases year to year through various payment methodologies. Our traditional drug reimbursement mechanisms do nothing to control costs.

America's problem is largely brand drug prices. Drug utilization is similar with other countries. Between 47-60% of adults in all countries report taking one or more prescription drug regularly. The United States is at 59%, within the range. In a survey of nine developed countries, the United States has among the highest uses of cheaper generic drugs. The survey covered all three forms of healthcare in the developed world—socialized, single-payer, and universal access systems.[34-8]

The drug business lacks transparency. It has a series of middlemen and distribution channels, some of them shadowy, each taking its piece of the pie and inflating prices. These include manufacturers, wholesale distributors, pharmacy benefits managers (PBMs), drug rebate aggregators, and more.

As I outlined in Chapter 28, America shoulders a disproportionate share of the price of innovation in drug spending, not only because it is the largest developed economy but also because single-payer systems in Europe and elsewhere practice price fixing and rationing.

The introductory costs of innovator drugs are exceedingly high. The Federal Drug Administration (FDA) regulatory approval process for new drug introduction is labyrinthine and time consuming, even with recent and slated reforms. Drug manufacturers have to recoup investments in development typically in only a few years. Patent protection starts on filing. The long approval time for drugs eats into the exclusivity period—after which generics can be launched by any manufacturer. At the same time, for every drug that makes it through the approval process, multiple drugs have failed. This investment needs to be recouped as well.

Brand drugmakers have used aggressive marketing tactics and advertise with abandon. These practices are focused squarely on consumers and doctors to push brand medications when long-standing legacy generics, on the market for decades, could control disease states just as well—sometimes better.

While reforms have been made, drugmakers still prevent cheaper generics from coming to market quickly, sometimes even paying generic firms off to not create the drug immediately. This means that insurers and the public continue to pay the price of high-cost brands even after the patent has expired. Although some reforms have occurred, brand drugmakers frequently file lawsuits against generic entry to extend their patent time.

On a related note, instead of staying true to an innovation mission, some brand drug manufacturers have poured resources into finding ways to create chemically similar knockoffs that give them whole new patent periods, essentially extending patent life for a drug that would otherwise go generic. Then, they invest millions in marketing to convert Americans to these similar, high-cost brand drugs (with no better efficacy) even though the former drug has become a low-cost generic.

In addition, a good share of innovation has focused on high-cost disease states and biologics. These clearly help those who are afflicted but has led to drugs that cost in the tens or hundreds of thousands of dollars per year. Brand drugmakers did so because it has had better success keeping these drugs on plan formularies (as the only medically necessary treatment) as opposed to what could happen with new and truly innovative brand drugs for other common disease states.

Finally, Americans tend to get on newer and higher priced drugs much more quickly than citizens in other countries. This is in part due to the advertising and the FDA having different standards than government drug regulators in other developed countries. Other countries look at the effectiveness of a proposed drug but also whether it is more effective than existing therapies in the marketplace. Some countries also look at cost-effectiveness.[34-8]

How Do Other Countries Control Prices?

Quite simply, other countries employ price controls, aggressive negotiations with drugmakers, and the threat of removing certain drugs from that country's health system's drug list. This is the case in the socialized, single-payer, and universal access healthcare system models. If drug companies are unwilling to negotiate or accept reasonable prices, the drug is not paid for by the healthcare system.

There is some price fixing for certain federal programs in the United States, such as the federal supply schedule (FSS) for certain healthcare programs and the Medicaid drug rebate program. There are also negotiations between health plans and drug manufacturers for rebates. However, for the most part, drugs are not price controlled in the United States. This leads to exorbitant prices and exceedingly high annual inflation. Drug companies can largely ask what they want and increase prices from year to year with impunity.

In the other developed world nations (across all three types of healthcare systems), the following practices are common:[34-8, 34-14, 34-15, 34-16]

- ○ Centralized price negotiations by public, quasi-public, or private entities
- ○ National formularies, excluding drugs from manufacturers who do not meet price expectations from the drug list
- ○ Comparative and cost-effectiveness research for determining whether a drug will be offered and its price ceilings
- ○ In some countries, individuals pay 100% of the difference between the drug allowed by the healthcare system and one that is not. That effectively kills that drug's market share in the country. This is known as reference pricing, which is a transparency initiative to guide individuals to cost-effective drugs or services. If they choose a higher cost drug or service, they pay the difference.
- ○ Many developed nations also have adopted international reference pricing (IRP) to supplement their efforts in negotiations. IRP should not be confused with reference pricing. Twenty-nine European nations and numerous other developed world nations use it. In this scheme, countries look at prices paid for the same drugs in a range of nations when negotiating with drugmakers, setting prices, and determining what drugs will be on formulary.

As noted above, negotiations do occur in the United States, but it is far less effective than what is in other countries. This is because it is fragmented, pricing is far too complex, and the system lacks transparency. The U.S. is also less willing to strike a hard bargain or exclude drugs from drug lists or programs. We see this in various state and federal regulations.[34-8]

What Should the U.S. Do about Drug Prices?

Here is my bold vision for taking a bite out of drug costs. Many of these items come from my study of the issue over the years. Where applicable, I cite sources for some of the suggestions.

Patent and Food and Drug Administration (FDA) Process Reform

The FDA and the drug patent process must be overhauled from top to bottom. On one hand, there are concerns that the FDA has too streamlined its process for early-clinical, early-study, and fast-track reviews of drugs. As a result, patients may be exposed to unsafe therapies with limited benefits. While I agree that patients deserve a chance at novel, life-saving drugs, a review must be undertaken both on safety and what the costs of these early entry drugs should be. They should not carry the high costs we see throughout the system. In other cases, there are many complaints that the FDA process is too lengthy, costly, and delays drug entry unnecessarily. Faster introduction of generics and biosimilars is clearly merited for consideration as well to reduce spending. This will also require education of both providers and consumers. A congressional bill passed in 2021 and signed into law begins this process.[34-7, 34-8, 34-10, 34-17, 34-18]

America should also adopt drug-approval conditions found in other countries. Drugs should be assessed not only on effectiveness and safety but also on the following, simple criteria:[34-8, 34-14, 34-15, 34-16]

- ○   Is the drug more effective than other drugs in the market?
- ○   Is the drug cost-effective?

This is similar to what other countries do with regard to looking at both efficacy and cost-effectiveness. The Biden Administration wants to limit launch prices of drugs that face no competition by establishing an independent review board to assess value and recommend reasonable prices.[34-19] A number of states have also passed drug affordability review laws.

Patent timeframes and prices should be linked in part on the compensation or benefit the drugmaker has received from public sources. The federal government should quantify the huge benefit drugmakers receive from both government funding and research in terms of benefit to intellectual property and market value of a drug.[34-18]

Patents also could be limited in favor of other compensation (e.g., government grants and support, royalties, tax benefits, etc.).

Patents might be tied to whether a drug is more effective than others as well as whether they are cost-effective.

Allowable prices during the exclusivity period also could be regulated based on the amount of investment (to ensure a reasonable return on investment) as well as the benefit received from other sources.

While I am not a proponent of this approach, *per se*, some have suggested that patents might actually be extended to incentivize lower pricing on introduction because brand drugmakers could recoup their investment over a longer period of time. This would have to be heavily regulated, however, as it would mean generics take longer to come to market and could be abused by drugmakers.

Drugmakers should not be allowed to cosmetically reformulate or change existing drugs in order to extend patents.

Drugmakers should be prohibited from compensating generic manufacturers to delay market entry of a generic drug or biosimilar. They have avoided competition by paying generic companies to delay the launch of lower-cost alternatives in the market. In addition, watch drugmaker consolidation closely to avoid anti-competitive behavior, including acquisition of generic firms by brands, which could lead to delays in generics coming to market. These agreements cost consumers and taxpayers $3.5 billion annually in higher drug costs.[34-18]

We should require that brand drugmakers provide brand drug samples needed for generic development.[34-18]

The FDA process should encourage earlier generic entry, further squelch lawsuits by PhRMA objecting to generic entry, and reform the "authorized generics" loophole.[34-10]

Distribution Channel Reform and Price Transparency

The drug distribution system should be significantly streamlined to remove the huge markup we see through various distributors and middlemen and to increase price transparency. Distribution channel reform is a must, including the amount that various entities are entitled to earn as compensation for their services. The various players involved in the distribution channel should be paid reasonable but modest fixed fees tied to the service and value they provide. All discounts or rebates should be passed through to the health plan and ultimately the consumer.

Health plans and PBMs must be required to disclose information about the average net prices paid for prescription drugs, cost-sharing, and rebates. In addition, as the Trump Administration tried to do, prices should be clearly displayed on all advertising done by drugmakers. A number of states have also passed price transparency laws.[34-10]

Point of Sale Pass-through of Rebates and Discounts

Drug rebates are given by brands and some generic drugmakers after the drug transaction is made. By and large, however, with the exception of some employer plans, most consumers do not benefit at the point of sale from what can be large discounts made to health plans and PBMs after the drug is sold. Here is an example of what happens to the so-called little guy in this situation:

> Take an elderly woman on Medicare, whom we will call Marge. One of her brand drugs each month is $200 at retail. Her cost-sharing is set by the inflated gross price of that drug. However, plans do receive rebates on that drug. Rebate percentages can vary significantly and are not based on the exact retail price. In this case, we will say that the rebate for Marge's drug is 30% of $200, or $60. If the drug is $200, Marge's co-insurance is higher than the $140 that Marge would have paid if the drug were to include the rebate at the point of sale. If her co-insurance is 30% because her drug is a non-preferred brand, she is paying $60 if the rebate is not passed through at the point of sale, as opposed to $42 if it were.
>
> A good percentage of plans have co-insurance on the preferred brand tier and almost all have it at the non-preferred tier. As well, if she paid a flat dollar co-pay, her flat dollar amount might be higher in the benefit design than it otherwise would be if the rebate were passed through at the point of sale. Perhaps this is most true for generic brands.

Proposals from the Trump Administration and others would convert the rebates to upfront discounts at the point of sale. In fact, in the twilight of his administration Trump finalized a rule to do just that, which might go into effect in 2023 for Medicare Part D (at the time of this writing, Congress was looking at delaying or repealing the provision). The rule eliminates the safe harbor in the anti-kickback statute for post-sale drug rebates in Medicare Part D but allows it to stay in other lines of business. The upfront discounts would meet the safe harbor test.[34-20]

Why shouldn't consumers—as opposed to the health plans—benefit from the discounts offered by drugmakers? This change would have profound results:

- The current rebate system tends to help support the use of higher-cost brands because they derive the greatest rebates.
- The current rebate system tends to drive higher costs along the way.
- Passing through rebates at the point of sale would shift the focus to the lowest cost and most efficacious drug.
- This would mean better price transparency and perhaps also encourage generic use.
- It might also promote better discounts in the future as well as reduce administrative costs.
- In time, it could also bring harmony for drug costs across all lines of business—Medicare, Medicaid, and commercial.

Philosophically, there is no reason why discounts at the point of sale should not be the rule, but it is not that simple.

Health plans reasonably use these discounts offered on the back end to reduce other costs of health insurance, such as premiums, cost-sharing, and to provide additional benefits. If drug rebates are passed through at the point of sale, there are fewer overall dollars for the plans to structure benefit packages and ensure low cost-sharing in other areas. Thus, high drug utilizers might benefit from the pass-through at the point of sale, but the majority of enrollees likely will not.

This is especially the case in Medicare Advantage (MA) and Part D, where retail drug costs are extremely high due to the enrollment of aged and disabled populations. And health plans not only use rebates to reduce other costs within the Part D retail prescription program (such as overall premiums, benefits, and other cost-sharing), but they also could use it to enrich benefits on the Part C medical side.

Thus, pass-through of rebates at the point of sale would have to be examined very closely, especially in MA and Part D. It is possible, however, to create different types of plans depending on an individual's drug expense—one that passes through rebates at the point of sale and another that does not. But remember, the change in policy still washes throughout the health plan's revenue allocation. So, there will be some impact to the majority of enrollees as only a minority benefits from the pass-through of rebates.[34-18]

Reform Reimbursement Structures

As outlined earlier, health plans and PBMs reimburse providers in the prescription drug world through a variety of mechanisms, including discounts from the average wholesale price (AWP), using maximum allowable cost (MAC) lists, and increases to the average sales price (ASP). But these reimbursement structures, perhaps with some exception for MAC, do not control costs. In fact, they allow drugmakers and other entities to increase prices from year to year and the increase is largely rolled out through the reimbursement structure.

One critical area in need of reform is medical drug pricing. As an example, Medicare pays ASP plus 6% for medical drugs. This scheme carries over into the commercial world. Benchmarking reimbursement to ASP is incredibly inflationary. It encourages providers to prescribe the highest cost brand medication since the reimbursement is usually ASP plus a percentage. Providers administering an injectable or infusible drug should be paid a flat fee for administration and be encouraged to prescribe the least costly, most efficacious medication.[34-18]

The Trump Administration proposed a number of reforms. They include:

- o   Creating private-sector pharmaceutical vendors for the current "buy and bill" system. Private vendors would procure drugs, distribute them to physicians and hospitals, and take on the responsibility of billing Medicare FFS.[34-18]
- o   Changing the ASP reimbursement system to a flat fee for the drug itself.
- o   Compensating the providers via a flat payment for administration, including storing, handling, and administering the drug.
- o   Lowering costs by implementing international reference pricing. While private vendors would negotiate price concessions, prices paid by the government over time would be based on the average prices for these drugs in developed countries.

See the section on international reference pricing below for changes to Part B reimbursement that the Trump Administration finalized in a rule in late 2020 and changes made by the Biden administration. This includes international reference pricing.

PBMs should also be barred from so-called spread pricing. This is where a PBM charges a health plan more for a drug than it actually pays a pharmacy. PBMs should pass through the lowest cost possible per drug, down to the actual cost paid. PBMs and health plans could then negotiate an overall fee for the PBM's services.

Utilization Management (UM) Techniques

Additional utilization management (UM) techniques should be allowed and practiced in the world of medical and retail drugs.

- o   Recently, step therapy (where trying other cost-effective drugs may be necessary before a more expensive one) was allowed in the medical drug world for Medicare Part B.
- o   Also, in Part D, indication-based formulary management was introduced for Medicare. In this case, plans can now include drugs on a

formulary for specific indications such as disease states or conditions. This gives plans greater ability to control high-cost medications in an evidence-based manner.

○ Additional reforms are needed to promote generics and loosen protected class requirements—where mandates exist for coverage of all drugs in a class—while at the same time protecting individuals on existing therapies.

○ As with Part D plans, state Medicaid agencies should be allowed to limit coverage of drugs for which there is inadequate evidence of clinical effectiveness—as is the case for both Medicaid FFS and managed care. There are reasonable protections in Medicare Part D that balance cost and protection of health. In Medicaid, to be eligible for the federal rebate program, state agencies must cover far more drugs. Consequently, generic penetration is far less than in Medicare.[34-18]

Direct Price Negotiations, Rebate Extension and Reform, and Inflation Controls

Lawmakers and policymakers should entertain direct price negotiations in various ways.

As noted earlier, many countries have public, quasi-public, and plan-collaborative negotiations with drugmakers. This leads to a huge reduction in the overall cost of retail and medical drugs. In addition, they also require drugs to be reviewed against numerous other factors, including whether drugs are more efficacious compared to others in a therapeutic class and therefore are worthy of inclusion or included at higher prices.[34-8, 34-14, 34-15, 34-16, 34-18, 34-21]

There is no reason that this could not succeed in the United States. Today, each health plan and PBM is on its own to fight drugmakers for the best rebates that can be obtained. True, some take advantage of rebate aggregators (PBMs themselves or outside entities) to increase volume and negotiating power, but this is still far short of what we see in other developed nations. The federal government already does do this in Medicaid through the rebate program, which derives greater savings than we see in the overall system today.

If a national price system is too big a leap for some, then direct price negotiation could begin in the Medicare world, where the lion's share of many brand drugs is consumed. Medicare Part B and D drug spending was about $129 billion in 2016.[34-5] It could be expanded to other lines of business.

Price negotiations and related price reforms could include:

Direct Medicare negotiations with drugmakers by the federal government. House Democrats have previously passed a bill in the House that would slowly roll this out in Medicare over several years. The bill would have the Department of Health and Human Services (HHS) negotiate prices for twenty-five drugs per year for Medicare, with the number eventually rising to fifty. Only a pre-set number of 250 drugs are eligible for such negotiation. Commercial plans could adopt the prices, as well. Additionally, drug prices would be limited annually, or plans would rebate the excess increase to Medicare. The latter provision would also apply more broadly to all commercial plans over time. At the time of this writing, Democrats in Congress were looking at whether they have the votes to pass some sort of Medicare drug negotiation bill.

Authorization for health plans and PBMs to negotiate together, through buying collaboratives, on drug price discounts.

Extending the Medicaid drug rebate program to Medicare, which would have the impact of increasing the number of rebates received compared with what currently are gained by individual plans or PBMs in negotiations. For years, in the Medicaid program the federal government has extracted rebates from both brand and generic manufacturers. Today, these concessions stand at 23% for brands and 13% for generics. In addition, the government is guaranteed the best price against non-federal program deals. Most states now have migrated to a program where bigger state discounts are demanded in addition to the national concessions. Big states and state collaboratives could add significantly to the federal discount, increasing the reduction by about double. And many states have now taken over the drug price negotiations of private managed care plans, either by carving out the drug benefit from managed care plans or deeming the health plan drug spending as part of the master state Medicaid rebate program. From my experience, and from estimates I have read, average rebates in the Part D program from drugmakers to plans is about 15%. This would mean an opportunity to push the discount to as high as 46%.

Deep discounts also occur in other federal programs, including the Federal Supply Schedule (FSS), the 340B pricing program, and the Federal Ceiling Price Program (FCP). These programs help support low drug costs in a series of federal health programs, such as the VA, as well as private non-profit hospitals, community entities, and programs. These include Ryan White AIDS programs and Federal Qualified Health Centers (FQHCs).

Change how rebates are protected as a safe harbor in the anti-kickback statute. This would help lower overall prices. It would be important to apply this rule across all lines of business.[34-7]

Rebates generally need reform. One area of major concern is stopping brand drugmakers from various pernicious activities that stop health plans and PBMs from adoption of lower-cost drugs. Brand drugmakers should be banned from so-called "rebate walls" in their rebate agreements, which may include retroactive recoupment of rebates if a health plan's or PBM's drug availability is changed through formulary changes or when generics come to market.

Increase transparency related to prices and price increases for drugs. Force drugmakers to publicly report any price increase of 7% or more and scale this threshold down to 3.5% over time.

Pass laws that severely limit the size of the annual inflationary factor for drugs. Why should a drug already on the market be allowed to inflate exorbitantly from year to year? As a good example, at the height of the COVID-19 pandemic, drugmakers increased the prices of a record 832 drugs in January 2021, nearly 200 more than in January 2020. This was the highest since 2014. List prices increased by an average of 4.6%. Half of the medications had increases in 2019 and 2020.[34-22]

The Biden Administration is known to support a tax penalty on drugmakers and barring them from participating in Medicare if prices on drugs are raised each year beyond the general inflation rate.[34-19]

Similarly, as in Medicaid, drugmakers should be required to pass the difference through as increased discounts or rebates if they violate the provision. Indeed, as part of the COVID-19 relief measure passed by Congress in early 2021, the current cap on Medicaid inflation rebates will be lifted in 2024.

International Reference Pricing (IRP) or Benchmarking to International Prices for Drugs

So, why not benchmark the prices Americans pay for drugs against the prices in the rest of the developed world? The Trump Administration toyed with the idea of international reference pricing in a series of announcements and executive orders over several years for both retail and medical drugs.

As noted, such a program has worked throughout Europe and in other developed nations. In this scheme, countries explicitly tie prices for drugs to international benchmarks or take them into consideration in determining price and whether a given drug will be on a formulary in that nation. Some require that the nation reimburse at the lowest cost in a comparable nation (also called a "most-favored nation" or MFN).

A study published in *Health Affairs* regarding potential adoption of external reference pricing found:[34-23]

- Prices in the United States, compared with the United Kingdom, Japan, and Ontario (Canada), were 3.2 to 4.1 times higher for single-source, brand-name drugs after rebates were considered.

- ○   The price difference for individual drugs varied from 1.3-70.1%.
- ○   The longer a drug remained on the market, the greater the price difference.
- ○   The Medicare Part D program could have saved $72.9 billion in 2018 by adopting the average price of drugs in the referenced countries.

Indeed, the Trump Administration finalized a rule for Part B medical drugs just before he left office that would reform Part B drug reimbursement and include international reference pricing. For fifty drugs (representing about 73% of Part B medical drug spend), reimbursement would be reduced over four years until the drug price hits the MFN price against an international benchmark for comparable developed countries. The reimbursement system would become a flat rate for the drug and a flat rate for administration by the provider. Providers would be left to negotiate prices with drugmakers during this seven-year innovation pilot. Trump's Administration said this will save $85 billion for the federal government and Medicare beneficiaries over seven years.[34-24]

The reason behind this:[34-24]

- ○   Medicare Part B spending was $30 billion in 2019.
- ○   From 2015 to 2019, the annual inflationary trends for Part B drugs were 11.5%.
- ○   Part B drugs represent about 14% of Part B spending, up from 11% in 2015.
- ○   Part B drug spending has accounted for 37% of the overall Part B spending increase from 2015 to 2019.
- ○   From 2006 to 2017, Part B drug spending grew at 8.1% annually. This is more than twice the inflation of the Part D program and more than three times overall retail drug increases.
- ○   Part B drugs were expected to grow by 8% annually from 2020 through 2027.

Although it is sympathetic to the approach, the Biden Administration has abandoned the rule, although it says it may implement a provision like this in the future. This should open up the drug pricing debate and lead to some reforms in the future.

However, states are now looking at international reference pricing as well. The National Academy of State Health Policy has created model international reference pricing legislation that state legislatures can pass. No bills have passed yet in legislatures as of this writing, but some base pricing on those in Canadian provinces. The bills could impact commercial and perhaps MA and Part D drug pricing in those states.[34-25]

Some worry that international reference pricing could mean withholding drugs for seniors, the disabled, and others with chronic co-morbidities because other nations use quality adjusted life year (QALY) assessments to determine drug availability and prices. These assessments essentially take into account the overall extended life and quality of life that would be derived from a given drug. I believe America could address these concerns and still use international reference pricing. In the alternative, some are looking at a domestic reference pricing concept, where the lowest available price in the nation would be passed through to all lines of business. Savings, especially in Medicare, would be significant.

Empower Health Plans and PBMs to Reduce Costs

Even as we explore price controls, rebates, and broader negotiations, it is important to continue to empower health plans and pharmacy benefit managers (PBMs) to control costs. Plans and PBMs have pushed America to low-cost generics. One example of this is the recent conclusion of the Kaiser Family Foundation (KFF) and Vanderbilt University researchers, finding that Medicare Part D plans do in fact design their drug lists around the cost-effective use of generic drugs. This contradicts the popular wisdom suggesting that somehow health plans and PBMs were in cahoots with drug manufacturers to push costly brand drugs through shadowy rebate programs, thereby increasing overall costs.

The researchers at the two groups found that 84% of the time only the generic drug was covered on the health plan or PBM drug list or formulary.

About 15% of the time, both the brand and generic drugs were covered. The brand drug alone was covered only about 1% of the time. The costs were low for both brand and generic drugs. More importantly, so-called UM (prior authorization, step therapy, and so on) was used rather infrequently when both brand and generic drugs were on the drug list.[34-26, 34-27]

The study points to a few things:

- Health plans and PBMs are constructing very cost-effective formularies that are keeping the overall cost and inflation down in the Part D program. Since the program's inception in 2006, costs have been consistently lower than anticipated spending benchmarks. Further, Part D premiums have remained consistently low, sometimes dropping year over year.

- The Centers for Medicare and Medicaid Services (CMS) have established strong requirements to ensure that plans cover drugs in every class. The study shows that strong regulations and private plan administration can ensure both quality and cost-effective coverage.

- The leveraging of private health plans is a big benefit of our current healthcare system. It is hard to imagine a government-administered prescription system in America coming anywhere close to this track record. It would not have the expertise or innovation. Without private plans deploying effective formulary and some utilization management (UM) techniques, drug costs would burgeon.

Importation or Reimportation

Each year, a reported 19 million Americans illegally import drugs from Canada in order to afford them. This number is probably much higher. In addition, in 2016, 36 million American adults did not fill a prescription due to high costs.[34-10]

If America cannot muster the courage to rein in drug prices in its own country, then it is hard to argue that Americans shouldn't at least have the right to import drugs legally from other countries. Notwithstanding the scare tactics from drugmakers, this can be done safely and securely from many developed nations. At the very least, this should be allowed for high-priced medications.[34-7]

The Trump Administration implemented a rule to allow states to create importation programs from Canada. Biden is known to support importation. As of this writing, several states, including Florida and Colorado, have passed legislation setting up the programs and are awaiting approval to begin importation.[34-28] The Biden administration has endorsed the importation programs moving forward. In addition, there are calls on Capitol Hill to allow for the personal importation of drugs, which is now technically illegal under most circumstances.

Advertising and Marketing Reforms

Despite some reforms, drugmakers continue to advertise and market with abandon. It is time to rein in outlandish advertising or even ban it. We must educate the public that the latest and the greatest drug may not always be needed. Advertising has become so outlandish that we are also having drugmakers play with our emotions for drugs to cure our pets' itchiness and anxiety.

The Biden Administration is known to be considering taking away tax breaks for brand drugmaker advertising.[34-19]

Foster Value-based Pricing to Reward True Clinical Efficacy

Slowly but surely, value-based payment is emerging in America. This holds great promise in the retail and medical drug world. There could come a day where our drug purchases are not purely transaction based but are exclusively or in some form based on the quality outcomes we see from effective and quality drug use. As an example, for cancer treatment, drugmakers could be rewarded a sliding, value-based reimbursement tied to how well the drug agent did in improving conditions, extending life, or preventing death, as well as the safety of the drug. Drugmakers could be required to rebate portions of costs of drugs for poor outcomes and safety. A number of drugmakers are beginning to introduce changes along these lines.

In a rule released late in 2020, the Trump Administration made changes to Medicaid rules effective January 1, 2022, to allow for value-based payment arrangements within the federal best price rebate program.[34-29]

Focus on Care Management, Adherence, and Safety

As with the rest of our healthcare system, we tend to approach healthcare from a UM standpoint. This is especially true for drugs. But as more and more drugs are used to tackle major and complex disease states and co-morbidities, it is essential that health plans and PBMs begin tying authorization, drug safety, adherence, and care management together. As an example, few plans and PBMs have mastered how to treat holistically someone on a specialty medication or cancer agent that costs tens of thousands if not hundreds of thousands per year. A health plan or PBM should be able to comprehensively manage and perform the following:

- Authorize therapy, initially and on an ongoing basis.
- Constantly monitor for effectiveness of the medication.
- Monitor for drug safety and interactions.
- Monitor for adherence to the regimen.
- Educate on correct dosing, administration, and adherence.
- Care manage the individual for the drug therapy in concert with other co-morbidities and drugs.

Conclusion

Fixing drug pricing represents a major reform agenda. So, what is the elephant in the room? Of course, it is price controls. The Republican in me shivers at the concept, but what is the alternative?

We hear much about the potential fallout on brand drugmakers if we go down this road. After all, Medicare is their most lucrative market. Billions could be lost. Drugmaker margins would drop dramatically. It is even possible that new innovation could be delayed or foregone. Simply put, less revenue to brand drugmakers would mean less margin, which would mean less in the research and development budgets.

However, a few key points need to be re-stated:

- Other countries negotiate huge discounts or price fix and have much lower prices and better health outcomes. There is not a lack of drug access in these countries.
- Americans have access to about 90% of all new drugs, while those with price controls in other developed countries have access to about 47%.
- There are drug list restrictions in these countries and the concept is also in place in the United States.
- Why should America continue to subsidize the world drug market and shoulder the primary innovation burden? Estimates suggest that America is responsible for about 70% of global drugmaker profits.[34-30]
- America must tackle price in its healthcare system across the board. Out of all its overall costs, retail and medical drugs account for about 16% and growing.
- America does have major penetration when it comes to generic drugs, but there is a huge mismatch between brand and generic drug costs. Thus, even a small percentage of brand utilization means that brand drug costs dominate drug spend and its growth.
- Aren't margins that are nearly 20% unreasonable for brand drug-makers?
- While drugs have made a huge difference in our quality of life for many diseases, it is also true that high drug prices create barriers to good health. The lack of affordability of some drugs has life and death consequences. Even if innovation lagged, might we be better off in the aggregate with lower prices?
- Expensive drugs have also had a perverse effect on spending, with high-cost medications prescribed when legacy drugs costing almost nothing might do the job. This is tremendously wasteful.

The question remains: Would innovation really be crippled by drug price reform? A Congressional Budget Office (CBO) analysis of the Democratic bill calling for Medicare price negotiations concludes that eight to fifteen fewer drugs would be launched over the decade from passage if the bill were to be adopted, with the loss growing to thirty fewer over the following decade. (CBO recently updated that study and concluded the bill would reduce drug innovation by two drugs in the first ten years, twenty-three in the following decade, and thirty-four in the decade after that.) About 300 drugs would come to market in the first ten-year period, which is a reduction of up to 5%. Industry-sympathetic and -aligned analysts have argued against this analysis, claiming the following:[34-30]

- It takes about fifteen years for a drug to come to market.
- The bill would not come into effect until three years into the first decade analyzed.
- Drugmakers will see the bill just as a start and would rein in further investment as a result.
- Drugmakers see bigger impacts on overall population health because drugmakers will abandon important work on drugs for Alzheimer's, diabetes, and the like.
- The CBO says a 1% reduction in price would reduce innovation— meaning the number of new drugs launched—by as little as 0.25% or as much as 4%. Drugmakers see an impact meaningfully higher.
- Price controls would mean life expectancy at older ages would be reduced by about 3%.
- Americans have access to about 90% of all new drugs, while those with price controls in other developed countries have access to about 47%.

The President of the PhRMA brand drugmaker trade group projected a trillion-dollar impact on drug manufacturers over a decade, with the annual impact far exceeding the entire investment in research and development.[34-31]

Not to be outdone, the White House Council of Economic Advisers under President Trump also attacked the CBO analysis, saying its estimates suggest 100 fewer drugs entering the United States market over the next decade, or about one-third of the total number of drugs expected to enter the market. It also said the bill would reduce Americans' average life expectancy by about four months—nearly one-quarter of the projected gains in life expectancy over the next decade.[34-32]

What seems to be lost on the PhRMA folks and the then-Trump White House (which seemed to have a schizophrenic view on drug price reform) is that we already suffer from among the lowest life expectancies in the developed world. This is very much tied to the lack of affordable, universal access and high overall costs. As Uwe Reinhardt declared in *Priced Out*, America has priced the average citizen out of quality healthcare, and we are suffering for it.

It may be that we have to trade some innovation for lower prices. But as I noted, a great deal of innovation comes from federal research. It could be that an economic investment to boost spending here would make up for any risk of less innovation by brand drugmakers. It may even be that we team up more closely with countries in the developed world to better advance research into drugs and disease prevention.

It is true that the entire paradigm for drugmakers could be upended, with vast implications on finances (company profits) and policy (the question of whether innovation will dry up). But I would argue good companies remake themselves. Drugmakers will adapt—as many other entities, including health plans, have done.

I will give credit to the Trump Administration for attempting to call attention to the problem. At the very least, the threat of moving to price fixing could bring drugmakers to the table. In late 2020, when President Trump relaunched his effort to bring international benchmark pricing to Medicare medical drugs, he challenged drugmakers to come back with a counterproposal. It did so, with an offer to save $100 billion over a decade. The proposal would have reduced medical drug (not retail) spending by about 10% compared with the 20% reduction that might have been seen through the international pricing benchmark. It would also have reduced Medicare beneficiary out-of-pocket costs. In addition, drugmakers would have picked up additional costs for Medicare beneficiaries who enter the catastrophic phase of the Medicare Part D program.[34-33]

This might be viewed as miserly, although it is in the range if not above the estimated savings of the original Trump proposal. And it showed drugmakers to be vulnerable. They are concerned about what could happen on drug pricing. (In the end, Trump rejected the offer and called for extending international benchmarking to retail drugs as well.)

During the presidential election, Joe Biden signaled that he supports price negotiations as well as the German system of drug price controls (which includes negotiations and international reference pricing). Democrats want to move on price negotiations as well. As of this writing, there was no movement yet, but reform is long overdue. I am encouraged by a recent Biden Executive Order that seeks regulatory reforms in many of the areas I have noted in the chapter, including value-based purchasing, swifter generic entry, pay-to-delay reforms, and drug importation.

CHAPTER 35

CHAPTER 35

The Aging of America Time Bomb

Tick, tick, tick. America is getting older by the day.

Unless we act, the inefficient healthcare system we have built will create huge financial problems for the nation. However, the aging of America will compound the woes we will face even further.

To some degree, aging and living longer is good and we should celebrate it—at least I hope so, as I am at that age where you begin thinking about these issues. Living longer and aging comes with being an advanced, developed country. It also seems that technological advancement pushes the potential to live longer even further each day. All those drug ads also lead us to believe there could be the equivalent of the Fountain of Youth out there.

But at the same time, if developed nations don't plan for aging of their societies, longer life creates both economic and quality-of-life complications. Without careful thought and action, the aging of America threatens to further cripple our already out-of-control healthcare spending. Given the sheer cost of long-term care, today and in the future, it also threatens to cripple the budget and well-being of individual families.

The aging of society is not just something felt here in the United States. The costs of aging tend to impact developed countries much more than others. Sadly, this is because people in the developing world do not live as long and do not have access to the life-saving technology and pharmaceuticals that tend to prolong life. With a healthcare system predicated on access to the very best, America's aging population will likely have an even greater impact on our costs than those in the government-run socialized medicine or single-payer countries, where access to life-saving services and technology is often explicitly or implicitly rationed.

The real cost crunch of aging comes in two ways, the first being the cost of acute care. Medical care tends to increase dramatically as the decades add up. Second, as we age, we often need access to some form of long-term care, from in-home support all the way to a nursing home for some of us. While a great deal of such care is provided informally—by family members and friends—a large share is not. Also, informal care has its societal and economic costs, including lower incomes for families who are caregivers and the need to tap other public assistance programs due to financial constraints.

The real problem is that only the wealthiest of those among us can possibly plan for and save for such care. With bills to pay in retirement, how can the broad base of Americans save tens or hundreds of thousands of dollars for potential long-term care costs or purchase long-term-care insurance? Thus, while the Medicaid program was initially fashioned for the truly destitute, it has increasingly become the payer of long-term care (and with it, some of the acute medical care later in life) for the poor and some middle-class Americans. Those who plan well are able to set up trusts or engage in other asset transfers. These protect the upper middle-class and even wealthy inheritances that go to children while still allowing parents to go on Medicaid for long-term care services. Those that don't plan so well end up "spending down" what little assets and income they have. Often, they quickly become eligible for Medicaid long-term care and acute services as well.

The aging of America is creating a ticking time bomb for state and national budgets. As the proportion of those over sixty-five increases each year, the resources needed for Medicaid and Medicare budgets in the outyears are greater. I mention both government programs because Medicare covers acute medical care as well as short-term, acute, rehabilitative stays and services. But Medicaid covers the secondary acute care costs and 100% (with federal revenue sharing in states) of the chronic long-term care bill. As bad as the unfunded liabilities of Medicare and Medicaid are projected to be now, they will only get worse as life expectancy and technological innovation increases.

Let's talk first about what long-term care (LTC) services are. They come in two forms—acute and chronic.

Acute LTC is largely funded by Medicare or a commercial health plan and constitutes stays in rehabilitation or skilled nursing facilities (SNFs) to help recover from an illness or accident. It also includes provision of care at home by nurses or health aides as you recover. In these cases, you are discharged from a hospital, have so-called LTC for several weeks or months, and you are back to functioning.

Chronic LTC is the provision of similar services because the individual in question has deficiencies in their activities of daily living (ADL) that do not allow them to live independently or be at home alone safely. These services are dependent on the severity of the ADL deficiencies and are furnished based on assessing the individual's independence and overall needs.

Chronic LTC services are funded either by a private, long-term care insurance policy (if you have the money to buy one) or Medicaid (if you qualify).

When Americans cannot afford LTC coverage, as noted they tend to "spend down" their assets—if they had not already transferred them to their children—and end up poor enough to qualify for Medicaid LTC coverage. In most states, qualifying for Medicaid LTC coverage is at higher incomes than the poverty standards for regular medical care. Eventually, many also end up on Medicaid for acute medical services.

In rough measure, chronic LTC services might be broken out as follows:

Level 1 Services include clinical and non-clinical support by a home healthcare agency. The number of hours can be scaled, based on need. They also include elderly, supportive, or congregate housing with non-clinical supports and clinical supports for some. Finally, Level 1 services include community adult day care in conjunction with the above.

Level 2 Services include assisted living, where tiered clinical and non-clinical supports are furnished twenty-four hours a day.

Level 3 Services include the use of chronic skilled nursing facilities due to major impairments and inability to live independently.

Here are two other definitions: Long-term services and supports (LTSS) is a blanket term often used for all LTC services. This is especially used in Medicaid. This includes institutional services, such as nursing homes. It also includes what are known as home and community-based services (HCBS), which includes home care, adult day care, congregate housing with supports, and assisted living, among others.

Here are a few rough facts on aging in the world and in America:

- According to the World Health Organization (WHO), between 2000 and 2050, the population of those over 60 will go from 605 million to 2 billion—a doubling, from 11% to 22% of the population. The number of people aged 80 years or older will almost quadruple between 2000 and 2050 and rise to 395 million.[35-1]

- In the United States, average life expectancy increased from 68 years in 1950 to 78.6 years in 2017. This was in large measure due to the reduction in mortality at older ages. The number of Americans aged 65 and older will almost *double*, from 52 million in 2018 to 95 million by 2060—from 16% to 23%. One-fifth of the population will be 65 or older by 2050. Other sources say the population of those 65 and older and those 85 and older will more than double and more than triple, respectively, by 2050. One interesting point: some developed nations are already older than the United States and will age much more dramatically than we will. This includes a number of European nations, Japan, Asia, and Brazil. This is in part due to lower fertility rates in those nations.[35-2, 35-3, 35-4, 35-5]

What is the cost of these LTC services that will threaten to bankrupt America and individual families?

Based on average costs for various services and studies I have reviewed, I estimate that the cost of lower-end, community-based solutions, such as moderate home care supports or adult day care, is between $20,000 and $25,000 per year, nationally, on average. The cost of intensive home care and assisted living is between $40,000 to $50,000 per year, on average. The cost of nursing home institutionalization is between $80,000 and $100,000 per year, on average.[35-4, 35-5, 35-6, 35-7, 35-8]

Who pays the freight for LTC services, and what will the tab be for government and individuals? Statistics are very much influenced by various factors so numbers sometimes can differ. That said, here are some facts: As of 2013, two sources say America spent about $310 billion and Medicaid covered about 51% of those expenditures. About 19% was out-of-pocket costs and 21% were other public costs. Just 8% was private insurance. Another source says that in 2016 about $366 billion was spent on formal long-term care services. This was about 13% of healthcare expenditures in that year. Medicaid covered about 42%, with almost two-thirds of all nursing home residents covered by Medicaid each day for chronic long-term care. About 22% of the bill was paid by Medicare's acute portion. About 6% of LTC costs was paid by other public sources, 16% out of pocket, 8% by private insurance, and another 7% by other private sources.[35-4, 35-5, 35-9, 35-10]

These costs are clearly an under-estimate, as tens of millions of Americans (over 34 million) already act as caregivers to the elderly today. This is usually at the lower end of the care continuum and will grow. About two-thirds of Americans receive all of their long-term care from family or friends. While this does not appear to have direct costs, it has huge impact on the economy and family income. This is not counted in the above estimates, which represents formal costs only. A quick estimate by me of the number of hours people spend taking care of elderly and disabled people and what that amounts to in lost wages verifies that this informal LTC cost in America could be more than the formal one. Studies peg this at between $234 and $470 billion, per year.[35-3, 35-4] And costs will explode over the next few decades.

Alzheimer's and dementia as diseases will increase dramatically over the next several decades. This will add tremendously to LTC costs. About one-third of all those over age eighty-five have Alzheimer's. The estimated lifetime cost of treating someone with dementia is $342,000.[35-4]

Aging and inflation will push the cost up by staggering levels. There is an expected 50% increase in Medicaid spending related to long-term care between 2016 and 2026.[35-4] In 2013, the Centers for Medicare and Medicaid Services (CMS) and the Congressional Budget Office (CBO) indicated that aging, inflation, cognition/impairment, and other changes could increase LTC costs from about 1.3% of the gross domestic product (GDP) to between 1.9-3.3% of GDP by 2050.[35-3]

While this varies by sex, Americans can expect to need a high-level of long-term care for at least two years over their life and that number will grow with the advent of new treatments and technology. Over 50% of those sixty-five and older will meet this need, with the number of individuals meeting the need projected to well more than double by 2050.[35-4] The CBO suggests that two-thirds of those over sixty-five will need LTC in their lifetime.[35-3]

So, the crushing burden is coming, and America simply does not have a plan to grapple with aging and the LTC bill. If healthcare reform has languished, generally speaking, implementing a coherent long-term care policy in America is all but non-existent. Polls consistently show that a majority of U.S. adults—both Democrats and Republicans—favor a national LTC program.

Have we made any progress over the years? Yes, some. But the progress is not enough. Here are some facts over time from various sources. Again, statistics can vary based on a number of factors, but I include them all here to give a broad understanding of the issue: [35-5, 35-6, 35-11, 35-12, 35-13, 35-14, 35-15]

Today about forty-five states have home- and community-based waiver programs for all populations (seniors, other adults with physical disabilities, adults with development disabilities, and other groups) through Medicaid.

From 1995 to 2014, Medicaid long-term services and supports (LTSS) spending on home- and community-based services for all populations went from 18% to 53%.

The number of seniors on Medicaid LTSS services in the community was about 50% in 2011.

In 2013, Medicaid spending on alternatives to institutionalization for all populations overall averaged about 46% of LTSS expenditures (up from 32% in 2002).

The percentage of institutional alternatives spending in Medicaid as a percentage of total LTSS expenditures has steadily increased over the last thirty years. Alternatives surpassed 50% of LTSS expenditures in 2013, hitting 56.1% in FY 2018.

There is huge variability in states' penetration of alternatives to institutions in the LTSS program for all populations, ranging from 21% of Medicaid LTSS spent on alternatives to institutions all the way to 78% in 2013.

In 2013, just ten states and the District of Columbia spent over 50% of Medicaid LTSS funding on alternatives for all populations, with sixteen states spending 41-50% and fourteen states spending 31-40%.

In 2018, at least thirty-four states spent 60.8% or less on alternatives as a percentage of Medicaid LTSS spending overall for all populations. For just older adults and others with physical disabilities, Medicaid LTSS alternatives spending was 37.4% or less in at least thirty-two states.

Total Medicaid spending on LTSS had reached $129 billion in federal fiscal year 2018.

Managed long-term care programs (MLTC, where private managed care plans offer LTSS services on behalf of state Medicaid programs) have increased dramatically over the last twenty years, with national spending increasing more than threefold from $6.7 billion in 2008 to over $30 billion in 2018. Eight states used MLTC in 2006 and twenty-five did in 2018.

As a brief aside, as of this writing, President Biden did propose increased investments in home- and community-based services in early 2021. Congress had not yet acted. Biden has recommended in two different announcements a total of about $950 billion in new funding over an eight-to- ten-year horizon as a down payment to expand home- and community-based services to both deinstitutionalize individuals from nursing homes and stop admissions through funding and enhancements for chronic home care and other community services. This would reduce wait lists that often exist in states as states cap these programs due to overall costs. If passed, this would increase such funding between 150-170% annually. If anything does pass, the likelihood is that funding will be far less, perhaps $150 to $250 billion over a decade.

Biden's proposal is not an aging plan by any means. It is at best the start of a necessary dialogue at the national and state levels. So, it is fair to ask every politician some pressing questions. What will I do when I am too old to take care of myself? Medicare covers acute LTC stays, but not chronic ones. Most Americans' incomes cannot support the expenditures seen above. Will sons and daughters continue to be asked to cover the costs, for as long as possible, at an increasing rate, and at substantially greater costs than today? Will everyone end up on Medicaid by running through their assets? Won't this bankrupt America anyway, whether it is Medicaid alone or in combination with LTC benefits in Medicare for All (if it were to pass—heaven forbid)? Finally, will we be able to support quality LTC services at relatively low Medicaid and Medicare rates?

Should America raise the white flag and surrender to its socialist temptations to create a high-tax welfare state to meet its long-term care needs? The answer, of course, is no. There is a better way if America plans it out and creates an incentive-based system for both long-term and acute care for the elderly.

As Connecticut's Budget and Policy Secretary in the late 1990s and early 2000s, I led a team of multi-disciplinary policymakers that fashioned a continuum of care for lower-income and middle-class residents that reaped both short-term savings and projected long-term ones.

So, here are some basic tenets to frame the debate and move toward a long-term care agenda for the nation:

> Keep private healthcare plans as they can drive efficiencies, quality, and innovation. They are doing so for LTC services in Medicare and Medicaid today and could play a role in the commercial realm in the future as well.

> It is wrong to tell Americans they should ignore their future long-term costs because Big Brother will save the day. People should be vested in their long-term care future, much like they should be for retirement income and healthcare and life insurance.

> Government could never shoulder the total cost burden of LTC over time. It must be a shared responsibility, one that is rooted in efficient delivery and personal responsibility.

> Civilized, developed nations do need a social safety net, and LTC is part of it. Both public and private investment in LTC, including Medicaid and other government funding, is a balanced approach to tackling the problem.

> Time is short. We will need to change the culture for younger Baby Boomers (those in their fifties, like me) and younger generations, in order to change the paradigm.

With these tenets laid out, what should America do to begin building an accountable, long-term care partnership with its citizens?

Educate the Broader Public about Planning for Their Long-term Care Future

Admittedly, it is hard enough to educate the American public on insurance for medical care and prevention. But the late Baby Boomers (it is not too late for people, even in their fifties) and younger generations must quickly understand that long-term care insurance is as important to the future as medical insurance, life insurance and saving for retirement.

One source suggests that in 2011, just 7-9 million had private long-term care insurance. The average premium was about $2,283 annually. Another source says that in 2014 only 7.25 million Americans—or 2-3% of the population—had long-term care insurance in 2014. Estimates suggest that just 13% of those age sixty-five or older have some form of LTC insurance.[35-3, 35-4, 35-5]

Buying long-term care insurance when you are young creates affordable payments and greater coverage amounts for the future. Late Baby Boomers and Generation Xers still have some time to be converted to believing in long-term care insurance before chronic co-morbidities set in and premium costs skyrocket.

Connecticut was one of the first four states to adopt a Long-Term Care Partnership (LTCP) waiver. Today, almost all states have implemented some form of it. These partnerships allow citizens to buy various financial levels of long-term care policies. These policies are then used to pay for the initial long-term care that is needed. In return, those who need additional care may go on Medicaid and shield their assets (generally equal to the amount of the original policy) from government recoupment.

Today, forty-five states have Medicaid LTCP plans active. In addition, most of those states also allow reciprocity. This means that if an elder lived in one state for many years and moved to another state to be closer to family, the asset protection would be honored in the new state.[35-16]

It is a strategy that can work in concert with the education campaign described previously. In essence, citizens save for their long-term care needs by purchasing policies and still have a partial Medicaid safety net to fall back on. Their children also receive an inheritance. The state saves a lot as private insurance is paying a good portion of the LTC bill.

The statistics for LTCP policies sadly are worse than for LTC policies in general. They number just in the hundreds of thousands nationwide.[35-3] We must drive toward the sale of millions of these LTCP policies nationwide.

Interestingly, Washington state has introduced what amounts to a public-funded long-term care policy. Residents pay a 0.58% payroll tax until they retire and can receive up to $36,500 in long-term care benefits over a lifetime. The amount will be adjusted for inflation. It is a small start but begins to raise awareness of the need to plan for such care. (https://wacaresfund.wa.gov/)

Build a Broad Range of Alternatives to Nursing Home Care

While I oppose a 100% funded, blanket government LTC coverage plan, Democrats do have it right that providing lower-level LTC care early could help save or at least prolong more expensive institutional care. Nursing homes are by far the most expensive form of long-term, chronic care. Few states have invested enough in alternatives to nursing homes such as home care, adult day care, congregate housing, supportive housing, independent living with supports, and assisted living. Even if they have, they may not be able to meet the demand in the future. It will mean the state and federal governments will need to focus not only on the traditional Medicaid matching fund entitlement for medical services but also add baskets of capital funding, rental subsidies, and various long-term care and medical support services in the community.

Skittish states tend to shy away from such dynamic changes in their long-term care approaches. It is true that more could become eligible or want such services. But even with the additions, these forms of care run between one-quarter and one-half the cost of nursing homes. And because few states invest in a true continuum, only the wealthy have real access to community-based alternatives. The poor and middle class are disproportionately forced into expensive nursing homes, due to the lack of cost-effective alternatives.

In Connecticut, overall we found that these alternatives were still much more cost-effective than the cost of nursing home care. This proved to be true whether in the federal Medicaid matching program (at lower income levels) or even 100% state-funded (at middle income levels). This supports the premise that, whatever the risks, all states need to start building their alternative long-term care infrastructure now so as to be ready for the aging boom.

Adopt Broad Buy-in Approaches for Alternatives to Income-based Nursing Homes

As noted earlier, covering LTC costs should be a government and individual partnership, in part based on what someone can afford. In Connecticut, we found that allowing higher asset eligibility thresholds and creating income-based, sliding- scale buy-ins to our Medicaid and state-financed LTC programs helped residents gain access to alternatives to nursing homes and still pay a fair share. It made it easier for the state to expand the programs up the income scale. More importantly, it restored the dignity of living in the community for as long as possible. Apart from investments in children's healthcare, a more fiscally sound and socially compassionate public policy simply does not exist.

As an alternative, a catastrophic government program could be paired with private long-term care insurance. In this instance, private insurance policies would pay for long-term care coverage for a set dollar amount or number of years. After that, the government would cover costs.

Use Managed Care to Coordinate Acute and Long-term Care to Further Reduce Costs

Today, even with broad, managed care in most states for Medicaid medical assistance, long-term care is often still captive to the inefficient fee-for-service (FFS) environment. Coordinating the services or even hiring one managed care plan to deliver both sets of services will reap savings on both sides. Better coordinated care reduces acute episodes. Focusing on an elder's medication management, healthy nutrition, and socialization and cognition tend to help maintain them in alternatives for longer periods.

For the naysayers, those who believe that managed care has enough trouble managing acute care for relatively healthy populations in Medicaid, one need only look at the promising results of Medicaid-only, managed, long-term care—as well as Medicare institutional special needs plans (SNPs). Interesting and accountable models are being built to control costs and boost quality. These should be expanded in Medicare and Medicaid. In addition, the typical FFS-type LTC insurance policies that exist today could over time leverage many of the same managed care techniques.

Make It Harder for Americans to Transfer Assets in the Future

This sounds draconian given what I said earlier, but the education campaign noted previously will only be effective if Americans understand that Uncle Sam may not be the absolute safety net it has been—simply because we can't afford it. In all but one state (California), the state Medicaid agency requires that asset transfers occur at least sixty months prior to the long-term care need (in California it is thirty months),[35-17] but additional safeguards need to be put in place.

Harsher rules could have dramatic impacts on those within a decade of needing such services. However, phasing in more draconian asset transfer rules for younger Americans, by enacting federal and state laws now, is key to ensuring that long-term care insurance will begin to be thought of as being like life and health insurance. Indeed, more restrictive asset transfer rules is an important complement to educating people on the need for long-term care insurance and building out the cost-effective continuum of care outlined previously.

I would note that the Medicaid and CHIP Payment and Access Commission (MACPAC), the congressional policy arm to Congress, is proposing to actually loosen such rules and even make estate recovery by states optional. They note that such recoveries could fall disproportionately on the poor and people of color. But I would argue there are ways to deal with this inequity rather than eliminating estate recovery.[35-18]

It is time for CMS and state Medicaid agencies to begin collecting the best practices from various states, in order to pursue a long-term care agenda for the nation. Some very progressive states have proven models and incubators already exist out there.

So, time is ticking, and the stakes are extremely high—not only for healthcare but the nation's economy as a whole. If we don't create a reasonable, cost-effective, national long-term care plan—one that leverages the private sector, personal responsibility, and government funding—then we will be in dire economic and healthcare shape.

Don't let the bomb go off.

Afterword:
What the COVID-19 Crisis Has Taught Us

This book was finalized as the COVID-19 pandemic was exacerbating due to the delta variant. As of this writing, the final infection totals and death counts for America were not known but had reached 45 million cases and over 700,000 deaths. However, even at the time of this epilogue's writing, COVID-19 had already shined a bright light on the nagging uninsured crisis in America and what it means to the health and welfare of our nation.

As the late, great healthcare economist Uwe Reinhardt clearly articulated in his book, *Priced Out*, America is the only developed nation that has yet to endorse universal access to healthcare as a social good. If COVID-19 teaches us anything, I hope we finally conclude that if healthcare is not a fundamental right, it is darn near one. It certainly should not be a privilege driven by income or class.

COVID-19 had a disproportionate impact on those with sporadic or no access to health coverage. Based on what we know about the profile of the uninsured, it also makes this a socio-economic issue, a racial one, and an ethnic one.

Why is this? First, the uninsured tend to be individuals who are not in jobs or positions that allow them to work from home or social distance. Their risk of contracting the virus is thus much higher. Second, the uninsured, if employed, tend to work for employers that either do not offer insurance or do so at costs that are simply too high. While many do take advantage of Medicaid and Exchanges, some are not eligible for truly affordable coverage. Third, their lack of access to good, consistent coverage also means that they often have undiagnosed or poorly maintained chronic conditions. This fact increases both the risk of contracting COVID-19 and the severity of the illness if contracted. Last, many face socio-economic barriers to good health. Studies show these social determinants have greater impact on health outcomes than do underlying clinical factors.

I hope COVID-19 has taught us that the lack of universal access to healthcare has real life and death implications. By the way, this happens every day for the tens of millions who lack consistent access to coverage. They forego preventive visits for themselves and their families because of the cost of care. Their disease states and conditions exacerbate. Their cancers go undiagnosed. If they receive treatment, often it is late in the life cycle of their disease or illness. This leads to major health impacts and mortality, costing the system as a whole tremendously more than it should. But on a day-to-day basis, all of this is largely hidden from most Americans who have that employer-based insurance connection or otherwise have insurance. While we care, the issue is largely ignored.

But with the scourge of COVID-19, a great inequity has been exposed. It has shown how vulnerable Americans without coverage struggle every day, now more so during the COVID-19 crisis. This is not to say that COVID-19 discriminates; it does not. People with gold-plated health coverage will fall ill and perhaps even die, but those without coverage are more likely to fall ill and die in greater numbers. Because we lack universal access to healthcare, any pandemic by nature has a much greater impact on all Americans—socially, financially, and economically. Early numbers demonstrate this. The final statistics will bear out these impacts over time.

None of this is to say we should retire the healthcare system we have today or endorse socialized medicine or single-payer. As you know, I believe these are not answers to the woes of the American health system. I believe that a private delivery system is the best way to go. But as a nation, we should view affordable universal access to healthcare as a social good and implement a system where every American is able to receive consistent healthcare coverage. The rest of the developed world has done so. Although sometimes they have fanciful views of what healthcare should be, the Democrats have done so. It is time the Republicans recognize the ethics of healthcare, too. Will the virus move my party? I hope so.

Acknowledgments

I have been blessed to have a great life, with parents who gave me every opportunity, a wonderful, loving, and supportive wife and family, and a career that has spanned government and the private sector.

My work on healthcare issues has been by far the most rewarding of my career. Whether in government or working in the industry, I always enjoyed the technical complexity combined with the real-life stories of the people who health plans serve.

As this book gets published, I wanted to thank a few people who have been so supportive, encouraging, and helped make a difference in my life and allowed me to accomplish so much over the years.

To my wife, Donna, who has known me longer and understands me better than anyone. You have brought me great joy. You wholeheartedly support me in all my endeavors and "followed me where I wanted to go."

To my three children, Christopher, Conor, and Kathleen, and my daughter-in-law, Kate. You are all incredibly talented kids who will continue to do great things in life.

To my parents, Dennis and Paulette Ryan, and my sister, Dawn Ryan, who gave me such a great, loving start in life. You did more for me throughout the years than anyone will ever know.

To my mother-in-law and father-in-law, Marge and the late Don Breslin. Thank you for being such supportive and loving people.

To my late grandparents, Paul and Helen Ryan and Paul and Lucy Langlais. They, along with my parents, have been my inspiration throughout life, rising from modest means and achieving the American dream.

To my friends, Eva and Chuck Bunnell. Your friendship has been life-changing for Donna and me. Eva, thanks for showing me what putting your heart into something really means. It changed my outlook on how to approach healthcare.

To my first real bosses, L. Brent Bozell III and Brent Baker. Thanks for setting me on my course.

To my boss at the Waterbury Republican-American, the late great Publisher William J. Pape II. You showed me what courage and conviction really are.

To former Governors John G. Rowland and M. Jodi Rell, who took a chance on a relatively unproven young man. The chance you took gave me such tremendous experience and opportunities.

To my friend Mary Ann Hanley, who mentored me throughout my government career and after. You made such a difference in my life and career. You taught me what fairness and equity is and what critical thinking is all about.

To my friend and mentor from across the political aisle, Peter Kelly. Your ongoing support of me was amazing. I remember our time in Poland with happiness.

To Don Downes, Pam Law, Anne Gnazzo, Mike Cicchetti, Anne Foley, Brenda Sisco, Jean Henry, and all the other people of the state of Connecticut Office of Policy and Management and Governor's Office at the time. In those early years, many of you mentored me and taught me so much. Our work together was amazing for the people of Connecticut.

To Mike Starkowski of the Connecticut Department of Social Services. You were one of the best partners I could have asked for to work on healthcare policy in Connecticut.

To Kevin Sullivan (then Connecticut President Pro Tempore of the Senate and later Lieutenant Governor), Moira Lyons (then Connecticut Speaker of the House), Lou Deluca (then Connecticut Senate Minority Leader) and Bob Ward (then Connecticut House Minority Leader). Your friendship and our unlikely alliances at critical times meant so much to moving Connecticut forward in a fiscally sound and compassionate fashion.

To former U.S. Rep. Nancy Johnson. From your perch as a subcommittee chair on the powerful U.S. House Ways and Means Committee, you taught me more about state and federal health policy and how Congress worked than you will ever know. You also taught me that study and compromise were essential to good healthcare policy.

To the most unlikely of friends, former state Sen. Edith Prague, who early on saw and nurtured the compassionate side of my healthcare policy. Edith, I will forever be an Edith Prague Republican.

To the late Al Solnit, renowned psychiatrist and friend. When you were mental health commissioner, you taught me all about mental illness and substance abuse and why such diseases should be treated the same as any physical illness lest we marginalize so many. You also helped me discover my fondness for Tabasco.

To all my health plan friends I have worked with over the years. I am continually amazed by the dedication and commitment each of you have to your members and transforming healthcare into a value-driven system. Special thanks to Liz Goodman, Bryan Baier, Zac Pruitt, Katie Zito, April Sharpe, Sonia Diaz, Ana Romany, and Amy Do who were with me for many special adventures in the health plan world.

To the people of the AIDS Healthcare Foundation, who showed me that compassion has to be a real part of healthcare. This is especially true of Donna Stidham, the long-time lead of managed care at the foundation. You showed me how compassion and managed-care principles can succeed together.

To MedHOK (MHK) co-founders Anil Kottoor and Vig Ponnusamy. Guys, —the MedHOK roller coaster ride was one of the most incredible I have been on and it reached such great heights. The two of you served as great inspiration.

To my friends and colleagues at MHK and the Hearst Health family for their commitment to mission-driven healthcare. I especially want to thank Steve Swartz, Greg Dorn, Frank Bennack, Jr., Richard Malloch, Eve Burton, Chuck Tuchinda, Jeff Rose, Denielle Dewynter, Michelle Bennett, Barin Rovzar, Mark Redman, and Jennifer Tancredi for all they do for me and for making both MHK and Hearst a special and renowned place to work. I am so proud of Hearst for being a true leader in how successful businesses can be run with a clear focus on associates, clients, and the public at large.

To my past and present MHK management team (Alex Pauloski, Vig Ponnusamy, Ryan Smith, Amit Sinha, Natalie Dougherty, Ashley Cabrera, Cori Godeke, David Bricker, Ken Balakrishnan, Kim Boulahanis, Christina Broyles, Caleb McMillen, Drew Deaton, and David Garrigan). We have come together to fashion a great, high-growth and accountable technology company. Every day, we make a difference in the lives of tens of millions of Americans.

To my "Co-Editors in Chief"—my wife Donna and my son Christopher. Thanks for running through page after page to make this product the best it could be. I think the competition worked! To my expert copy editor, Kathleen Ryan. Thanks Kitty!

To my "Editors At Large"—my good friends David Bricker and Ashley Cabrera. Thanks for your editing and keen healthcare insights. Dave, you have been a great friend for many years now and your friendship and mentorship is a treasured gift. Ashley, you are becoming a tremendous healthcare IT executive and will have an incredible future.

To the entire crew at Amplify and RealClear Publishing, including Naren Aryal, Hobbs Allison, Nina Spahn, Kristin Perry, Nicole Hall, John Parsons, Becca Andersen, and Carl Cannon. It has been a pleasure to work with such professional and caring people.

Citations

Chapter 1:

1-1 Reinhardt, Uwe, Priced Out: The Economic and Ethical Costs of American Health Care, Princeton University Press, 2019, page xxiii

1-2 Cussen, Mark P., "Top 5 Reasons Why People Go Bankrupt," *Investopedia*, June 25, 2019, https://www.investopedia.com/financial-edge/0310/top-5-reasons-people-go-bankrupt.aspx, cites Harvard Study as to medical expenses being leading cause of bankruptcy and a majority have some form of health insurance.

Chapter 2:

2-1 Barkin, Kenneth, "Otto von Bismarck (1815-1898)," The Latin Library, http://www.thelatinlibrary.com/imperialism/notes/bismarck.html

2-2 Guthrie, Jr., Palmer. "Otto Von Bismarck," https://789839655772307049.weebly.com/realpolitik.html

2-3   Boissoneault, Lorraine, "Bismarck Tried to End Socialism's Grip—By Offering Government Healthcare," July 14, 2017, https://www.smithsonianmag.com/history/bismarck-tried-end-socialisms-grip-offering-government-healthcare-180964064/

2-4   History.com Editors, "Otto Von Bismarck," June 7, 2019, https://www.history.com/topics/germany/otto-von-bismarck

2-5   PrussianHistory.com Editors, "Bismarck and State Socialism," April 14, 2019, https://prussianhistory.com/bismarck-and-state-socialism/

2-6   Bauernschuster, Stefan and Anastasia Driva and Erik Hornung, "Bismarck's Health Insurance and the Mortality Decline," September 1, 2016, https://pdfs.semanticscholar.org/acd1/8a49068adb15b24a5e1c3e73453712131de1.pdf

2-7   Guyton, Gregory P. "A Brief History of Workers' Compensation," The Iowa Orthopaedic Journal, 1999; 19: 106–110, https://www.ncbi.nlm.nih.gov/pmc/articles/PMC1888620/

2-8   Guinnane, Timothy and Jochen Streb, "Incentives That Saved Lives: Government Regulation of Accident Insurance Associations in Germany, 1884-1914," Yale University, Economic Growth Center, 2012, https://ideas.repec.org/p/ags/yaleeg/130879.html

2-9   "Otto Von Bismarck," Social Security History, https://www.ssa.gov/history/ottob.html

2-10   "Seventy Years of Social Market Economy, June 18, 2018 , https://www.deutschland.de/en/topic/business/social-market-economy-in-germany-growth-and-prosperity

2-11   Sally, Razeen, Ludwig Ehrhard's social market economy – a liberal, not a social democratic concept," Institute of Economic Affairs, April 15, 2016, https://iea.org.uk/blog/ludwig-erhards-social-market-economy-a-liberal-not-a-social-democratic-concept

2-12   "The Social Market Economy in a Globalised World," Congress Document adopted by the European People's Party Statutory Congress Bonn, 9-10 December 2009, https://www.epp.eu/files/uploads/2015/11/The_Social_Market_Economy_in_a_Globalised_World.pdf

Chapter 3:

3-1   Nespor, Carrie, "19th Century Doctors in the U.S., Melnick Medical Museum, March 11, 2009, https://melnickmedicalmuseum.com/2009/03/11/19th-century-doctors-in-the-us/

3-2   Breslaw, Elaine G., 'What Was Healthcare Like in the 1800s?," History News Network, Columbian College of Arts and Sciences at George Washington University, December 10, 2012, https://historynewsnetwork.org/article/149661

3-3   "The Early 19th Century American Medical Worldview," University of Pennsylvania, https://www.sas.upenn.edu/~rogert/19wv.html

3-4   "History of Hospitals," University of Pennsylvania School of Nursing, https://www.nursing.upenn.edu/nhhc/nurses-institutions-caring/history-of-hospitals/

3-5   Healthcare Crisis: Healthcare Timeline, PBS.org, https://www.pbs.org/healthcarecrisis/history.htm

3-6   Moseley III, George, The U.S. Health Care Non-System, 1908-2008, AMA Journal of Ethics, May 2008, https://journalofethics.ama-assn.org/article/us-health-care-non-system-1908-2008/2008-05

3-7   Scofea, Laura, "The development and Growth of Employer-Provided Health Insurance," Monthly Labor Review, March 1994, https://www.bls.gov/opub/mlr/1994/03/art1full.pdf

3-8   Rosner, David and Gerald Markowitz, "The Struggle Over Employee Benefits: The Role of Labor in Influencing Modern Health Policy," The Milbank Quarterly, March 2003, https://www.ncbi.nlm.nih.gov/pmc/articles/PMC2690201/

3-9   "Chapter 2: Origins and Evolution of Employment-Based Health Benefits," Employment and Health Benefits: A Connection at Risk, National Center for Biotechnology Information, U.S. National Library of Medicine, National Academy of Sciences, 1993, https://www.ncbi.nlm.nih.gov/books/NBK235989/

3-10   Fox PhD, Peter D. and Peter R. Kongstvedt, MD, "Ch. 1: A History of Managed Health Care and Health Insurance in the United States," The Essentials of Managed Health Care, 2013, https://samples.jbpub.com/9781284043259/Chapter1.pdf

3-11   Blue Cross and Blue Shield A Historical Compilation, Consumer Reports Advocacy, https://advocacy.consumerreports.org/wp-content/uploads/2013/03/yourhealthdollar.org_blue-cross-history-compilation.pdf

3-12   "How it all started," Kaiser Permanente website, https://about.kaiserpermanente.org/our-story/our-history/how-it-all-started

3-13   "An Industry Pioneer," Blue Cross Blue Shield Association Website, https://www.bcbs.com/about-us/industry-pioneer

3-14   Thomasson, Melissa. "Health Insurance in the United States". EH.Net Encyclopedia, edited by Robert Whaples. April 17, 2003. http://eh.net/encyclopedia/health-insurance-in-the-united-states/

3-15   Conover, Christopher J., "How Private Health Insurance slashed the uninsured rate for Americans," American Enterprise Institute, September, 16, 2011, http://www.aei.org/publication/how-private-health-insurance-slashed-the-uninsured-rate-for-americans/

3-16   Fletcher, Nicole, "The History of American Health Insurance: A Look Back In Time To Understand How We Got To Where We Are," Pokitdok Blog, July 1, 2015, https://blog.pokitdok.com/the-history-of-american-health-insurance-a-look-back-in-time-to-understand-how-we-got-to-where-we-are/index.html

3-17   "Theodore Roosevelt: A Champion For Progressive Reform," Families USA website, December 9, 2010, https://familiesusa.org/blog/theodore-roosevelt-a-champion-for-progressive-reform

3-18   Woolner, David, "Special interests to FDR: 'National healthcare is un-American, a threat to capitalism, nay. Slavery!' (Sound familiar?)", Roosevelt Institute Blog, Roosevelt Institute, August 21, 2009, https://rooseveltinstitute.org/special-interests-fdr-national-health-care-un-american-threat-capitalism-nay-slavery-sound-familiar/

3-19   Markel, Howard, "69 years ago, a president pitches his idea for national health care," PBS NewsHour, November 19, 2014, https://www.pbs.org/newshour/health/november-19-1945-harry-truman-calls-national-health-insurance-program

3-20   Anderson Steve, A brief history of Medicare in America, Medicareresources.org, May 1, 2019, https://www.medicareresources.org/basic-medicare-information/brief-history-of-medicare/

3-21   Seervai, Shanoor and David Blumenthal, MD, "Lessons on Universal Coverage from and Unexpected Advocate: Richard Nixon," The Commonwealth Fund, November 2, 2017, https://www.commonwealthfund.org/blog/2017/lessons-universal-coverage-unexpected-advocate-richard-nixon

3-22   Gruber, Lynn R., Maureen, Shadle, and Cynthia L. Polic, "From Movement to Industry: The Growth of HMOs," Health Affairs, Summer 1988, https://www.healthaffairs.org/doi/full/10.1377/hlthaff.7.3.197

3-23   Tobin, Christine, "What is Managed Health Care?", Reprinted from AADE News, American Association of Diabetes Educators, January 1997, https://nfb.org/images/nfb/publications/vodold/mngdcare.htm

3-24   "Private Payers Serving Individuals With Disabilities and Chronic Conditions. Characteristics of Managed Care," Office of the Assistant Secretary for Planning and Evaluation, January 1, 2000, https://aspe.hhs.gov/report/private-payers-serving-individuals-disabilities-and-chronic-conditions/characteristics-managed-care

3-25   "Health Plans and Benefits: ERISA," Department of Labor, https://www.dol.gov/general/topic/health-plans/erisa

3-26   Seitz-Wald, Alex, "Reagan's Healthcare Mandate," Salon, July 5, 2012, https://www.salon.com/2012/07/05/reagans_healthcare_mandate/

3-27   Andreas, Jonathan, Ronald Reagan is one of the main architects of the U.S. welfare system," Medianism, August 17, 2015, https://medianism.org/2015/08/17/ronald-reagan-is-one-of-the-main-architects-of-the-us-welfare-system/

3-28   Amadeo, Kimberly, "Hillarycare, the Health Security Act of 1993. Hillarycare: What It Was and Why It Failed," The Balance, March 13, 2019, https://www.thebalance.com/hillarycare-comparison-to-obamacare-4101814

3-29   "When Was HIPAA Enacted?," HIPAA Journal, March 9, 2018, https://www.hipaa-journal.com/when-was-hipaa-enacted/

3-30   Burak, Elizabeth Wright, 'What Every Policy Maker Needs to Know about the Children's Health Insurance Program (CHIP) – A Refresher," Georgetown University Health Policy Institute Center for Children and Families, August 3, 2017, https://ccf.georgetown.edu/2017/08/03/what-every-policy-maker-needs-to-know-about-the-childrens-health-insurance-program-chip-a-refresher/

3-31   "Part D / Prescription Drug Benefits," Center for Medicare Advocacy, https://www.medicareadvocacy.org/medicare-info/medicare-part-d/

3-32   "Obamacare Explained / An Explanation of Obamacare," November 16, 2018, https://obamacarefacts.com/obamacare-explained/

Chapter 4:

4-1   Frack, Bill, Andrew Garibaldi, and Andrew Kadar, "Why Medicare Advantage Is Marching Toward 70% Penetration," L.E.K., https://www.lek.com/sites/default/files/insights/pdf-attachments/1969_Medicare_AdvantageLEK_Executive_Insights_1.pdf

4-2   "Managed Care Fact Sheets: National Managed Care Penetration," Data for 2017, http://www.mcol.com/managed_care_penetration

4-3   "Total Medicaid MCO Enrollment," Kaiser Family Foundation, July 2017 data, https://www.kff.org/other/state-indicator/total-medicaid-mco-enrollment/?current-Timeframe=0&sortModel=%7B%22colId%22:%22Location%22,%22sort%22:%22as-c%22%7D

Chapter 5:

5-1   "Generic Drug Competition Lowers Prescription Drug Cost to $6 on Average, Study Finds," Association of Accessible Medicines, July 10, 2018, https://accessiblemeds.org/resources/press-releases/generic-drug-competition-lowers-prescription-cost-6-average-study-finds

5-2   "Average Brand-Name Drug Price Now Over 18 Times Higher Than Average Generic Drug Price, New AARP Report Shows," April 4, 2019, https://press.aarp.org/2019-4-4-Rx-Price-Watch-Report-Generic-Prescription-Drugs

Chapter 6:

6-1   Moffit, Robert E., "Trump's Expansion of Health Reimbursement Accounts Improve Health Care Choices," The Heritage Foundation, June 14, 2019, https://www.heritage.org/health-care-reform/commentary/trumps-expansion-health-reimbursement-accounts-improves-health-care

Chapter 7:

7-1   "Avoiding Surprises in Your Medical Bills A Guide for Consumers," Healthcare Financial Management Association, November 2018, https://www.aha.org/system/files/2018-11/Avoiding-Surprise-Bills-FINAL.pdf

7-2   Davis, Elizabeth, "Balance Billing in Health Insurance," VeryWell Health, June 27, 2019, https://www.verywellhealth.com/balance-billing-what-it-is-how-it-works-1738460

7-3   Hellman, Jessie, "Study: 4 in 10 patients faced surprise bills in 2016 after visiting in-network hospitals," The Hill, August 12, 2019, https://thehill.com/policy/healthcare/457159-study-4-in-10-patients-faced-surprise-bills-in-2016-after-visiting-in

7-4   Pollitz, Karen P, Lunna Lopes, Audrey Kearney, et al., "US Statistics on Surprise Medical Billing," JAMA Network, February 11, 2020, https://jamanetwork.com/journals/jama/fullarticle/2760721

7-5   Appleby, Julie, "Surprise! Congress Takes Steps to Curb Unexpected Medical Bills," Kaiser Health News, December 22, 2020, https://khn.org/news/article/surprise-congress-takes-steps-to-curb-unexpected-medical-bills/

7-6   Hoadley, Jack, Kevin Lucia, and Maanasa Kona, "State Efforts To Protect Consumers From Balance Billing," The Commonwealth Fund, January, 18, 2019, https://www.commonwealthfund.org/blog/2019/state-efforts-protect-consumers-balance-billing

7-7   Kona, Maanasa, "State Balance Billing Protections," The Commonwealth Fund, November 30, 2020, https://www.commonwealthfund.org/publications/maps-and-interactives/2020/nov/state-balance-billing-protections

7-8   Albright, Matthew, "Senate Bill and State Balance Billing Laws Lean On Providers," Zelis, https://www.zelis.com/resource/senate-bill-and-state-balance-billing-laws-lean-on-providers/

7-9   Shen, Wen, "Balance Billing: Current Legal Landscape and Proposed Federal Solutions," Congressional Research Service, April 15, 2019, https://fas.org/sgp/crs/misc/LSB10284.pdf

7-10   Komisar, Harriet, "Medicare's Financial Protections for Consumers: Limits on Balance Billing and Private Contracting by Physicians, America Association of Retired Persons Public Policy Institute, January 2017, https://www.aarp.org/content/dam/aarp/ppi/2017-01/medicare-limits-on-balance-billing-and-private-contracting-ppi.pdf

7-11   Cuppett, Trina, "Medicaid Billing Guidelines," American Academy of Professional Coders," https://www.aapc.com/blog/5190-medicaid-billing-guidelines/

7-12   "Interstate Medicaid Billing Problems: Helping Medicaid Beneficiaries Who Get Care Out of State," Families USA, https://familiesusa.org/sites/default/files/product_documents/Interstate%20Medicaid%20Billing%20Problems.pdf

Chapter 8:

8-1   "Why Public Health Is Necessary to Improve Healthcare," National Association of Chronic Disease Directors, https://cdn.ymaws.com/www.chronicdisease.org/resource/resmgr/white_papers/cd_white_paper_hoffman.pdf

Chapter 9:

9-1 Fox PhD, Peter D. and Peter R. Kongstvedt,MD, "Ch. 1: A History of Managed Health Care and Health Insurance in the United States," The Essentials of Managed Health Care, 2013, https://samples.jbpub.com/9781284043259/Chapter1.pdf

9-2 Tatar, Margaret, Julia Paradise, and Rachel Garfield, "Medi-Cal Managed Care: An Overview and Key Issues," Kaiser Family Foundation, March 2, 2016, https://www.kff.org/medicaid/issue-brief/medi-cal-managed-care-an-overview-and-key-issues/

9-3 "Managed Care Fact Sheets: National Managed Care Penetration," Data for 2017, http://www.mcol.com/managed_care_penetration

9-4 "Total Medicaid MCO Enrollment," Kaiser Family Foundation, July 2017 data, https://www.kff.org/other/state-indicator/total-medicaid-mco-enrollment/?current-Timeframe=0&sortModel=%7B%22colId%22:%22Location%22,%22sort%22:%22asc%22%7D

9-5 Patel, Yash M. and Stuart Guterman, "The Evolution of Private Plans in Medicare," The Commonwealth Fund, December 8, 2017, https://www.commonwealthfund.org/publications/issue-briefs/2017/dec/evolution-private-plans-medicare

9-6 Tobin, Christine, "What is Managed Health Care?", Reprinted from AADE News, American Association of Diabetes Educators, January 1997, https://nfb.org/images/nfb/publications/vodold/mngdcare.htm

9-7 "Private Payers Serving Individuals With Disabilities and Chronic Conditions. Characteristics of Managed Care," Office of the Assistant Secretary for Planning and Evaluation, January 1, 2000, https://aspe.hhs.gov/report/private-payers-serving-individuals-disabilities-and-chronic-conditions/characteristics-managed-care

9-8 Farnham, Will, "Managed Care Plans and Common Acronyms," Healthlinks.net, https://healthlinks.net/archive/will4.html

9-9 Pinkovskiy, Maxim L., "The Impacts of the Managed Care Backlash on Health Care Costs: Evidence From State Regulation of Managed Care Cost Containment Practices," Federal Reserve Bank of New York, October 17, 2013, https://economics.mit.edu/files/8448

9-10 Catlin, Aaron C. and Cathy A. Cowan, "History of Health Spending in the United States, 1960-2013," Centers for Medicare and Medicaid Services, November 19, 2015, https://www.cms.gov/Research-Statistics-Data-and-Systems/Statistics-Trends-and-Reports/NationalHealthExpendData/Downloads/HistoricalNHEPaper.pdf

9-11   Lagoe, Ronald, Deborah L. Aspling, and Gert P. Westert, "Current and future developments in managed care in the United States and implications for Europe," Health research Policies and Systems, U.S. National Library of Medicine, National Institutes of Health, March 17, 2005, https://www.ncbi.nlm.nih.gov/pmc/articles/PMC1079919/

9-12   Centers for Medicare and Medicaid Services National Health Expenditure data website, https://www.cms.gov/Research-Statistics-Data-and-Systems/Statistics-Trends-and-Reports/NationalHealthExpendData/index.html

9-13   Blendon, Robert J., Mollyann Brodie, John M. Benson, Drew E. Altman, Larry Levitt, Tina Hoff, and Larry Hugick, "Understanding the Managed Care Backlash," Health Affairs, July/August 1998, https://www.healthaffairs.org/doi/full/10.1377/hlthaff.17.4.80

9-14   Mechanic, David, "The Managed Care Backlash: Perceptions and Rhetoric in Health Care Policy and the Potential for Health Care Reform, Rutgers University, The Milbank Quarterly, March 2001, https://www.ncbi.nlm.nih.gov/pmc/articles/PMC2751184/

Chapter 10:

10-1   "Understanding Your Insurance Plan: Usual, Customary and Reasonable Charges," Cancer Connect, https://news.cancerconnect.com/treatment-care/understanding-your-insurance-plan-usual-customary-and-reasonable-charges-2bv8PwBmU0C-5fo92usJXuw/

10-2   "Large Employers Double Down on Efforts to Stem Rising U.S> Health Benefit Costs which are Expected to Top $15,000 per Employee in 2020," National Business Group on Health, Press Release, August 13, 2019, https://www.businessgrouphealth.org/news/nbgh-news/press-releases/press-release-details/?ID=361

Chapter 11:

11-1   "2017 Employer Health Benefits Survey," Kaiser Family Foundation, September 19, 2017, https://www.kff.org/report-section/ehbs-2017-section-10-plan-funding/

11-2   "Health Plans and Benefits: ERISA," Department of Labor, https://www.dol.gov/general/topic/health-plans/erisa

11-3 "Appeal a Health Plan Decision: External Review," Healthcare.Gov, Centers for Medicare and Medicaid Services, https://www.healthcare.gov/appeal-insurance-company-decision/external-review/

11-4 "State Health Facts: State External Appeals Review Processes," Kaiser Family Foundation, May 16, 2018, https://www.kff.org/health-reform/state-indicator/external-appeals-review-processes/?currentTimeframe=0&sortModel=%7B%22colId%22:%22Location%22,%22sort%22:%22asc%22%7D

11-5 "Affordable Care Act: Working with States to Protect Consumers," Centers for Medicare and Medicaid Services, May 16, 2018, https://www.cms.gov/CCIIO/Resources/Files/external_appeals.html

11-6 "Quality of Care External Quality Review," Medicaid.gov, Centers for Medicare and Medicaid Services, https://www.medicaid.gov/medicaid/quality-of-care/medicaid-managed-care/external-quality-review/index.html

11-7 "Quality Improvement Organizations," Centers for Medicare and Medicaid Services, https://www.cms.gov/Medicare/Quality-Initiatives-Patient-Assessment-Instruments/QualityImprovementOrgs/index.html

11-8 "File a Complaint," Quality Improvement Organizations, https://qioprogram.org/file-complaint

Chapter 12:

12-1 Senterfitt, Barry, "Material differences exist in HMO vs. Insurer regulations, Managed Healthcare Executive, May 1, 2005, https://www.managedhealthcareexecutive.com/letter-law/material-differences-exist-hmo-vs-insurer-regulations

12-2 "Accountable Care Organizations (ACOs): General Information," Centers for Medicare and Medicaid Services, https://innovation.cms.gov/initiatives/aco/

12-3 National Association of ACOs website, https://www.naacos.com/

12-4 "CMS Provider Incentive (PIP) Regulations and Stop Loss Reinsurance Requirements," FRG, https://frgsystems.com/healthcare-finance-news/cms-pip-regulations-stop-loss-reinsurance-requirements

Chapter 13:

13-1   Centers for Medicare and Medicaid Services National Health Expenditure data website, https://www.cms.gov/Research-Statistics-Data-and-Systems/Statistics-Trends-and-Reports/NationalHealthExpendData/index.html

13-2   "CMS Office of the Actuary Releases 2019 National Health Expenditures," Centers for Medicare and Medicaid Services, December 16, 2020, https://www.cms.gov/newsroom/press-releases/cms-office-actuary-releases-2019-national-health-expenditures

13-3   Berchick, Edward R., Emily Hood, and Jessica C. Barnett "Health Insurance Coverage in the United States: 2017 Current Population Reports," United States Census Bureau, U.S. Department of Commerce, September 2018, https://www.census.gov/content/dam/Census/library/publications/2018/demo/p60-264.pdf

13-4   Minemyer, Paige, "Uninsured rates among young people dropped under ACA: Urban Institute," Fierce Healthcare, February 18, 2021, https://www.fiercehealthcare.com/payer/uninsured-rates-among-young-people-dropped-under-aca-urban-institute

13-5   Artiga, Samantha and Kendal Orgera, "Changes in Health Coverage by Race and ethnicity since implementation of the ACA, 2013-2017," Kaiser Family Foundation, February 13, 2019, https://www.kff.org/disparities-policy/issue-brief/changes-in-health-coverage-by-race-and-ethnicity-since-implementation-of-the-aca-2013-2017/

13-6   Chaudry, Ajay, Adlan Jackson, and Sherry A. Glied, "Did the Affordable Care Act Reduce Racial and Ethnic Disparities in Health Insurance Coverage?", Commonwealth Fund Issue Brief, August 2019, https://www.commonwealthfund.org/sites/default/files/2019-08/Chaudry_did_ACA_reduce_racial_disparities_ib_v3.pdf

13-7   Bivens, Josh and Ben Zipperer, "Health insurance and the COVID-19 shock," The Economic Policy Institute, August 26, 2020, https://www.epi.org/publication/health-insurance-and-the-covid-19-shock/

13-8   King, Robert, "Deloitte: Greater consumer agency will decelerate healthcare spending over next 20 years," Fierce Healthcare, February 8, 2021, https://www.fiercehealthcare.com/payer/deloitte-greater-consumer-agency-will-decelerate-healthcare-spending-over-next-20-years

13-9   Gebreyes, Kulleni, Andy Davis, Steve Davis, Maulesh Shukla, and Brian Rush, "Breaking the cost curve," Deloitte, February 9, 2021, https://www2.deloitte.com/us/en/insights/industry/health-care/future-health-care-spending.html

Chapter 14:

14-1   Centers for Medicare and Medicaid Services National Health Expenditure data website, https://www.cms.gov/Research-Statistics-Data-and-Systems/Statistics-Trends-and-Reports/NationalHealthExpendData/index.html

14-2   Fuglesten Biniek, Jeannie and John Hargraves, "2017 Health Care Cost and Utilization Report," Health Care Cost Institute, February 2019, https://www.healthcostinstitute.org/images/easyblog_articles/276/HCCI-2017-Health-Care-Cost-and-Utilization-Report-02.12.19.pdf

14-3   https://www.cms.gov/research-statistics-data-and-systems/statistics-trends-and-reports/cms-fast-facts/index.html

14-4   "Medicare Spending Per Enrollee, By State," Kaiser Family Foundation, https://www.kff.org/medicare/state-indicator/per-enrollee-spending-by-residence/?currentTimeframe=0&sortModel=%7B%22colId%22:%22Location%22,%22sort%22:%22asc%22%7D

14-5   "An Overview of Medicare," Kaiser Family Foundation, February 13, 2019, https://www.kff.org/medicare/issue-brief/an-overview-of-medicare/

14-6   Allen, Kristin, "Medicaid Managed Care Spending in 2017," Health Management Associates Blog, April 2, 2018, https://www.healthmanagement.com/blog/medicaid-managed-care-spending-2017/

14-7   "State Health Facts: Distribution of Medicaid Spending by Service, FY 2017" Kaiser Family Foundation, https://www.kff.org/medicaid/state-indicator/distribution-of-medicaid-spending-by-service/?currentTimeframe=0&sortModel=%7B%22colId%22:%22Location%22,%22sort%22:%22asc%22%7D

14-8   Rudowitz, Robin, Rachel Garfield, and Elizabeth Hinton, "10 Things to Know about Medicaid: Setting the Facts Straight," Kaiser Family Foundation, March 6, 2019, https://www.kff.org/medicaid/issue-brief/10-things-to-know-about-medicaid-setting-the-facts-straight/

14-9   "Medicaid Facts and Figures," Centers for Medicare and Medicaid Services, January 30, 2020, https://www.cms.gov/newsroom/fact-sheets/medicaid-facts-and-figures

Chapter 15:

15-1   Bannow, Tara, "Dems villainize insurers, even as pharma profits dominate," Modern
         Healthcare, August 1, 2019, https://www.modernhealthcare.com/finance/dems-vil-
         lainize-insurers-even-pharma-profits-dominate?utm_source=modern-healthcare-am-fri-
         day&utm_medium=email&utm_campaign=20190802&utm_content=article1-head-
         line

Chapter 16:

16-1   Barrette, PhD, Eric and Niall Brennan, MPP, "The Value of Health Insurance through
         Price Discounts, NEJM Catalyst, New England Journal of Medicine, November 20,
         2017, https://catalyst.nejm.org/value-health-insurance-price-discounts/

16-2   Myers, Lynn, "Determining discounts," Milliman White Paper, 2012, http://www.
         milliman.com/uploadedFiles/insight/healthreform/pdfs/determining-discounts.pdf

16-3   Pelech, Daria, "An Analysis of Private-Sector Prices for Physicians' Services," Working
         Paper Series, Working Paper, 2018-01, Congressional Budget Office, January
         2018, https://www.cbo.gov/system/files/115th-congress-2017-2018/workingpa-
         per/53441-workingpaper.pdf

Chapter 17:

17-1   Centers for Medicare and Medicaid Services National Health Expenditure data website,
         https://www.cms.gov/Research-Statistics-Data-and-Systems/Statistics-Trends-and-Re-
         ports/NationalHealthExpendData/index.html

17-2   "2020 Employer Health Benefits Survey," Kaiser Family Foundation, October 8, 2020,
         https://www.kff.org/report-section/ehbs-2020-section-1-cost-of-health-insurance/

17-3   Harding, Leslie, "What's the Difference Between Small Group and Large Group Health
         Insurance," Gusto Blog, November 1, 2019, https://gusto.com/blog/health-insurance/
         small-vs-large-group-health-insurance

17-4   Norris, Louise, "How Obamacare changed group health insurance," Healthinsurance.
         org, November 28, 2016, https://www.healthinsurance.org/group-health-insurance/

17-5　Cauchi, Richard, "ACA Requirements for Medium and Large Employers to Offer Health Coverage," National Conference of State Legislatures, June 22, 2016, https://www.ncsl.org/documents/health/aca_requirements_for_employers.pdf

17-6　"Grandfathered Status Fact Sheet," Cigna website, August 2018, https://www.cigna.com/assets/docs/about-cigna/informed-on-reform/grandfathered-plan-fact-sheet.pdf?WT.z_nav=health-care-reform%2Ffaqs%3Baccordion%3BWhat%20are%20grandfathered%20plans%3F%3BGrandfathered%20Plan%20Fact%20Sheet

17-7　"What It Means To Be Grandfathered," Medical Mutual website, https://www.medmutual.com/Healthcare-Reform/The-Basics/Grandfathered-Status.aspx

17-8　King, Robert, "DOL, HHS finalize rule to give more flexibility to ACA grandfathered plans," Fierce Healthcare, December 11, 2020, https://www.fiercehealthcare.com/payer/dol-hhs-finalize-rule-to-give-more-flexibility-to-aca-grandfathered-plans

17-9　Appold, Karen, "The State of Employer-Sponsored Healthcare," Managed Healthcare Executive, March 6, 2019, https://www.managedhealthcareexecutive.com/business-strategy/state-employer-sponsored-healthcare

Chapter 18:

18-1　https://www.cms.gov/Medicare-Medicaid-Coordination/Medicare-and-Medicaid-Coordination/Medicare-Medicaid-Coordination-Office/Downloads/MMCO_Factsheet.pdf

18-2　"Dual-Eligible Beneficiaries Under Medicare and Medicaid," Centers for Medicare and Medicaid Services, May 2018, https://www.cms.gov/Outreach-and-Education/Medicare-Learning-Network-MLN/MLNProducts/downloads/Medicare_Beneficiaries_Dual_Eligibles_At_a_Glance.pdf

Chapter 19:

19-1　Frack, Bill, Andrew Garibaldi, and Andrew Kadar, "Why Medicare Advantage Is Marching Toward 70% Penetration," L.E.K., https://www.lek.com/sites/default/files/insights/pdf-attachments/1969_Medicare_AdvantageLEK_Executive_Insights_1.pdf

19-2   Centers for Medicare and Medicaid Services National Health Expenditure data website, https://www.cms.gov/Research-Statistics-Data-and-Systems/Statistics-Trends-and-Reports/NationalHealthExpendData/index.html

19-3   "An Overview of Medicare," Kaiser Family Foundation, February 13, 2019, https://www.kff.org/medicare/issue-brief/an-overview-of-medicare/

19-4   https://www.medicare.gov/supplements-other-insurance/how-to-compare-medigap-policies

19-5   https://www.cms.gov/Medicare/Eligibility-and-Enrollment/OrigMedicarePartABEligEnrol/index

19-6   "When to Apply for Medicare: Late-Enrollment Penalties," eHealth Medicare, https://www.ehealthmedicare.com/medicare-enrollment-articles/when-to-apply-medicare-late-enrollment-penalties/

19-7   "What You Need To Know About Medicare's Late Enrollment Penalty," Aging in Place, February 2020, https://www.aginginplace.org/what-you-need-to-know-about-medicares-late-enrollment-penalties/

19-8   https://www.cms.gov/files/document/2020-medicare-trustees-report.pdf

19-9   Cubanski, Juliette and Tricia Neuman, "FAQs on Medicare Financing and Trust Fund Solvency, Kasier Family Foundation, March 16, 2021, https://www.kff.org/medicare/issue-brief/faqs-on-medicare-financing-and-trust-fund-solvency/

19-10   "The benefit period," Medicare Interactive, Medicare Rights Center, https://www.medicareinteractive.org/get-answers/medicare-covered-services/inpatient-hospital-services/the-benefit-period

19-11   "Medicare and You, "2021 Edition, Centers for Medicare and Medicaid Services, https://www.medicare.gov/Pubs/pdf/10050-Medicare-and-You.pdf

19-12   "Medicare Part A covered services," Medicare Interactive, Medicare Rights Center, https://www.medicareinteractive.org/get-answers/medicare-covered-services/medicare-coverage-overview/summary-of-part-a-covered-services

19-13   https://www.cms.gov/newsroom/fact-sheets/2021-medicare-parts-b-premiums-and-deductibles#:~:text=The%20standard%20monthly%20premium%20for,deductible%20of%20%24198%20in%202020.

19-14   "SNF basics," Medicare Interactive, Medicare Rights Center, https://www.medicareinteractive.org/get-answers/medicare-covered-services/skilled-nursing-facility-snf-services/snf-basics

19-15   https://www.medicare.gov/coverage/skilled-nursing-facility-snf-care

19-16   https://www.medicare.gov/coverage/home-health-services

19-17   https://www.medicare.gov/coverage/hospice-care

19-18   https://www.medicare.gov/your-medicare-costs/medicare-costs-at-a-glance

19-19   "Medicare Part B covered services," Medicare Interactive, Medicare Rights Center, https://www.medicareinteractive.org/get-answers/medicare-covered-services/medi-care-coverage-overview/summary-of-part-b-covered-services

19-20   What is CMMI? And 11 other FAQs about the CMS Innovation Center," Kaiser Family Foundation, February 27, 2018, https://www.kff.org/medicare/fact-sheet/what-is-cmmi-and-11-other-faqs-about-the-cms-innovation-center/

19-21   LaPointe, Jacqueline, "36% of Payments Tied to Alternative Payment Models in 2018," Rev Cycle Intelligence, Xtelligent Healthcare Media, October 24, 2019, https://revcy-cleintelligence.com/news/36-of-payments-tied-to-alternative-payment-models-in-2018

Chapter 20:

20-1   Frack, Bill, Andrew Garibaldi, and Andrew Kadar, "Why Medicare Advantage Is Marching Toward 70% Penetration," L.E.K., https://www.lek.com/sites/default/files/insights/pdf-attachments/1969_Medicare_AdvantageLEK_Executive_Insights_1.pdf

20-2   Freed, Meredith, Anthony Damico, and Tricia Neuman, "A Dozen Facts About Medi-care Advantage in 2020," Kaiser Family Foundation, January 13, 2021, https://www.kff.org/medicare/issue-brief/a-dozen-facts-about-medicare-advantage-in-2020/

20-3   "Trump Administration Announces Historically Low Medicare Advantage Premiums and New Payment Model to Make Insulin Affordable Again for Seniors," Press Release, CMS Newsroom, CMS.gov, September 24, 2020, https://www.cms.gov/newsroom/press-releases/trump-administration-announces-historically-low-medicare-advan-tage-premiums-and-new-payment-model

20-4   "Announcement of Calendar Year (CY) 2020 Medicare Advantage Capitation Rates and Medicare Advantage and Part D Payment Policies and Final Call Letter," Centers for Medicare and Medicaid Services, April 1, 2019, https://www.cms.gov/Medicare/Health-Plans/MedicareAdvtgSpecRateStats/Downloads/Announcement2020.pdf

20-5 "Fact Sheet - 2020 Part C and D Star Ratings," Centers for Medicare and Medicaid Services, October 8, 2020, https://www.cms.gov/files/document/2021starratingsfact-sheet-10-08-2020.pdf

20-6 https://www.cms.gov/research-statistics-data-and-systems/statistics-trends-and-reports/cms-fast-facts/index.html

20-7 "Medicare and You, " 2021 Edition, Centers for Medicare and Medicaid Services, https://www.medicare.gov/Pubs/pdf/10050-Medicare-and-You.pdf

20-8 https://bettermedicarealliance.org/news/analysis-medicare-advantage-supplemental-benefits-grew-in-36-out-of-41-categories-for-2021/
https://bettermedicarealliance.org/wp-content/uploads/2021/02/2-10-21-cy-2021-ma-supplemental-benefits-v1.ashx_.pdf

20-9 https://www.medicare.gov/sign-up-change-plans/types-of-medicare-health-plans/medicare-advantage-plans

20-10 "Understanding Medicare Advantage Plans," Centers for Medicare and Medicaid Services, https://www.medicare.gov/Pubs/pdf/12026-Understanding-Medicare-Advantage-Plans.pdf

20-11 "Types of Medicare Advantage Coverage," Medicare Interactive, Medicare Rights Center, https://www.medicareinteractive.org/get-answers/types-of-medicare-advantage-coverage

20-12 "Employer Group Waiver Plans," White Paper, Better Medicare Alliance, March 2018, https://www.bettermedicarealliance.org/sites/default/files/2018-03/BMA_Employer-GroupWaiverPlans_WhitePaper_2018_03_02_FINAL.pdf

20-13 https://www.medicare.gov/sign-up-change-plans/when-can-i-join-a-health-or-drug-plan/special-circumstances-special-enrollment-periods

20-14 MedPAC presentation, December 3, 2020, http://medpac.gov/docs/default-source/meeting-materials/ma-status-medpac-dec-2020.pdf?sfvrsn=0

20-15 "Executive Summary and Chapter 12," Report to Congress: Medicare Payment Policy, MedPAC, March 2021, http://medpac.gov/docs/default-source/reports/mar21_medpac_report_to_the_congress_sec.pdf?sfvrsn=0

20-16 Holahan, John and Stacey McMorrow, "Slow Growth in Medicare and Medicaid Spending per Enrollee Has Implications for Policy Debates," Urban Institute, February 2019, https://www.urban.org/sites/default/files/publication/99748/rwjf451631_1.pdf

20-17   "Chapter 13 -- The Medicare Advantage program: status report," Report to Congress: Medicare Payment Policy, MedPAC, March 2020, http://www.medpac.gov/docs/default-source/reports/mar20_medpac_ch13_sec.pd

20-18   King, Robert, "MedPAC supports changes to the development of MA plan payment benchmarks," Fierce Healthcare, October 2, 2020, https://www.fiercehealthcare.com/payer/medpac-supports-changes-to-development-ma-plan-payment-benchmarks

20-19   Brady, Michelle, "MedPAC likely to recommend an effective cut in Medicare Advantage spending," Modern Healthcare, March 5, 2021, https://www.modernhealthcare.com/medicare/medpac-likely-recommend-effective-cut-medicare-advantage-spending

20-20   MedPAC presentation, April 1, 2021, http://www.medpac.gov/docs/default-source/meeting-materials/ma-benchmarks-medpac-april-2021.pdf?sfvrsn=0

20-21   "Chapter 1 -- Rebalancing Medicare Advantage benchmark policy," Report to the Congress, Medicare and the Health Care Delivery System," MedPAC, June 2021, http://www.medpac.gov/docs/default-source/reports/jun21_medpac_report_to_congress_sec.pdf?sfvrsn=0

20-22   "Chapter 3 -- Replacing the Medicare Advantage quality bonus program," Report to the Congress: Medicare and the Health Care Delivery System," MedPAC, June 2020, http://www.medpac.gov/docs/default-source/reports/jun20_reporttocongress_sec.pdf

20-23   Bannow, Tara, "Little change in regional Medicare spending differences, despite attention," Modern Healthcare, November 28, 2020, https://www.modernhealthcare.com/medicare/little-change-regional-medicare-spending-differences-despite-attention

Chapter 21:

21-1   King, Robert, "Seniors on Medicare Advantage Less Likely to Have Issues Paying Medical Bills: CDC Study," Fierce Healthcare, February 13, 2020, https://www.fiercehealthcare.com/payer/seniors-ma-less-likely-than-traditional-medicare-to-have-issues-paying-medical-bills-cdc

21-2   Cha, Ph.D., M.P.H., Amy E., Robin A. Cohen, Ph.D "Problems Paying Medical Bills, 2018," NCHS Data Brief, No. 357, National Center for Health Statistics, Centers for Disease Control and Prevention, Department of Health and Human Services, February 2020 https://www.cdc.gov/nchs/data/databriefs/db357-h.pdf

21-3 "Medicare Advantage Provides Key Financial Protections to Low- and Modest Income Populations, Analysis by Anne Tumlinson Innovations, Better Medicare Alliance, July 2019, https://www.bettermedicarealliance.org/sites/default/files/2019-07/BMA_Research%20Brief_2019_07_09_Income%20Populations.pdf

21-4 Minemyer, Paige, "UnitedHealth study: Medicare Advantage members spend 40% less per year than fee-for-service beneficiaries," Fierce Healthcare, April 12, 2021, https://www.fiercehealthcare.com/payer/unitedhealth-study-medicare-advantage-members-spend-40-less-per-year-than-fee-for-service

21-5 King, Robert, "Medicare Advantage plans achieve better outcomes than traditional Medicare, BMA analysis finds," Fierce Healthcare, December 9, 2020, https://www.fiercehealthcare.com/payer/medicare-advantage-plans-achieve-better-outcomes-than-traditional-medicare-bma-analysis-finds

21-6 Minemyer, Paige, Study: Higher MA star ratings associated with improvements in members' outcomes, "Fierce Healthcare, February 2, 2021, https://www.fiercehealthcare.com/payer/study-higher-ma-star-ratings-associated-improvements-members-outcomes

21-7 "New Study: Medicare Advantage Serves Beneficiaries with Higher Social Risk Factors," Better Medicare Alliance, September 8, 2020, https://www.bettermedicarealliance.org/news/new-study-medicare-advantage-serves-beneficiaries-with-higher-social-risk-factors/

21-8 https://bettermedicarealliance.org/news/poll-medicare-advantage-satisfaction-hits-new-high-amid-covid-19-crisis/ https://bettermedicarealliance.org/wp-content/uploads/2021/01/BMA_Seniors-on-Medicare-Memo_.pdf

21-9 Jacobson, Gretchen, Rachel Fehr, Cynthia Cox, Tricia Newman, "Financial Performance of Medicare Advantage, Individual and Group Health Insurance Markets, Kaiser Family Foundation, August 5, 2019, https://www.kff.org/report-section/financial-performance-of-medicare-advantage-individual-and-group-health-insurance-markets-issue-brief/

Chapter 22:

22-1 https://www.cms.gov/Medicare-Medicaid-Coordination/Medicare-and-Medicaid-Co-ordination/Medicare-Medicaid-Coordination-Office/Downloads/MMCO_Factsheet.pdf

22-2 https://www.cms.gov/Medicare/Health-Plans/SpecialNeedsPlans/Downloads/Special-Need-Plans-SNP-Frequently-Asked-Questions-FAQ.pdf

22-3 Nicholas Johnson, Christopher Kunkel, and Annie Hallum, "Changing how Medicare and Medicaid talk to each other," Milliman, March 18, 2020, https://www.milliman.com/en/insight/changing-how-medicare-and-medicaid-talk-to-each-other

Chapter 23:

23-1 Funk, Allyson, Five Things You Might Not Know About Medicare Part D," The Catalyst, PhRMA Website, October 15, 2014, https://catalyst.phrma.org/five-things-you-might-not-know-about-medicare-part-d

23-2 McCaughan, Mike, "Medicare Part D," Health Affairs, August 10, 2017, https://www.healthaffairs.org/do/10.1377/hpb20171008.000172/full/

23-3 "Medicare Part D," PhRMA Website, https://www.phrma.org/en/Advocacy/Medicare/PartD?utm_campaign=2020-q1-phb&utm_medium=pai-cpc-blg-ggl-adf&utm_source=ggl&utm_content=awr-cli-pat-scl-beh-usa-all-nap-tgt-pai-cpc-blg-ggl-adf-WhatIsPartD-acc-edu-inf-lrh-lpg-std-vra-adf&utm_term=nap&gclid=Cj0KCQiA1-3yBRCmARIsAN7B4H3D4xR78Qk5e-jpHVuNb5gcdwTFYzfQR90qYtsNx4K0mCIDy9Z0bu80aApLMEALw_wcB

23-4 "An Overview of the Medicare Part D Prescription Drug Benefit," Kaiser Family Foundation, October 13, 2021, https://www.kff.org/medicare/fact-sheet/an-overview-of-the-medicare-part-d-prescription-drug-benefit/

Cubanski, Juliette and Anthony Damico, "Medicare Part D: A First Look at Medicare Prescription Drug Plans in 2021," Kaiser Family Foundation, October 29, 2020, https://www.kff.org/medicare/issue-brief/medicare-part-d-a-first-look-at-medicare-prescription-drug-plans-in-2021/

23-5 "10 Essential Facts About Medicare and Prescription Drug Spending," Kaiser Family Foundation, January 29, 2019, https://www.kff.org/infographic/10-essential-facts-about-medicare-and-prescription-drug-spending/

23-6   "State Pharmaceutical Assistance Programs," Medicare Rights Center, https://www.medicareinteractive.org/pdf/SPAP-Chart.pdf

23-7   "Part D/Prescription Drug Benefits," Center for Medicare Advocacy, https://www.medicareadvocacy.org/medicare-info/medicare-part-d/#retiree%20subsidy

23-8   "2021 Medicare Part D Outlook," q1 Medicare.com, https://q1medicare.com/PartD-The-2021-Medicare-Part-D-Outlook.php

23-9   "Part D Payment System," MedPAC, October 2016, http://www.medpac.gov/docs/default-source/payment-basics/medpac_payment_basics_16_partd_final.pdf

23-10   https://secure.ssa.gov/poms.nsf/lnx/0603001005

23-11   "Medicare Low Income Subsidy: Get Extra Help Paying for Part D," Center for Benefits Access, National Council on Aging, https://www.ncoa.org/economic-security/benefits/prescriptions/lis-extrahelp/

23-12   O'Neill Hayes, Tara, "More Evidence of The Need for Structural Reform in Medicare Part D," Insight, American Action Forum, January 25, 2019, https://www.american-actionforum.org/insight/evidence-for-structural-reform-part-d/

23-13   Cubanski, Juliette, and Tricia Neuman, "How Will The Medicare Part D Benefit Change Under Current Law and Leading Proposals?," Kaiser Family Foundation, October 11, 2019, https://www.kff.org/medicare/issue-brief/how-will-the-medicare-part-d-benefit-change-under-current-law-and-leading-proposals/

Chapter 24:

24-1   "Total Medicaid Spending," Kaiser Family Foundation, FY 2018, https://www.kff.org/medicaid/state-indicator/total-medicaid-spending/?currentTimeframe=0&sortModel=%7B%22colId%22:%22Location%22,%22sort%22:%22asc%22%7D

24-2   Centers for Medicare and Medicaid Services National Health Expenditure data website, https://www.cms.gov/Research-Statistics-Data-and-Systems/Statistics-Trends-and-Reports/NationalHealthExpendData/index.html

24-3   https://www.cms.gov/research-statistics-data-and-systems/statistics-trends-and-reports/cms-fast-facts/index.html

24-4   "Managed care authorities," Medicaid.gov, Centers for Medicare and Medicaid Services, https://www.medicaid.gov/medicaid/managed-care/authorities/index.html

24-5 "Home & Community-Based Services 1915(c)," Medicaid.gov, Centers for Medicare and Medicaid Services, https://www.medicaid.gov/medicaid/hcbs/authorities/1915-c/index.html

24-6 "Eligibility, Medicaid.gov, Centers for Medicare and Medicaid Services, https://www.medicaid.gov/medicaid/eligibility/index.html

24-7 "Mandatory and Optional Medicaid Benefits, Medicaid.gov, Centers for Medicare and Medicaid Services, https://www.medicaid.gov/medicaid/benefits/list-of-benefits/index.html

24-8 "Federal Medical Assistance Percentage (FMAP) for Medicaid and Multiplier," Kaiser Family Foundation, https://www.kff.org/medicaid/state-indicator/federal-matching-rate-and-multiplier/?currentTimeframe=0&sortModel=%7B%22colId%22:%22Location%22,%22sort%22:%22asc%22%7D

24-9 "Medicaid Financing: An Overview of the Federal Medicaid Matching Rate (FMAP)," Kaiser Family Foundation, September 30, 2012, https://www.kff.org/health-reform/issue-brief/medicaid-financing-an-overview-of-the-federal/

24-10 Mitchell, Alison, "Medicaid's Federal Medical Assistance Percentage (FMAP)," Congressional Research Service, April 25, 2018, https://fas.org/sgp/crs/misc/R43847.pdf

24-11 Rudowitz, Robin, Kendal Orgera, and Elizabeth Hinton, "Medicaid Financing: The Basics," Kaiser Family Foundation, March 21, 2019, https://www.kff.org/report-section/medicaid-financing-the-basics-issue-brief/

24-12 "Managed Care Fact Sheets: National Managed Care Penetration," Data for 2017, http://www.mcol.com/managed_care_penetration

24-13 "Total Medicaid MCO Enrollment," Kaiser Family Foundation, July 2017 data, https://www.kff.org/other/state-indicator/total-medicaid-mco-enrollment/?currentTimeframe=0&sortModel=%7B%22colId%22:%22Location%22,%22sort%22:%22asc%22%7D

24-14 Lieberman, Richard and Bradley Bruce Armstrong, FSA, MAAA, "Session 65 L, Medicaid Risk Adjustment: Role of Encounter Data and Understanding Model-Specific Nuances," 2017 SOA Health Meeting, Hollywood, FL, Society of Actuaries, June 12-14, 2017, https://www.soa.org/globalassets/assets/files/e-business/pd/events/2017/health-meeting/pd-2017-06-health-session-065.pdf

Chapter 25:

25-1   Weissmann, Jordan, "Enrolling Americans in Medicaid Is Now Cheaper Than Subsidizing Their Obamacare Coverage," Slate, August 10, 2018, https://slate.com/business/2018/08/medicaid-expansion-is-now-more-cost-effective-than-obamacare-exchanges.html

25-2   https://www.cms.gov/research-statistics-data-and-systems/statistics-trends-and-reports/cms-fast-facts/index.html

25-3   Marketplace Enrollment, 2014-2021, Kaiser Family Foundation, https://www.kff.org/health-reform/state-indicator/marketplace-enrollment/?currentTimeframe=4&sortModel=%7B%22colId%22:%22Location%22,%22sort%22:%22asc%22%7D

25-4   https://www.hhs.gov/about/news/2021/09/15/biden-harris-administration-announces-2-8-million-people-gained-affordable-health-coverage-during-2021-special-enrollment.html

25-5   Galewicz, Phil, "Nearly Half of U.S. Births Are Covered by Medicaid, Study Finds," Kaiser Health News, September 3, 2013, https://khn.org/news/nearly-half-of-u-s-births-are-covered-by-medicaid-study-finds/

25-6   Benz, Christine, "75 Must-Know Statistics About Long-Term Care: 2018 Edition," Morningstar, August 20, 2018, https://www.morningstar.com/articles/879494/75-mustknow-statistics-about-longterm-care-2018-ed

25-7   https://www.cms.gov/Medicare-Medicaid-Coordination/Medicare-and-Medicaid-Coordination/Medicare-Medicaid-Coordination-Office/Downloads/MMCO_Factsheet.pdf

25-8   Snyder, Laura and Robin Rudowicz, "Medicaid Enrollment Snapshot: December 2013," Kaiser Family Foundation, June 3, 2014, https://www.kff.org/medicaid/issue-brief/medicaid-enrollment-snapshot-december-2013/

25-9   https://www.medicaid.gov/about-us/program-history/medicaid-50th-anniversary/?entry=47688

25-10   "Status of State Medicaid Expansion Decision: Interactive Map," Kaiser Family Foundation, March 12, 2021, https://www.kff.org/medicaid/issue-brief/status-of-state-medicaid-expansion-decisions-interactive-map/

25-11   Rudowitz, Robin, "5 Key Questions: Medicaid Block Grants and Per Capita Caps" Kaiser Family Foundation, January 31, 2017, https://www.kff.org/medicaid/issue-brief/5-key-questions-medicaid-block-grants-per-capita-caps/

Chapter 26:

26-1 "The Children's Health Insurance Program," Georgetown University Health Policy Institute, February 6, 2017, https://ccf.georgetown.edu/2017/02/06/about-chip/

26-2 https://www.cms.gov/research-statistics-data-and-systems/statistics-trends-and-reports/cms-fast-facts/index.html

26-3 Brooks, Tricia, Lauren Roygardner, and Samantha Artiga, Medicaid and CHIP Eligibility, enrollment, and Cost Sharing Policies as of January 2019: Findings from a 50-State Survey," Kaiser Family Foundation, March 27, 2019, https://www.kff.org/medicaid/report/medicaid-and-chip-eligibility-enrollment-and-cost-sharing-policies-as-of-january-2019-findings-from-a-50-state-survey/

26-4 "CHIP financing," MACPAC, https://www.macpac.gov/subtopic/financing/

26-5 Brooks, Tricia, "CHIP Funding Has Been Extended, What's Next For Children's Health Coverage?," Health Affairs, January 30, 2018, https://www.healthaffairs.org/do/10.1377/hblog20180130.116879/full/

26-6 Schneider, Andy, "The End-of-Year COVID Relief Package: Medicaid and CHIP Highlights," Center for Children and Families, Georgetown University Health Policy Institute, January 6, 2021, https://ccf.georgetown.edu/2021/01/06/the-end-of-year-covid-relief-package-medicaid-and-chip-highlights/

26-7 The Children's Health Insurance Program, Families USA, September 2019, https://familiesusa.org/wp-content/uploads/2019/09/CHIP_101.fin_.pdf

Chapter 27:

27-1 Centers for Medicare and Medicaid Services National Health Expenditure data website, https://www.cms.gov/Research-Statistics-Data-and-Systems/Statistics-Trends-and-Reports/NationalHealthExpendData/index.html

27-2 "Status of State Medicaid Expansion Decision: Interactive Map," Kaiser Family Foundation, March 21, 2021, https://www.kff.org/medicaid/issue-brief/status-of-state-medicaid-expansion-decisions-interactive-map/

27-3 "Medicaid enrollment changes following the ACA," MACPAC, https://www.macpac.gov/subtopic/medicaid-enrollment-changes-following-the-aca/

27-4   "Health Coverage Under the Affordable Care Act: Enrollment Trends and State Esti-
        mates," Office of Health Policy, ASPE, Department of Health and Human Services,
        June 5, 2021, https://aspe.hhs.gov/system/files/pdf/265671/ASPE%20Issue%20Brief-
        ACA-Related%20Coverage%20by%20State.pdf

27-5   Marketplace Enrollment, 2014-2021, Kaiser Family Foundation, https://www.kff.org/
        health-reform/state-indicator/marketplace-enrollment/?currentTimeframe=4&sort-
        Model=%7B%22colId%22:%22Location%22,%22sort%22:%22asc%22%7D

27-6   https://www.hhs.gov/about/news/2021/09/15/biden-harris-administration-an-
        nounces-2-8-million-people-gained-affordable-health-coverage-during-2021-special-en-
        rollment.html

27-7   "Are you eligible to use the Marketplace?" healthcare.gov, https://www.healthcare.gov/
        quick-guide/eligibility/

27-8   "State Health Insurance Marketplace Types, 2021," Kaiser Family Foundation,
        https://www.kff.org/health-reform/state-indicator/state-health-insurance-mar-
        ketplace-types/?currentTimeframe=0&sortModel=%7B%22colId%22:%22Loca-
        tion%22,%22sort%22:%22asc%22%7D

27-9   "Building the Health Insurance Marketplace," National Conference of State Legis-
        latures, https://www.ncsl.org/research/health/american-health-benefit-exchanges.
        aspx#acabasic

27-10   Claxton, Gary, Cynthia Fox, and Matthew Rae, "The Cost of Care with Marketplace
        Coverage," Kaiser Family Foundation, February 11, 2015, https://www.kff.org/health-
        costs/issue-brief/the-cost-of-care-with-marketplace-coverage/

27-11   "Explaining Health Care Reform: Questions About Health Insurance Subsidies,"
        Kaiser Family Foundation, January 16, 2020, https://www.kff.org/health-reform/
        issue-brief/explaining-health-care-reform-questions-about-health/

27-12   "Poverty Guidelines 2021," HHS website, https://aspe.hhs.gov/poverty-guidelines

27-13   "Unsubsidized Enrollment on the Individual Market Dropped 45 Percent from 2016
        to 2019, CMS Newsroom, Centers for Medicare and Medicaid Services, October 9,
        2020, https://www.cms.gov/newsroom/press-releases/unsubsidized-enrollment-indi-
        vidual-market-dropped-45-percent-2016-2019-0

27-14   Norris, Louise, "The ACA's cost-sharing subsidies," Healthinsurance.org, September
        23, 2019, https://www.healthinsurance.org/obamacare/the-acas-cost-sharing-subsidies/

27-15 "Cost-sharing reductions," Healthcare.gov, https://www.healthcare.gov/lower-costs/save-on-out-of-pocket-costs/

27-16 https://www.healthcare.gov/small-businesses/choose-and-enroll/shop-marketplace-overview/

27-17 https://www.healthcare.gov/small-businesses/provide-shop-coverage/small-business-tax-credits/

27-18 https://www.cms.gov/CCIIO/Programs-and-Initiatives/Health-Insurance-Marketplaces/SHOP

27-19 Holt, Christopher, "The American Rescue Plan and Health Policy," Insight, American Action Forum, February 11, 2021, https://www.americanactionforum.org/insight/the-american-rescue-plan-and-health-policy/

27-20 Lotven, Amy, Senate Dems' Bill would Enhance, Fund ACA's Cost-Sharing Reductions," Inside Health Policy, March 10, 2021, https://insidehealthpolicy.com/daily-news/senate-dems%E2%80%99-bill-would-enhance-fund-aca%E2%80%99s-cost-sharing-reductions

27-21 Liss, Samantha, "Average marketplace premiums for 2020 show smallest increases ever," Healthcare Dive, August 13, 2019, https://www.healthcaredive.com/news/average-marketplace-premiums-for-2020-show-smallest-increase-ever/560866/

27-22 Waddell, Kelsey, "ACA Premiums Will Fall 4% and 20 Payers Join Marketplace in 2020," Health Payer Intelligence, October 25, 2019, https://healthpayerintelligence.com/news/aca-premiums-will-fall-4-and-20-payers-join-marketplace-in-2020

27-23 Fehr, Rachel, Rabah Kamal, and Cynthia Cox, "How ACA Marketplace Premiums Are Changing by County in 2020," Kaiser Family Foundation, November 7, 2019, https://www.kff.org/health-costs/issue-brief/how--marketplace-premiums-are-changing-by-county-in-2020/

27-24 McDermott, Daniel and Cynthia Cox, How ACA Marketplace Premiums Are Changing by County in 2021," Kaiser Family Foundation, November 11, 2020, https://www.kff.org/private-insurance/issue-brief/how-aca-marketplace-premiums-are-changing-by-county-in-2021/#:~:text=Premiums%20for%20ACA%20Marketplace%20benchmark,for%20the%20third%20consecutive aca %20year.&text=Because%20insurers%20load%20additional%20costs,the%20cost%20of%20silver%20plans.

27-25   King, Robert, "Cigna plans to expand its ACA exchange presence in 2021," Fierce Healthcare, September 9, 2020, https://www.fiercehealthcare.com/payer/cigna-will-expand-aca-presence-by-27-2021

27-26   Japsen, Bruce, "Cigna Will Expand Obamacare To More Than 200 Counties In 10 States For 2021," Forbes, September 9, 2020, https://www-forbes-com.cdn.ampproject. org/c/s/www.forbes.com/sites/brucejapsen/2020/09/09/cigna-will-expand-obamacare-plans-to-300-counties-in-10-states-for-2021/amp/

27-27   Japsen, Bruce, "Centene Will expand Obamacare To 400 New Counties For 2021,", Forbes, September 11, 2020, https://www-forbes-com.cdn.ampproject.org/c/s/www. forbes.com/sites/brucejapsen/2020/09/11/centene-will-expand-obamacare-to-400-new-counties-for-2021/amp/

27-28   McDermott, Daniel and Cynthia cox, "Insurer Participation on ACA Marketplaces, 2014-2021,"Kaiser Family Foundation, November 23, 2020, https://www.kff.org/private-insurance/issue-brief/insurer-participation-on-the-aca-marketplaces-2014-2021/

27-29   "Plan Year 2021 Qualified Health Plan Choice and Premiums in HealthCare.gov States," Centers for Medicare and Medicaid Services, November 23, 2020, https://www.cms. gov/CCIIO/Resources/Data-Resources/Downloads/2021QHPPremiumsChoiceReport.pdf

27-30   Waddell, Kelsey, "Aetna to Re-Enter ACA Individual Health Insurance Marketplace," Health Payer Intelligence, February 17, 2021, https://healthpayerintelligence.com/news/aetna-to-re-enter-aca-individual-health-insurance-marketplace

Chapter 28:

28-1   Reinhardt, Uwe, Priced Out: The Economic and Ethical Costs of American Health Care, Princeton University Press, 2019, page xxiii

28-2   Centers for Medicare and Medicaid Services National Health Expenditure data website, https://www.cms.gov/Research-Statistics-Data-and-Systems/Statistics-Trends-and-Reports/NationalHealthExpendData/index.html

28-3 Mossialos, Elias, Ana Djordjevic, Robin Osborn, and Dana Sarnak (editors), "International Profiles of Health Care Systems," The Commonwealth Fund, May 2017, https://www.commonwealthfund.org/sites/default/files/documents/___media_files_publications_fund_report_2017_may_mossialos_intl_profiles_v5.pdf

28-4 Roosa Tikkanen, Multinational Comparisons of Health Systems Data, 2018," The Commonwealth Fund, https://www.commonwealthfund.org/sites/default/files/2018-12/Multinational%20Comparisons%20of%20Health%20Systems%20Data%202018_RTikkanen_final.pdf

28-5 "The U.S. Health Care System: An International Perspective,"2016 Fact Sheet, Department for Professional Employees, AFL-CIO, August 15, 2016, https://www.dpeaflcio.org/factsheets/the-us-health-care-system-an-international-perspective

28-6 Kamal, Rabah, Giorlando Ramirez, and Cynthia Cox, "How does health spending in the U.S. compare to other countries?" Peterson-KFF Health System Tracker, December 23, 2020, https://www.healthsystemtracker.org/chart-collection/health-spending-u-s-compare-countries/#item-spendingcomparison_health-consumption-expenditures-per-capita-2019

28-7 Rae, Matthew, Rebecca Copeland, and Cynthia Cox, "Tracking the rise in premium contributions and cost-sharing for families with large employer coverage," Peterson-KFF Health System Tracker, Access an Affordability Briefs, August 14, 2019, https://www.healthsystemtracker.org/brief/tracking-the-rise-in-premium-contributions-and-cost-sharing-for-families-with-large-employer-coverage/

28-8 "Medical cost trend: Behind the numbers 2020," Health Research Institute, PwC, June 2019, https://www.pwc.com/us/en/industries/health-industries/assets/pwc-hri-behind-the-numbers-2020.pdf

28-9 Minemyer, Paige, "Report: Premiums, deductibles take up growing portion of workers' incomes," Fierce Healthcare, November 30, 2020, https://www.fiercehealthcare.com/payer/report-premiums-deductibles-take-up-growing-portion-workers-incomes

28-10 https://www.worldometers.info/demographics/life-expectancy/

28-11 Tikkanen, Roosa and Melinda K. Abrams, "U.S. Health Care from a Global Perspective, 2019: Higher Spending, Worse Outcomes?" The Commonwealth Fund, January 30, 2020, https://www.commonwealthfund.org/publications/issue-briefs/2020/jan/us-health-care-global-perspective-2019

28-12   "America's Health Rankings: 2018 Annual Report," United Health Foundation, Published 2020, https://www.americashealthrankings.org/learn/reports/2018-annual-report

28-13   "The expanding universal: The fix for American health care can be found in Europe," The Economist, August 10, 2017, https://www.economist.com/united-states/2017/08/10/the-fix-for-american-health-care-can-be-found-in-europe

28-14   Tolbert, Jennifer, Kendal Ortega, and Anthony Damico, "Key Facts about the Uninsured Population," Kaiser Family Foundation, November 6, 2020, https://www.kff.org/uninsured/issue-brief/key-facts-about-the-uninsured-population/

28-15   "Medicaid enrollment changes following the ACA," MACPAC, https://www.macpac.gov/subtopic/medicaid-enrollment-changes-following-the-aca/

28-16   "Health Coverage Under the Affordable Care Act: Enrollment Trends and State Estimates," Office of Health Policy, ASPE, Department of Health and Human Services, June 5, 2021, https://aspe.hhs.gov/system/files/pdf/265671/ASPE%20Issue%20Brief-ACA-Related%20Coverage%20by%20State.pdf

28-17   Garfield, Rachel, Kendal Ortega, and Anthony Damico, "The Coverage Gap: Uninsured Poor Adults in States that Do Not Expand Medicaid," Kaiser Family Foundation, January 21, 2021, https://www.kff.org/medicaid/issue-brief/the-coverage-gap-uninsured-poor-adults-in-states-that-do-not-expand-medicaid/

28-18   Collins, Sara R., Herman K. Bhupal, and Michelle M. Doty, "Health Insurance Coverage Eight Years After the ACA," The Commonwealth Fund, February 7, 2019, https://www.commonwealthfund.org/publications/issue-briefs/2019/feb/health-insurance-coverage-eight-years-after-aca

28-19   Pomerleau. Kyle, "The United States' Corporate Income Tax Rate is Now More in Line with Those Levied by Other Major Nations," The Tax Foundation, February 12, 2018, https://taxfoundation.org/us-corporate-income-tax-more-competitive/

28-20   Asen, Elke, "Corporate Income Tax Rates in Europe," The Tax Foundation, February 7, 2019, https://taxfoundation.org/corporate-tax-rates-europe-2019/#:~:text=The%20countries%20with%20the%20lowest,between%2019%20and%2025%20percent.

28-21   https://worldpopulationreview.com/countries/countries-by-national-debt

28-22   Amin, Krutika, Gary Claxton, Giorlando Ramirez, and Cynthia Cox, "How does cost affect access to care?," Peterson-KFF Health System Tracker, January 5, 2021, https://www.healthsystemtracker.org/chart-collection/cost-affect-access-care/#item-start

28-23   "Bipartisan Rx for America's Health Care: A Practical Path To Reform," Bipartisan Policy Center, February 2020, https://bipartisanpolicy.org/wp-content/uploads/2020/02/43530-BPC-FHC-Report-Proof.pdf

28-24   Minemyer, Paige, "Private plans pay 247% more for hospital services than Medicare does, study finds," Fierce Healthcare, September 18, 2020, https://www.fiercehealthcare.com/payer/private-plans-pay-247-more-for-hospital-services-than-medicare-study-finds

28-25   Miller, Emily, "U.S. Drug Prices vs. The World," Drug Watch, July 27, 2020, https://www.drugwatch.com/featured/us-drug-prices-higher-vs-world/#:~:text=%E2%80%-9CList%20prices%20for%20U.S.%20drugs,in%20other%20high%2Dincome%20countries.

28-26   "A Painful Pill to Swallow: U.S. vs. International Prescription Drug Prices," U.S. House of Representatives Ways and Means Committee, September 2019, https://waysand-means.house.gov/sites/democrats.waysandmeans.house.gov/files/documents/U.S.%20vs.%20International%20Prescription%20Drug%20Prices_0.pdf

28-27   Levey, Noam N., "A primary-care physician for every American, science panel urges," Modern Healthcare/Kaiser Health News, May 4, 2021, https://www.modernhealth-care.com/physicians/primary-care-physician-every-american-science-panel-urges

28-28   Landi, Heather, "Physician shortage could hit 139K by 2033, AAMC projects," Fierce Healthcare, October 22, 2020, https://www.fiercehealthcare.com/practices/physician-shortage-could-hit-139k-by-2033-aamc-projects

28-29   "QUICK COVID-19 PRIMARY CARE SURVEY SERIES 19 FIELDED AUGUST 21 –24, 2020," https://www.pcpcc.org/sites/default/files/news_files/C19%20Series%20 19%20National%20Executive%20Summary.pdf

28-30   "Why Public Health Is Necessary to Improve Healthcare," National Association of Chronic Disease Directors, https://cdn.ymaws.com/www.chronicdisease.org/resource/resmgr/white_papers/cd_white_paper_hoffman.pdf

28-31   https://www.cdc.gov/chronicdisease/about/costs/index.htm

28-32   Tepper, Nona, "Five chronic conditions cost employers $2.5 billion over two years, study shows," Modern Healthcare, February 18, 2021, https://www.modernhealthcare.com/insurance/five-chronic-conditions-cost-employers-25-billion-over-two-years-study-shows

28-33   McIlvennan, Collen K., DNP, ANP, Zubin J. Eapen, MD, MHS, and Larry A. Allen, MD, MHS, "Hospital Readmissions Reduction Program," U.S, National Library of Medicine, National Institutes of Health, May 19, 2016, https://www.ncbi.nlm.nih. gov/pmc/articles/PMC4439931/

28-34   Shrank, William, MD, MSHS, Teresa L. Rogstad, MPH, and Natasha Parekh, MD, MS, "Waste in the U.S. Health Care System: Estimated Costs and Potential for Savings," JAMA Network, October 7, 2019, https://jamanetwork.com/journals/jama/article-abstract/2752664

28-35   Mitchell, Emily M. PhD, "Statistical Brief #533: Concentration of Health Expenditures and Selected Characteristics of High Spenders, U.S. Civilian Noninstitutionalized Population, 2018," Agency for Healthcare Research and Quality, January 2021, https:// meps.ahrq.gov/data_files/publications/st533/stat533.shtml

28-36   Schneider, Eric C., Arnav Shah, Michelle M. Doty, Roosa Tikkanen, Katharine Fields, and Reginald D. Williams II, "Mirror, Mirror 2021: "Reflecting Poorly: Health Care in the U.S. Compared to Other High-Income Countries," The Commonwealth Fund, August 2021, https://www.commonwealthfund.org/sites/default/files/2021-08/ Schneider_Mirror_Mirror_2021.pdf

Chapter 29:

29-1   https://www.cms.gov/Medicare-Medicaid-Coordination/Medicare-and-Medicaid-Co-ordination/Medicare-Medicaid-Coordination-Office/Downloads/MMCO_Factsheet. pdf

29-2   "Why Public Health Is Necessary to Improve Healthcare," National Association of Chronic Disease Directors, https://cdn.ymaws.com/www.chronicdisease.org/resource/ resmgr/white_papers/cd_white_paper_hoffman.pdf

29-3   Minemyer, Paige, "Humana saved $4B through its value-based care programs last year," Fierce Healthcare, October 7, 2020, https://www.fiercehealthcare.com/payer/ humana-saved-4b-through-its-value-based-care-programs-last-year

29-4   Minemyer, Paige, Aetna, Cleveland Clinic launching co-branded health plan," Fierce Healthcare, August 19, 2020, https://www.fiercehealthcare.com/payer/aetna-cleveland-clinic-launching-co-branded-health-plan

29-5   Minemyer, Paige, "CMS finalizes physician fee schedule, including controversial updates to E/M visits," Fierce Healthcare, December 1, 2020, https://www.fiercehealthcare.com/practices/cms-finalizes-physician-fee-schedule-including-controversial-updates-to-e-m-visits

29-6   Appleby, Julie, "Surprise! Congress Takes Steps to Curb Unexpected Medical Bills," Kaiser Health News, December 22, 2020, https://khn.org/news/article/surprise-congress-takes-steps-to-curb-unexpected-medical-bills/

29-7   "Updated Physician Practice Acquisition Study: National and Regional Changes in Physician Employment 2012-2018," Physicians Advocacy Institute, February 2019, http://www.physiciansadvocacyinstitute.org/Portals/0/assets/docs/021919-Avalere-PAI-Physician-Employment-Trends-Study-2018-Update.pdf?ver=2019-02-19-162735-117

29-8   Livingston, Shelby, "Cigna joins other insurers in limiting MRIs, CT scans at hospitals, Modern Healthcare, October 12, 2020, https://www.modernhealthcare.com/payment/cigna-becomes-third-major-payer-restrict-mris-ct-scans-hospitals

29-9   Bannow, Tara, "Hospitals fight UnitedHealthcare policies over lab test, specialty drug payments," Modern Healthcare, February 5, 2021, https://www.modernhealthcare.com/payment/hospitals-fight-unitedhealthcare-policies-over-lab-test-specialty-drug-payments

29-10 King, Robert, "CMS finalizes hospital OPPS rule that phases out inpatient-only list, preserves 340B cuts," Fierce Healthcare, December 2, 2020, https://www.fiercehealthcare.com/hospitals/cms-finalizes-hospital-opps-rule-preserves-cuts-to-340b-phasing-out-inpatient-only-list

29-11 "CMS Proposes New Rules to Address Prior Authorization and Reduce Burden on Patients and Providers," Centers for Medicare and Medicaid Services, December 10, 2020, https://www.cms.gov/newsroom/press-releases/cms-proposes-new-rules-address-prior-authorization-and-reduce-burden-patients-and-providers

29-12 King Robert, "House bill mandates Medicare Advantage plans adopt electronic prior authorization," Fierce Healthcare, May 14, 2021, https://www.fiercehealthcare.com/practices/house-bill-mandates-ma-plans-adopt-electronic-prior-authorization-among-other-reforms

29-13   Hellmann, Jessie and Nona Tepper, "Bipartisan bill would revamp Medicare Advantage prior authorization," Modern Healthcare, May 13, 2021, https://www.modernhealthcare.com/insurance/bipartisan-bill-would-revamp-medicare-advantage-prior-authorization

29-14   https://delbene.house.gov/uploadedfiles/prior_auth.pdf

29-15   King, Robert, "Biden infrastructure package includes $400B to expand Medicaid home services," Fierce Healthcare, March 31, 2021, https://www.fiercehealthcare.com/payer/biden-infrastructure-package-includes-400b-to-expand-medicaid-home-services

29-16   Hellmann, Jessie and Ginger Christ, "Biden pushes for home health Medicaid coverage, $400 billion in funding," Modern Healthcare, March 31, 2021, https://www.modernhealthcare.com/politics-policy/biden-pushes-home-health-medicaid-coverage-400-billion-funding

29-17   https://www.whitehouse.gov/wp-content/uploads/2021/04/FY2022-Discretionary-Request.pdf

Chapter 30:

30-1   "The expanding universal: The fix for American health care can be found in Europe," The Economist, August 10, 2017, https://www.economist.com/united-states/2017/08/10/the-fix-for-american-health-care-can-be-found-in-europe

30-2   Centers for Medicare and Medicaid Services National Health Expenditure data website, https://www.cms.gov/Research-Statistics-Data-and-Systems/Statistics-Trends-and-Reports/NationalHealthExpendData/index.html

30-3   "Compare Medicare-for-all and Public Plan Proposals," Kaiser Family Foundation, May 15, 2019, https://www.kff.org/interactive/compare-medicare-for-all-public-plan-proposals/

30-4   Neuman, Tricia, Karne Pollitz and Jenifer Tolbert, "Medicare-for-All and Public Plan Buy-In Proposals: Overview and Key Issues," Kaiser Family Foundation, October 9, 2018, https://www.kff.org/medicare/issue-brief/medicare-for-all-and-public-plan-buy-in-proposals-overview-and-key-issues/

30-5   "Compare Proposals to Replace the Affordable Care Act," Kaiser Family Foundation, https://www.kff.org/interactive/proposals-to-replace-the-affordable-care-act/

Chapter 31:

31-1 "Compare Medicare-for-all and Public Plan Proposals," Kaiser Family Foundation, May 15, 2019, https://www.kff.org/interactive/compare-medicare-for-all-public-plan-proposals/

31-2 Cubanski, Juliette and Tricia Neuman, "FAQs on Medicare Financing and Trust Fund Solvency, Kasier Family Foundation, March 16, 2021, https://www.kff.org/medicare/issue-brief/faqs-on-medicare-financing-and-trust-fund-solvency/

31-3 Centers for Medicare and Medicaid Services National Health Expenditure data website, https://www.cms.gov/Research-Statistics-Data-and-Systems/Statistics-Trends-and-Reports/NationalHealthExpendData/index.html

31-4 LaPointe, Jacqueline, "36% of Payments Tied to Alternative Payment Models in 2018," Rev Cycle Intelligence, Xtelligent Healthcare Media, October 24, 2019, https://revcycleintelligence.com/news/36-of-payments-tied-to-alternative-payment-models-in-2018

31-5 LaPointe, Jacqueline, "Medicare, Medicaid Reimbursement $76.8B Under Hospital Costs," Rev Cycle Intelligence, Xtelligent Healthcare Media, January 7, 2019, https://revcycleintelligence.com/news/medicare-medicaid-reimbursement-76.8b-under-hospital-costs

31-6 Frack, Bill, Andrew Garibaldi, and Andrew Kadar, "Why Medicare Advantage Is Marching Toward 70% Penetration," L.E.K., https://www.lek.com/sites/default/files/insights/pdf-attachments/1969_Medicare_AdvantageLEK_Executive_Insights_1.pdf

Chapter 32:

32-1 Reinhardt, Uwe, Priced Out: The Economic and Ethical Costs of American Health Care, Princeton University Press, 2019

32-2 https://fas.org/sgp/crs/misc/RS20946.pdf

32-3 Levey, Noam N., "A primary-care physician for every American, science panel urges," Modern Healthcare/Kaiser Health News, May 4, 2021, https://www.modernhealthcare.com/physicians/primary-care-physician-every-american-science-panel-urges

32-4 Artiga, Samantha and Elizabeth Hinton, "Beyond Health Care: The Role of Social Determinants in Promoting Health and Health Equity," Kaiser Family Foundation, May 10, 2018, https://www.kff.org/disparities-policy/issue-brief/beyond-health-care-the-role-of-social-determinants-in-promoting-health-and-health-equity/#:~:text=Determinants%20of%20Health%3F-,Social%20determinants%20of%20health%20are%20the%20conditions%20in%20which%20people,health%20care%20(Figure%201).

32-5 "Bipartisan Rx for America's Health Care: A Practical Path To Reform," Bipartisan Policy Center, February 2020, https://bipartisanpolicy.org/wp-content/uploads/2020/02/43530-BPC-FHC-Report-Proof.pdf

32-6 Blumberg, Linda J., John Holahan, Stacey McMorrow, and Michael Simpson, "Estimating the Impact of a Public Option or Capping Provider Payment Rates," Urban Institute, March 2020, https://www.urban.org/sites/default/files/2020/03/23/estimating-the-impact-of-a-public-option-or-capping-provider-payment-rates.pdf

32-7 Liu, Jodi, Zachary M. Levinson, Nabeel Shariq Qureshi, and Christopher M. Whaley, "Impact of Policy Options for Reducing Hospital Prices Paid by Private Health Plans," RAND Corporation, February 18, 2021, https://www.rand.org/pubs/research_reports/RRA805-1.html

32-8 Schwartz, Karyn, Jeannie Fuglesten Biniek, Matthew Rae, Tricia Newman, and Larry Levitt, "Limiting Private Insurance Reimbursement to Medicare Rates Would Reduce Health Spending by About $350 Billion in 2021," Kaiser Family Foundation, March 1, 2021, https://www.kff.org/medicare/issue-brief/limiting-private-insurance-reimbursement-to-medicare-rates-would-reduce-health-spending-by-about-350-billion-in-2021/

32-9 https://onepercentsteps.com/policy-briefs/

32-10 https://www.dartmouthatlas.org/faq/https://atlasdata.dartmouth.edu/

32-11 Appleby, Julie, "Surprise! Congress Takes Steps to Curb Unexpected Medical Bills," Kaiser Health News, December 22, 2020, https://khn.org/news/article/surprise-congress-takes-steps-to-curb-unexpected-medical-bills/

32-12 "Who Went Without Health Insurance in 2019, and Why?," Congressional Budget Office, September 2020, https://www.cbo.gov/system/files/2020-09/56504-Health-Insurance.pdf

32-13 "Reforming America's Health Care Through Choice and Competition," U.S. Departments of Health and Human Services, Treasury, and Labor, Report pursuant to Executive Order 13813, Page 7

32-14 Schwartz, Nelson, D., "Swiss Health Care Thrives Without Public Option," The New York Times, September 30, 2009, https://www.nytimes.com/2009/10/01/health/policy/01swiss.html?pagewanted=all

32-15 Slaybaugh, Chris, FSA, MAAA "International Healthcare Systems: The US Versus the World," Axene Health Partners, https://axenehp.com/international-healthcare-systems-us-versus-world/

32-16 Seervai, Shanoor and David Blumenthal, "Lessons on Universal Coverage from an Unexpected Advocate: Richard Nixon," The Commonwealth Fund, November 2, 2017, https://www.commonwealthfund.org/blog/2017/lessons-universal-coverage-unexpected-advocate-richard-nixon

32-17 Nixon, Richard, "Special Message to the Congress Proposing a Comprehensive Health Insurance Plan," February 6, 1974, https://www.presidency.ucsb.edu/documents/special-message-the-congress-proposing-comprehensive-health-insurance-plan

Chapter 33:

33-1 "The great consolidation: The potential for rapid consolidation of health systems, ," Deloitte Report, November 12, 2014, https://www2.deloitte.com/us/en/pages/life-sciences-and-health-care/articles/great-consolidation-health-systems.html#:~:-text=Health%20systems%20are%20on%20the,financial%20pressures%20and%20market%20dynamics.&text=All%20three%20estimates%20independently%20converged,likely%20remain%20in%2010%20years. 33-2

33-2 "Hospital M&A: When done well, M&A can achieve valuable outcomes," Deloitte Report, 2017, https://www2.deloitte.com/content/dam/Deloitte/us/Documents/life-sciences-health-care/us-lshc-hospital-mergers-and-acquisitions.pdf

33-3 "Bipartisan Rx for America's Health Care: A Practical Path To Reform," Bipartisan Policy Center, February 2020, https://bipartisanpolicy.org/wp-content/uploads/2020/02/43530-BPC-FHC-Report-Proof.pdf

33-4   Kacik, Alex, "Hospital M&A activity rebounds in Q4," Modern Healthcare, January 19, 2021, https://www.modernhealthcare.com/mergers-acquisitions/hospital-ma-activity-rebounds-q4

33-5   Kacik, Alex, "Mergers and acquisitions among regional hospitals are on the rise," Modern Healthcare, July 8, 2021, https://www.modernhealthcare.com/mergers-acquisitions/mergers-and-acquisitions-among-regional-hospitals-are-rise?adobe_mc=MCMID%3D564237775737261103721643999535443368753%7CMCORGID%3D138FFF2554E6E7220A4C98C6%2540AdobeOrg%7CTS%3D1626179980&CSAuthResp=1%3A%3A954992%3A1317%3A24%3Asuccess%3A3AF90976BA7760936D-1ABF96F75A72B5

33-6   "INSIGHT: Health-Care Consolidation Strong in 2019—Expect Even Stronger 2020, Bloomberg Law, January 27, 2020, https://news.bloomberglaw.com/health-law-and-business/insight-health-care-consolidation-strong-in-2019-expect-even-stronger-2020

33-7   "Updated Physician Practice Acquisition Study: National and Regional Changes in Physician Employment 2012-2018," Physicians Advocacy Institute, February 2019, http://www.physiciansadvocacyinstitute.org/Portals/0/assets/docs/021919-Avalere-PAI-Physician-Employment-Trends-Study-2018-Update.pdf?ver=2019-02-19-162735-117

33-8   Bannow, Tara, "Nearly 70% of U.S. physicians now employed by hospitals or corporations, report finds," Modern Healthcare, June 29, 2021, https://www.modernhealthcare.com/providers/nearly-70-us-physicians-now-employed-hospitals-or-corporations-report-finds

33-9   Muoio, Dave, "Hospitals, corporations own nearly half of medical practices, spurred by COVID-19 disruption: report," Fierce Healthcare, June 29, 2021, https://www.fiercehealthcare.com/practices/practice-consolidation-private-practice-departures-skyrocketed-during-covid-19

33-10   Livingston, Shelby, "Reigniting the physicians arms race, insurers are buying practices, Modern Healthcare, June 2, 2018, https://www.modernhealthcare.com/article/20180602/NEWS/180609985/reigniting-the-physicians-arms-race-insurers-are-buying-practices

Chapter 34:

34-1 "Generic Drug Competition Lowers Prescription Drug Cost to $6 on Average, Study Finds," Association of Accessible Medicines, July 10, 2018, https://accessiblemeds.org/resources/press-releases/generic-drug-competition-lowers-prescription-cost-6-average-study-finds

34-2 "Average Brand-Name Drug Price Now Over 18 Times Higher Than Average Generic Drug Price, New AARP Report Shows," April 4, 2019, https://press.aarp.org/2019-4-4-Rx-Price-Watch-Report-Generic-Prescription-Drugs

34-3 Centers for Medicare and Medicaid Services National Health Expenditure data website, https://www.cms.gov/Research-Statistics-Data-and-Systems/Statistics-Trends-and-Reports/NationalHealthExpendData/index.html

34-4 Neuman, Tricia and Juliette Cubanski, "Most People Are Unlikely to See Drug Cost Savings From President Trump's "Most Favored Nation" Proposal," Kaiser Family Foundation, August 27, 2020, https://www.kff.org/policy-watch/most-people-are-unlikely-to-see-drug-cost-savings-from-president-trumps-most-favored-nation-proposal/

34-5 "10 Essential Facts About Medicare And Prescription Drug Spending," Kaiser Family foundation, January 29, 2019, https://www.kff.org/infographic/10-essential-facts-about-medicare-and-prescription-drug-spending/

34-6 Kamal, Rabah, Cynthia Cox, and Daniel McDermott, "What are the recent and forecasted trends in prescription drug spending?," Peterson-Kaiser Family Foundation Health System Tracker, February 20, 2019, https://www.healthsystemtracker.org/chart-collection/recent-forecasted-trends-prescription-drug-spending/#item-nominal-and-inflation-adjusted-increase-in-rx-spending_2017

34-7 "Medical cost trend: Behind the numbers 2020," Health Research Institute, PwC, June 2019, https://www.pwc.com/us/en/industries/health-industries/assets/pwc-hri-behind-the-numbers-2020.pdf

34-8 Sarnak, Dan O., David Squires, and Shawn Bishop, "Paying for Prescription Drugs Around the World: Why is the U.S. an Outlier?," The Commonwealth Fund, October 5, 2017," https://www.commonwealthfund.org/publications/issue-briefs/2017/oct/paying-prescription-drugs-around-world-why-us-outlier

34-9 "Medical Pharmacy Trend Report: 2019 Tenth Edition," Magellan Rx Management, https://issuu.com/magellanrx/docs/mptr2019?fr=sMmE2MTk0MDI3Nw

34-10 Miller, Emily, "U.S. Drug Prices vs. The World," Drug Watch, July 27, 2020, https://www.drugwatch.com/featured/us-drug-prices-higher-vs-world/#:~:text=%E2%80%-9CList%20prices%20for%20U.S.%20drugs,in%20other%20high%2Dincome%20countries.

34-11 Marsh, Tori, MPH, "Prices for Prescription Drugs Rise Faster Than Any Other Medical Good or Service," GoodRx, September 17, 2020, https://www.goodrx.com/blog/prescription-drugs-rise-faster-than-medical-goods-or-services/

34-12 "A Painful Pill to Swallow: U.S. vs. International Prescription Drug Prices," U.S. House of Representatives Ways and Means Committee, September 2019, https://waysandmeans.house.gov/sites/democrats.waysandmeans.house.gov/files/documents/U.S.%20vs.%20International%20Prescription%20Drug%20Prices_0.pdf

34-13 Langreth, Robert, Blacki Migliozzi, and Ketaki Gokhale, "The U.S. Pays a Lot More for Top Drugs Than Other Countries," Forbes, December 18, 2015, https://www.bloomberg.com/graphics/2015-drug-prices/

34-14 Robinson, James C, Patricia Ex, and Dimitra Panteli, "How Drug Prices Are Negotiated in Germany," The Commonwealth Fund, June 13, 2019, https://www.commonwealthfund.org/blog/2019/how-drug-prices-are-negotiated-germany

34-15 Robinson, James C, Dimitra Panteli, and Patricia Ex, "Reference Pricing in Germany: Implications for U.S. Pharmaceutical Purchasing," The Commonwealth Fund, February 4, 2019, https://www.commonwealthfund.org/publications/issue-briefs/2019/jan/reference-pricing-germany-implications

34-16 Capretta, James C., A Closer Look at International Reference Pricing for Prescription Drugs," Real Clear Policy, March 29, 2019, https://www.realclearpolicy.com/articles/2019/03/29/a_closer_look_at_international_reference_pricing_for_prescription_drugs_111142.html

34-17 Wechsler, Jill, "Too Fast or Too Slow? Debate Intensifies over FDA Regulatory Requirements," Applied Clinical Trials, July 9, 2019, https://www.appliedclinicaltrialsonline.com/view/too-fast-or-too-slow-debate-intensifies-over-fda-regulatory-requirements

34-18 "Bipartisan Rx for America's Health Care: A Practical Path To Reform," Bipartisan Policy Center, February 2020, https://bipartisanpolicy.org/wp-content/uploads/2020/02/43530-BPC-FHC-Report-Proof.pdf

34-19 Goldberg, Stephanie, "Why Biden worries Big Pharma," Modern Healthcare, November 23, 2020, https://www.modernhealthcare.com/politics-policy/why-biden-worries-big-pharma

34-20 "HHS Finalizes Rule to Bring Drug Discounts Directly to Seniors at the Pharmacy Counter," Department of Health and Human Services, November 20, 2020, https://www.hhs.gov/about/news/2020/11/20/hhs-finalizes-rule-bring-drug-discounts-direct-ly-seniors-pharmacy-counter.html#:~:text=Today%2C%20in%20response%20to%20President,D%2C%20in%20order%20to%20create

34-21 Kost, Danielle, "Why Germany's Approach To Drug Pricing Offers Lessons To U.S.," Forbes, December 23, 2019, https://www.forbes.com/sites/hbsworkingknowl-edge/2019/12/23/why-germanys-approach-to-drug-pricing-offers-lessons-to-us/#-789c50a93f55

34-22 Marsh, Tori, "800+ Drugs Became More Expensive This January — The Largest Number of Increases in Years," GoodRx Blog, February 2, 2021, https://www.goodrx.com/blog/january-2021-drug-increases-recap/

34-23 Kang, So-Yeon, Michael J. DiStefano, Mariana P Socal, and Gerard F. Anderson, "Using External Reference Pricing In Medicare Part D To Reduce Drug Price Differentials With Other Countries," Health Affairs, May 2019, https://www.healthaffairs.org/doi/full/10.1377/hlthaff.2018.05207

34-24 "Trump Administration Announces Prescription Drug Payment Model to Put American Patients First," Department of Health and Human Services, November 20, 2020, https://www.cms.gov/newsroom/press-releases/trump-administration-announces-pre-scription-drug-payment-model-put-american-patients-first

34-25 Sachs, Rachel, "The National Academy for State Health Policy's Proposal for State-Based International Reference Pricing for Prescription Drugs," National Academy for State Health Policy, August 10, 2020, https://www.nashp.org/the-national-acad-emy-for-state-health-policys-proposal-for-state-based-international-reference-pric-ing-for-prescription-drugs/

34-26 Dusetzina, Stacie D., Juliette Cubanski, Leonce Nshuti, Sarah True, Jack Hoadley, Drew Roberts, and Tricia Neuman, "Medicare Part D Plans Rarely Cover Brand-Name Drugs When Generics Are Available," Health Affairs, August 2020, https://www.healthaffairs.org/doi/full/10.1377/hlthaff.2019.01694

34-27 Minemyer, Paige, "Part D plans don't push beneficiaries to take brand-name drugs over generics: study," Fierce Healthcare, August 4, 2020, https://www.fiercehealthcare.com/payer/part-d-plans-don-t-push-beneficiaries-to-take-brand-name-drugs-over-generics-study

34-28 Sullivan, Thomas, "States Moving Forward with Canadian Drug Importation Plans, Despite No Clear Instruction from Biden Administration," PolicyMed, February, 28, 2021, https://www.policymed.com/2021/03/states-moving-forward-with-canadian-drug-importation-plans-despite-no-clear-instruction-from-biden-administration.html

34-29 "CMS Issues Final Rule to Empower States, Manufacturers, and Private Payers to Create New Payment Methods for Innovative New Therapies Based on Patient Outcomes," Centers for Medicare and Medicaid Services, December 21, 2020, https://www.cms.gov/newsroom/press-releases/cms-issues-final-rule-empower-states-manufacturers-and-private-payers-create-new-payment-methods

34-30 Goodman, Dana, "CBO estimate on Pelosi drug bill misses its long-term impact on health," STAT, October 16, 2019, https://www.statnews.com/2019/10/16/cbo-estimate-pelosi-drug-bill-misses-long-term-impact/#:~:text=CBO%20estimate%20on%20Pelosi%20drug,long%2Dterm%20impact%20on%20health&text=The%20CBO%20estimated%20that%20the,in%20the%20rate%20of%20innovation.

https://www.cbo.gov/system/files/2021-08/57010-New-Drug-Development.pdf

Ciarametaro, Michael, Craig Garthwaite, Craig Mitton, Sue Peschin, and Joel White, "Reforms Are Needed To Rein in Health Spending, But Reference pricing Isn't Worth The Risk," Health Affairs, October 8, 2021, https://www.healthaffairs.org/do/10.1377/hblog20211004.561448/full/

34-31 Ubl, Stepen J., "Pelosi's drug pricing plan puts medical innovation at risk, STAT, October 17, 2019, https://www.statnews.com/2019/10/17/pelosi-bill-drug-costs-medical-innovation-risk/

34-32 "House Drug Pricing Bill Could Keep 100 Lifesaving Drugs from American Patients," Press Release, The White House, December 3, 2019, https://www.whitehouse.gov/articles/house-drug-pricing-bill-keep-100-lifesaving-drugs-american-patients/

34-33 Owermohle, Sarah and Susannah Luthi, "Drugmakers deliver counteroffer to Trump international pricing plan," Politico, August 25, 2020, https://www-politico-com.cdn. ampproject.org/c/s/www.politico.com/amp/news/2020/08/25/trump-drug-pricing-pharma-401775

Chapter 35:

35-1 "Facts about ageing," World Health Organization, September 30, 2014, https://www. who.int/ageing/about/facts/en/

35-2 Mather, Mark, Paola Scommegna, Lilian Kilduff, "Fact Sheet: Aging in the United States," Population Reference Bureau, July 15, 2019, https://www.prb.org/aging-unitedstates-fact-sheet/

35-3 "Rising Demand for Long-Term Services and Supports for Elderly People," Congressional Budget Office, June 2013, https://www.cbo.gov/sites/default/files/113th-congress-2013-2014/reports/44363-ltc.pdf

35-4 Benz, Christine, "75 Must-Know Statistics About Long-Term Care: 2018 Edition," Morningstar, August 20, 2018, https://www.morningstar.com/articles/879494/75-mustknow-statistics-about-longterm-care-2018-ed

35-5 Reaves, Erica L. and MaryBeth Musumeci, "Medicaid and Long-Term Services and Supports: A Primer," Kaiser Family Foundation, December 15, 2015, https://www. kff.org/medicaid/report/medicaid-and-long-term-services-and-supports-a-primer/

35-6 Thach, Nga T. and Joshua M. Wiener, TCI International, "An Overview of Long-Term Services and Supports and Medicaid: Final Report," ASPE, HHS, https://aspe. hhs.gov/basic-report/overview-long-term-services-and-supports-and-medicaid-final-report#LTSSRole

35-7 "Costs of care," October 10, 2017, Longtermcare.acl.gov, https://longtermcare.acl. gov/costs-how-to-pay/costs-of-care.html

35-8 "Cost of Care Survey 2019," Genworth Financial, https://www.genworth.com/aging-and-you/finances/cost-of-care.html

35-9 Colello, Kirsten J., "Who Pays for Long-Term Services and Supports?," Congressional Research Service In Focus, August 22, 2018, https://fas.org/sgp/crs/misc/IF10343.pdf

35-10 Houser, Ari, "Nursing Homes," AARP Public Policy Institute, October 2007, https:// assets.aarp.org/rgcenter/il/fs10r_homes.pdf

35-11   "Long-Term Services and Supports Expenditures on Home & Community-Based Services," https://www.medicaid.gov/state-overviews/scorecard/ltss-expenditures-on-hcbs/index.html

35-12   Murray, Caitlin, Alena Tourtellotte, Debra Lipson, and Andrea Wysocki. "Medicaid Long Term Services and Supports Annual Expenditures Report: Federal Fiscal Years 2017 and 2018." Mathematica, January 7, 2021, for Centers for Medicare and Medicaid Services, January 7, 2021, https://www.medicaid.gov/medicaid/long-term-services-supports/downloads/ltssexpenditures-2017-2018.pdf

35-13   King, Robert, "Biden infrastructure package includes $400B to expand Medicaid home services," Fierce Healthcare, March 31, 2021, https://www.fiercehealthcare.com/payer/biden-infrastructure-package-includes-400b-to-expand-medicaid-home-services

35-14   Hellmann, Jessie and Ginger Christ, "Biden pushes for home health Medicaid coverage, $400 billion in funding," Modern Healthcare, March 31, 2021, https://www.modernhealthcare.com/politics-policy/biden-pushes-home-health-medicaid-coverage-400-billion-funding

35-15   https://www.whitehouse.gov/wp-content/uploads/2021/04/FY2022-Discretionary-Request.pdf

35-16   "The Partnership States," Partnership for Long Term Care, https://www.partnershipforlongtermcare.com/partnershipmaps.html

35-17   "Understanding Medicaid's Look-Back Period; Penalties, Exceptions and State Variances," American Council on Aging, July 21, 2019, https://www.medicaidplanningassistance.org/medicaid-look-back-period/

35-18   https://www.macpac.gov/publication/medicaid-estate-recovery-improving-policy-and-promoting-equity/

Acronym and Style Guide

A

accountable care organizations (ACOs)

administrative services only (ASO) fee

Affordable Care Act (ACA)

ambulatory surgery centers

American Hospital Association

American Medical Association

American Left (the Left)

American Right (the Right)

annual notice of change (ANOC)

B

Band-Aids

Prince Otto Eduard Leopold von Bismarck (Uncle Otto)

Bismarckian Socialism (or State Socialism)

Blue Cross Plans

C

care management (CM)

catastrophic plan

Centers for Medicare and Medicaid Services (CMS)

chronic care special needs plans (C-SNPs)

co-insurance

co-pay

Consolidated Omnibus Budget Reconciliation Act (COBRA)

Communist Manifesto

Congressional Budget Office (CBO)

conservative political movement

consumer-driven health plan (CDHP)

consumer-directed health plans (CDHPs)

cost-sharing

cost-sharing reduction (CSR) subsidies

COVID-19 (not Coronavirus, COVID)

D

departments of insurance (DOIs)

Democratic Congress

Democrats (when referencing members of one of American's main political parties), but democrat (when referencing an individual who supports democratic societies)

Diagnosis Related Groups (DRGs)

disproportionate share hospital (DSH) program

downstream

drugmaker (au preference)

dual eiligibles

dual eligibility (no hyphen, au preference)

dual eligible special needs plans (D-SNPs)

durable medical equipment (DME)

E

Economic Policy Institute (EPI)

Emergency Medical Treatment and Labor Act (EMTALA)

Employee Retirement Security Act (ERISA)

employer group waiver plans (EGWPs)

employer-employee bureaus

employer-sponsored coverage

employer-sponsored insurance (ESI)

end-stage renal disease (ESRD)

essential health benefits (EHBs)

exclusive provider organizations (EPOs)

external review/appeals entities (EREs)

external quality review organizations (EQROs)

F

federal-state partnership

Federal Employees Health Benefit Plans (FEHBP)

Federal Medical Assistance Percentage (FMAP)

fee-for-service (FFS)

flexible spending account (FSA)

forte

fraud, waste, and abuse (FWA)

full benefit dual eligibles (FBDEs)

fully integrated dual eligible SNP (FIDE SNP)

G

gatekeeper

give-and-take

gross domestic product (GDP)

H

Health Insurance Portability and
  Accountability Act (HIPAA)

health maintenance organizations
  (HMOs)

health plan-negotiated discounts

health reimbursement account (HRA)

healthcare

Health Care Cost Institute (HCCI)

Healthcare Effectiveness Data and Information Sets (HEDIS)

Healthcare Revolution with MHK
  (podcast)

Hearst Corporation

hierarchical condition category (HCC)
  system

high-deductible health plans (HDHPs)

highly integrated dual eligible SNP
  (HIDE SNP)

Hippocratic oath

I

independent practice associations (IPAs)

independent review entities (IREs)

independent review organizations
  (IROs)

initial coverage limit (ICL)

initial enrollment period

interoperability rule

Iron Curtain

K

Kaiser Family Foundation (KFF)

L

laissez faire free market economics

lifeblood

local coverage determinations (LCDs)

low-income subsidy (LIS) program
  (known as Extra Help)

M

Machiavelli

managed long-term care (MLTC)

maximum out-of-pocket (MOOP) cost

MCG Health

Medical House of Knowledge
  (MedHOK or, more recently, MHK)

medical loss ratio (MLR)

Medicare Administrative Contractors (MACs)

Medicare Advantage (MA)

Medicare Part A Hospital Insurance
  Trust Fund

Medicare-Medicaid Plan (MMP)

Medicare savings programs (MSP)

Medicare Star quality program

minimum medical loss ratio (MLR)

mandate

model of care (MOC)

N

National Association of Insurance Commissioners (NAIC)

National Committee for Quality Assurance (NCQA)

national coverage determinations (NCDs)

National Health Expenditure Data (NHED)

New Deal Programs

no-balance-bill (adj.)

non-elderly

O

Office of Personnel Management (OPM)

open access health maintenance organization (OA-HMO)

opioid

out-of-pocket costs

out-of-network costs

over-the-counter drugs

P

per-member-per-month (PMPM)

personally identifiable information (PII)

pharmacy benefit managers (PBMs)

physician-hospital organizations (PHOs)

physician incentive plan (PIP)

Physicians Advocacy Institute

places of service

point of service(s) (POS) plans

policymaker

pre-COVID-19 (adj.)

preferred provider organizations (PPOs)

prepaid

prescription drug plans (PDPs)

program of all-inclusive care for the elderly (PACE) plans

protected health information (PHI)

primary care case management (PCCM)

primary care physicians (PCPs)

private fee-for-service (PFFS) plans

provider sponsored networks (PSNs)

public-private partnership

Q

qualified Medicare beneficiary (QMB)

quality improvement organizations (QIOs)

quasi-public

R

Realpolitik

Reichstag (parliament)

Republican in Name Only (RINO)

risk adjustment data validation (RADV)
  audit

Roman Catholic

S

sliding-scale premium

Social Security *(when generally referencing the benefit)*

Social Security Administration

Social Security Act

social-safety-net program

socialist

special needs plans (SNPs)

specified low-income Medicare beneficiary (SLMB)

State Children's Health Insurance Program (SCHIP)

State Fair Hearing

Supplementary Medical Insurance (SMI) Trust Fund

Supplemental Security Income (SSI)

Summary of Benefits and Coverage (SBC)

T

third-party administrator (TPA)

U

usual and customary rate (UCR)

utilization management (UM)

V

value based insurance design (VBID)

versus

vice versa

W

well-being

well-off (adj)

King Wilhelm I

wrap-around benefits

Numbers

1115 Waivers

1900s

1915(b) waivers

2000 BC

January 1